2

PROGRESS
IN CARDIOLOGY

2

PROGRESS
IN CARDIOLOGY

Edited by

PAUL N. YU, M.D.

Sarah McCort Ward Professor of Medicine and Head,
Cardiology Unit, University of
Rochester School of Medicine and Dentistry,
Rochester, New York

and

JOHN F. GOODWIN, M.D.

Professor of Clinical Cardiology,
Royal Postgraduate Medical School,
London, England

LEA & FEBIGER • *Philadelphia, 1973*

OTHER BOOKS IN THE SERIES

Progress in Cardiology 1—1972

Library of Congress Cataloging in Publication Data
Main entry under title:

Progress in cardiology.

Includes bibliographies.
1. Cardiology. I. Yu, Paul N., 1915–   ed.
II. Goodwin, John F., ed. [DNLM: 1. Cardiology—
Yearbooks. W1 PR667P]
RC667.P75   616.1'2   77–157474
ISBN 0-8121-0326-2 (v. 1)

ISBN 0-8121-0409–9

Published in Great Britain by Henry Kimpton Publishers, London

Library of Congress Catalog Card Number 77–157474

Printed in the United States of America

PREFACE

The second volume of *Progress in Cardiology* follows the pattern laid down for the first. It is an attempt to present important new aspects of, and advances in, cardiovascular disease, concentrating upon current vital issues. The chapters have been selected because of their immediate importance, rather than with a desire to produce a survey of any special group of topics. The editors have been fortunate in obtaining contributions from leaders in their fields, who have written essentially for the committed readers but have not hesitated to explore the finer points of their subjects and explain the basic principles clearly and authoritatively on behalf of readers less interested in details.

The second volume opens with two important chapters on genetics and immunological aspects of cardiovascular disease respectively, followed by a chapter on cardiac glycoside assay techniques. It then proceeds to cover recent advances in congenital heart disease and cardiac dysrhythmias in children. New aspects of electrophysiology of the heart are discussed in the ensuing chapter on the bundle of His electrogram. Pathophysiology of and medical therapy for shock in acute myocardial infarction are dealt with next. The volume concludes with two chapters on substrate utilization by skeletal muscle during exercise and the effects of physical training on the heart, both by authorities from Scandinavia.

Six of the contributions have been drawn from the United States, two from Great Britain, and two from continental Europe. For Volume 3, which is now in preparation, the editors have cast their net wider and promise an even more international flavor.

Rochester, New York   Paul N. Yu
London, England   John F. Goodwin

v

CONTRIBUTORS

Mark V. Barrow, M.D., Ph.D.
Assistant Professor of Medicine
College of Medicine
University of Florida
Gainesville, Florida

Jay N. Cohn, M.D.
Professor of Medicine
Georgetown University School of Medicine
Chief, Hypertension and Clinical Hemodynamics
Veterans Administration Hospital
Washington, D.C.

Anthony N. Damato, M.D.
Chief, Cardiovascular Program
U.S.P.H.S. Hospital
Staten Island, New York

Kathryn Hawes Ehlers, M.D.
Associate Professor of Pediatrics
Associate Director, Pediatric Cardiology
The New York Hospital—
   Cornell Medical Center
New York, New York

Mary Allen Engle, M.D.
Professor of Pediatrics
Head, Division of Pediatric Cardiology
The New York Hospital—
   Cornell Medical Center
New York, New York

Joseph A. Franciosa, M.D.
Instructor in Medicine
Georgetown University School of Medicine
Chief, Medical Intensive Care Unit
Veterans Administration Hospital
Washington, D.C.

Gunnar Grimby, M.D.
Associate Professor, Departments of Clinical
   Physiology and Rehabilitation Medicine
University of Göteborg
Göteborg, Sweden

Edgar Haber, M.D.
Chief, Cardiac Unit
Massachusetts General Hospital
Professor of Medicine
Harvard Medical School
Boston, Massachusetts

Donald C. Harrison, M.D.
Chief, Cardiology Division
Professor of Medicine
Stanford University School of Medicine
Stanford, California

Sun H. Lau, M.D.
Deputy Chief, Cardiovascular Program
U.S.P.H.S. Hospital
Staten Island, New York

M. H. Lessof, M.D., F.R.C.P.
Physician and Professor of Medicine
Guy's Hospital
London, England

Celia M. Oakley, M.D., F.R.C.P., F.A.C.C.
Consultant Cardiologist
Hammersmith Hospital
Honorary Lecturer
Royal Postgraduate Medical School
London, England

Mark G. Perlroth, M.D.
Assistant Professor of Medicine
Stanford University School of Medicine
Stanford, California

C. I. Roberts, B.M., M.R.C.P.
Clinical Tutor and Honorary Physician
Guy's Hospital
London, England

Robert N. Schnitzler, M.D.
Research Associate
U.S.P.H.S. Hospital
Staten Island, New York

Thomas W. Smith, M.D.
Assistant Professor of Medicine
Harvard Medical School and
Massachusetts General Hospital
Boston, Massachusetts

W. Jape Taylor, M.D.
Professor of Medicine
Chief, Division of Cardiology
College of Medicine
University of Florida
Gainesville, Florida

John Wahren, M.D.
Assistant Professor of Clinical Physiology
Karolinska Institute
Acting Head, Department of Clinical Physiology
Serafimer Hospital
Stockholm, Sweden

CONTENTS

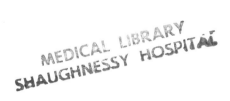

Chapter 1

RECENT ADVANCES IN GENETICS

OF CARDIOVASCULAR DISEASE

W. Jape Taylor, M.D., and Mark V. Barrow, M.D., Ph.D.

During the past two decades solutions at the molecular level have been found for many of the fundamental problems of genetics. The utilization of microorganisms in a variety of sophisticated biochemical techniques led to the delineation of the genetic code and the manner in which it is transcribed from DNA through a variety of RNAs to the ultimate step of peptide and protein synthesis. The mechanisms by which the entire system is integrated and modulated remain to be unraveled in the future.

The mechanism by which the sequential and appropriate activation of the genetic material, which apparently is identical throughout the body, leads to differentiation of the various tissues and organs is one of the more fundamental—and unanswered—questions in genetic research. How are the orderly appearance and disappearance of specific proteins programmed? At times, it might be desirable to reactivate synthesis of a particular protein after the period when it is ordinarily phased out; for example, to continue the production of fetal hemoglobin in those individuals who make a disordered adult hemo-

globin, as in sickle-cell anemia, might prevent major illness. Conceivably, too, a continual phasing out of active synthesis is the ultimate pathway to aging and senility. Abundant quantities of excess and presumably redundant DNA are present in the chromosomes of most animals and may, indeed, serve as a large pool for potential genetic modeling if mechanisms for appropriate activation of this apparently functionless DNA are discovered.[31,188]

In a broad sense, control systems must be involved in the very different responses to environmental stimuli which characterize organisms on various evolutionary planes. Elucidation of some of the mechanisms by which some bacteria can respond to a given medium by the production of a specific enzyme while others cannot led to the elaboration by Jacob and Monod of the scheme of regulator genes in addition to structural ones.[94] A dramatic example in a mammalian species is the ability of sheep with hemoglobin-A genotype to produce hemoglobin C with an entirely new beta chain in response to anemic stress, while sheep of hemoglobin-B

1

genotype do not have this ability.[18,134] The production of specific antibodies following contact with foreign antigens is virtually taken for granted, but the means by which the system is activated remain elusive.

The common cardiovascular diseases, such as arteriosclerosis and hypertension, result from complex interrelationships between the genetic background of the individual and the environmental milieu which surrounds him. Inability to recognize potential differences in individual responses has made it necessary to promote widespread changes in dietary habits, which has led to confusion, apathy, and, on occasion, to active resistance to what is undoubtedly a desirable goal.

In addition to looking at a few diseases where genetic influences will override virtually any environmental influences, this review will primarily examine examples of genetically determined differences in response to a common stimulus. Variant drug effects are extremely important, not only because they influence therapeutic effects but also because they represent a type of controlled situation which can serve as a model for examination of other types of relationships between genes and environment. Animal models which shed light on such problem areas will be discussed, as will methods for early identification of high-risk individuals.

GENETIC INFLUENCES ON RESPONSES TO CARDIO-VASCULAR DRUGS

Unanticipated drug responses may be due to a number of genetically determined variations from the usual. The effect of an agent may be accentuated or reduced, as the case may be, by a mutation in the enzymes which leads to breakdown or inactivation of the drug, thereby altering either its concentration or persistence. A related but more complicated factor which influences drug metabolism is the responsiveness of microsomal enzymes, which may degrade the drug, to concomitant environmental influences, such as

the administration of a second drug. Modification of the usual activity may be related to a heritable mutation in the end-organ, perhaps at a receptor site through which its effect is mediated. Finally, an unusual drug effect may be due to an immunological response to the agent or to a chemical interaction with a mutant protein which is not necessarily concerned with the drug's primary actions, such as methemoglobin production by certain drugs in hemoglobin variants in which an amino acid has been substituted in the vicinity of the heme crevices.

Examples of almost all of the types of genetically determined unusual drug responses which have been delineated in recent years have been ascribed to commonly used cardiovascular drugs. Examination of these known variant responses may provide clues for similar but as yet unrecognized heritable factors which influence the usage of many medications currently applied in a largely empirical fashion.

Oral Anticoagulants

Perhaps because the administration of these agents is routinely monitored by a laboratory determination of their effectiveness, a number of responses which vary significantly from those of the population at large have been detected. The competition of warfarin with vitamin K, which results in a decreased synthesis of clotting factors V, VII, IX, and X and an anticoagulant effect, is thought to be related to unaltered warfarin rather than to any of its metabolites. This view is based on the fact that the major metabolites of warfarin in the rat are hydroxylated compounds which have no hypoprothrombinemic effect[118] and on a correlation of plasma half-life of the drug with pharmacological effect.[148] Alterations in this concept may be required by the recent demonstration that, in addition to hydroxywarfarins, warfarin alcohols can be identified as metabolites of the drug in man.[116] These warfarin compounds are very similar to biologically potent phenprocoumon and raise the theoretical possibility that increased sensitivity to warfarin can be based on genetically determined enzyme activity which may result in high concentrations of these metabolites. To date no examples of this phenomenon have been described and mechanisms which alter warfarin disappearance rates or end-organ responsiveness to the drug must be considered as the only known causes for varying effectiveness. The extensive review by O'Reilly and Aggeler examines in detail the environmental and genetic factors responsible for such variations.[146]

Following the administration of Dicumarol to an unselected human population, Motulsky found that the plasma half-lives for this drug were distributed in a unimodal fashion which he interpreted as evidence for polygenic determination of the metabolism of the drug.[135] Pyörälä and Nevanlinna demonstrated a similar plasma half-life distribution curve for warfarin in domestic rats, but selective breeding of animals at either end of the distribution curve for four generations produced two strains with quite different rates of warfarin metabolism.[160] Crossbreeding of these sensitive and resistant strains suggested that only a few genes are responsible for the production of the hydroxylases and other enzymes which catabolize warfarin.

The importance of genetic determinants for plasma disappearance rates of oral anticoagulants has also been demonstrated in man. In a study of identical and nonidentical twins, Vesell and Page demonstrated a marked similarity in the plasma decay curves of Dicumarol in identical twins, while fraternal twins were more variable.[192] However, no convincing reports have been presented of genetically determined shortening of plasma half-lives of coumarin anticoagulants in man with sufficient resistance to the drug to be of therapeutic importance. Patients have been reported in whom the plasma half-lives were greatly shortened but no familial aggregation, other than the distribution curve noted above, has been described

and associated disease seems a more likely explanation.[115]

It is clear, however, that genetically determined differences may secondarily influence rates of drug metabolism and, accordingly, their therapeutic effectiveness. Many drugs are catabolized by enzymes within the liver microsomes, the quantity of which can be either increased or decreased by a variety of influences. The barbiturates were among the first microsomal-inducing agents studied in man, and resistance to coumarin drugs after the administration of these agents is now well known; however, it is not always recognized that this resistance is quite variable in degree. Experiments of Vesell and Page demonstrated that the responsiveness of the microsomal system was under genetic control by studying the degree to which antipyrine half-lives were shortened after phenobarbital administration to identical and nonidentical twins.[193] The identical twins had virtually uniform responses to phenobarbital enzyme induction while the fraternal twins were more disparate. Interestingly, a greater decrease in the longer half-lives than in the shorter ones after phenobarbital brought the responses of the entire group within a more narrow range. A large number of chemicals, ranging from insecticides to caffeine or chloral hydrate, can serve as enzyme inducers. Discontinuation of one of these agents in a patient whose anticoagulant regimen was stabilized while the enzyme inducer was being administered can lead to excessive anticoagulation if the genotype of the individual had promoted marked enzyme induction. An excellent review of this entire area has been presented by Conney.[38]

Marked resistance to warfarin from an entirely different mechanism has been described by O'Reilly.[145,147] In two families, index members were found to require an extremely large warfarin dose to induce an anticoagulant effect. Pedigrees indicated an autosomal dominant inheritance of this trait. Lack of responsiveness due to more rapid metabolism of the drug or to a metabolic alteration, such as increased protein binding or altered distribution within the body, was excluded by detailed studies of the involved individuals. A marked sensitivity to vitamin K was also present, so that O'Reilly and colleagues postulated a dominant inheritance of a receptor site for a protein with altered affinity for, or permeability to, vitamin K. Interestingly, the same type of resistance to warfarin was demonstrated in wild rats, which were noted to be immune to warfarin applied as a pesticide. In these rodents, the anticoagulant resistance is also inherited as an autosomal dominant trait.[149]

In circumstances of increased sensitivity to warfarin, a mutant hydroxylase can be envisioned which cannot metabolize the drug as rapidly as normal, resulting in a long plasma half-life. Indeed, Solomon has reported a man with marked sensitivity to warfarin in association with delayed degradation of the agent.[180] It was suggested that a similar defect was present in the man's mother, who had sustained a major hemorrhage while on low-dosage anticoagulant therapy, but studies to confirm this in her or other members of the family are not available.

In summary, it can be seen from evidence both in man and rat that the anticoagulant effect of warfarin may be altered by genetic differences in the metabolism of the drug, either directly or through the induction of microsomal enzymes. Furthermore, resistance to warfarin due to a binding-site mutation can be transmitted in a dominant fashion in both species.

Cholinesterase Deficiency

Even if cardiologists were not frequently involved in the care of patients undergoing surgical procedures, discussion of heritable variants of serum cholinesterase would be appropriate because of the principles of genetically determined drug interactions which they illustrate.

Serum cholinesterase (formerly termed pseudocholinesterase) hydrolyzes a large number of esters, including cholinesters and benzoic-acid derivatives, in contrast to true cholinesterase, which is virtually specific for acetylcholine and is active primarily at the neuromuscular junction. In the blood, true cholinesterase is found in erythrocytes. Medical interest in serum cholinesterase was aroused shortly after the widespread introduction of the muscle relaxant suxamethonium (succinylcholine) into anesthetic practice. A few cases were soon described in which the usual dose of succinylcholine was followed by apnea persisting for several hours, instead of the brief period which is customary and which has made the drug so convenient as an adjunct to anesthesia.[22,57] Subsequent pedigree studies utilizing serum assays led to the definition of three phenotypes with normal, low, and intermediate enzyme activities and the suggestion that the deficient individuals were homozygous for a recessive gene.[4]

Although the basic framework for the inheritance of serum-cholinesterase levels was provided by the above early observations, it remained unclear whether the enzyme deficiency was related to a quantitative decrease in the normal enzyme or to the production of a less efficient mutant protein. Three additional approaches aided in the demonstration that the "recessive" gene is actually a "codominant" gene which programs for a defective cholinesterase. The first of these was the demonstration that the cholinesterase from the deficient individual not only hydrolyzes less substrate but acts more slowly than the normal enzyme.[45] Secondly, resistance to cholinesterase inhibitors was markedly different and, indeed, the use of differential inhibitors allowed the definition of a number of cholinesterase phenotypes. Originally, the local anesthetic dibucaine was utilized for this purpose after the demonstration that the atypical variant is more resistant to dibucaine at a standard concentration than is the normal enzyme.[99] Later, fluoride inhibition was used in the same fashion and permitted the recognition of additional phenotypes.[82] Finally, electrophoresis on starch gel demonstrated an additional phenotype which did not seem to segregate in the usual allelic pattern when categorized by selective inhibition as well as by electrophoretic migration. Harris and colleagues considered that this phenotype provided evidence for at least two gene loci controlling the production of cholinesterase.[81] Accordingly, classification of the cholinesterase phenotypes utilized not only deficiencies in enzyme function but also variations in a secondary characteristic and evidence for structural differences in the protein.

As might be expected, the mutant cholinesterases are associated with varying degrees of succinylcholine sensitivity. Statistically, the two most important are the normal and atypical phenotypes originally described. However, two others are of particular note because of additional insights which they lend. A so-called silent gene, which is quite rare in most areas of the world and is associated with exquisite succinylcholine sensitivity, has been found in relatively high frequency in Eskimos of a particular locale in southern Alaska, demonstrating that genes uncommon in one population may be concentrated in racial isolates.[78] Accordingly, extreme caution should be used, both theoretically and in practice, in extrapolation of information regarding biological characteristics from one group to another. Recently, evidence has been presented that two or more "silent" alleles may exist.[165]

Like most other inborn metabolic errors, the mutant cholinesterases were originally recognized because their reduced effectiveness led to an undesired effect. Rarely have more efficient deviant proteins been recognized, so that the recent description of a cholinesterase with increased activity is of great interest.[138] The true incidence of such "beneficial" mutations and their potential importance are unknown.

It is unclear if any drug interactions other than those to succinylcholine may be important in the cholinesterase variants, since the physiological role of the enzyme is not known.

However, in view of the fact that all local anesthetic agents are cholinesterase inhibitors to varying degrees, unusual reactions to lidocaine may be anticipated in some of the cholinesterase variants as the use of this agent as an antiarrhythmic drug increases.

Immune Responses to Cardiovascular Drugs

Among the more dramatic of drug reactions is the lupus syndrome which follows a number of agents, among which cardiovascular drugs are prominent. Since all patients do not respond adversely, it is evident that the host provides critical ingredients for the interaction. Theoretically, these ingredients could range from specific haptene carriers of the drug or its metabolic products to an ability to recognize the foreign antigen or to responsiveness of the immunoglobulin system of the host. For most untoward drug reactions, it is not possible to determine the area at fault.

These syndromes are important to the cardiologist, not only because they are often superimposed on an underlying cardiovascular problem but also because they may occur with pericarditis and other manifestations of a vasculitis, including myocarditis.

HYDRALAZINE

Shortly after the introduction of hydralazine as an antihypertensive agent, it was recognized that a febrile illness with arthritis, skin reactions, pleuritis, and other features of spontaneous systemic lupus erythematosus developed in some patients receiving the drug. Serological evidence of an auto-immune state was manifested by positive LE cell tests and the presence of antinuclear antibodies. More recently, these laboratory abnormalities have been found in patients receiving hydralazine who have no symptoms of the lupus syndrome.

A recent observation may help to link a genetic mechanism with the view of some investigators that the auto-immune response follows only large doses of hydralazine. Perry and co-workers reported that the incidence of the development of antinuclear antibodies in patients receiving hydralazine appeared to be related to the rate at which the patients were able to degrade hydralazine by acetylation.[152] In their study of 55 patients on long-term hydralazine therapy, 8 out of 10 individuals who had received a total dose in excess of 1200 gm had antinuclear antibodies, while 5 of 21 patients demonstrated this serological finding at doses less than 400 gm. In the intermediate total dose ranges between 400 and 1200 gm, 3 of 9 individuals who metabolized hydralazine rapidly and 13 of 15 who acetylated it slowly developed antinuclear antibodies.

Two populations of individuals with genetically determined different rates of isoniazid acetylation have been known for almost two decades.[88] In those patients who acetylate slowly, a higher percentage of the drug is excreted unchanged in the urine and the incidence of toxicity from a standard dose of isoniazid is considerably higher than in rapid acetylators, although the therapeutic efficacy of the drug remains adequate in the latter group. Pedigree studies revealed that rapid acetylation is inherited as an autosomal dominant while slow acetylation is a recessive trait. The geographical distribution of the genotypes is variable.[183] The most likely explanation is that the slow acetylators produce a mutant acetylase which is less effective than the normal enzyme. Further studies revealed that other drugs, including sulfamethazine and hydralazine, share the same acetyl transferase with isoniazid and, accordingly, have genetically determined differences in disappearance rates.[56] It has also been suggested that the conversion of digitoxin into digoxin may be seen in rapid acetylators; however, detailed information in this regard is not available.[96] At least one other drug-acetylation pathway exists in man, since para-aminosalicylic acid and sulfanilamide do not demonstrate the same segregation into fast and slow acetylators.

If further studies demonstrate that acetyla-

tion rate is indeed the major determinant of the development of the lupus phenomena in patients on long-term hydralazine therapy, determination of acetylation phenotype would appear to be required for proper planning of therapy with this agent; this can be done readily by using a test of sulfamethazine acetylation.[56]

Other genetic factors may be of importance, also, in that Alarcón-Segovia and colleagues, following a careful study of 50 cases of the hydralazine syndrome and a review of the literature, suggested that an underlying lupus diathesis was dormant in these patients until it was unmasked by the inducing drug.[2,3] Their evidence was that antecedent rheumatic manifestations were present in 74 per cent of the patients who developed the lupus syndrome following hydralazine but in only 13 per cent of a control group. Furthermore, in 34 per cent of the patients with the lupus syndrome, the family history was positive for rheumatic disease. In this regard, it is of note that Pollak has reported serum antinuclear antibodies in family members in 25 of the 43 lupus kinships which he investigated.[158] Finally, persistence of antinuclear antibodies has been reported, on the basis of the development of the lupus syndrome, for as long as nine years after hydralazine administration was stopped. Clearly, caution should be observed in the long-term usage of hydralazine therapy in an individual with a family history of rheumatic diseases.

Procainamide

Fewer than 100 cases of procainamide-induced lupus have been reported since the initial observation in 1962, but laboratory surveys for auto-immune phenomena have revealed a high incidence following procainamide.[111,133] Indeed, the combination of extensive use of the drug and a high incidence of reaction make procainamide one of the most prominent of the lupus-inducing drugs. Except for a lack of renal manifestation and somewhat less skin and lymph-node involvement, procainamide-induced illness is very much like spontaneous lupus erythematosus. Generally symptoms abate shortly after discontinuation of the drug but may occasionally persist for months; in the series reviewed by Dubois, laboratory abnormalities, which customarily are slow to resolve, demonstrated a median length of 16 weeks of positivity after cessation of exposure to procainamide.[49]

As yet no specific genetic interrelationship has been determined for the procainamide-induced auto-immune phenomena similar to the difference in acetylation rates which was discussed in the case of hydralazine. However, other observations suggest the possibility that procainamide produces difficulty only in individuals with a particular genetic set of the immune system. In a survey for LE cells, antinuclear antibodies, and rheumatoid factor in 22 asymptomatic patients on procainamide, Molina et al. found that 77 per cent were positive for one or more of these lupus-associated laboratory tests.[133] In the four patients who demonstrated positivity early after administration ($1\frac{1}{2}$ to 4 months), three had a background of rheumatic disease aside from rheumatic heart disease. As further evidence that procainamide may unmask an underlying diathesis, Lappat and Cawein reported a survey of relatives of patients with procainamide-induced lupus which yielded a number of asymptomatic family members with positive antinuclear antibodies.[113] Although such observations suggest that caution should be exercised in the administration of procainamide on a long-term basis in patients with evidence of a rheumatic diathesis in either themselves or close family members, Blomgren et al. have expressed the view that the high percentages of reactors mitigate against a genetic predisposition.[17] In their prospective study of 16 patients who received procainamide, 8 developed antinuclear antibodies and 2 of these had clinical lupus.

Dilantin (diphenylhydantoin)

Although Dilantin is a second-echelon antiarrhythmic drug, it is used frequently enough by cardiologists to merit comment, particu-

larly since it is an example of another type of genetically determined drug reaction. Although Dilantin is metabolized by parahydroxylation—and isoniazid is acetylated, as described previously—evidence has been presented that the metabolism of each may be influenced by the simultaneous administration of both of these agents. Brennan and colleagues reported Dilantin intoxication with confusion and ataxia in patients who were receiving both drugs; they then demonstrated that the involved individuals were slow isoniazid deactivators and that approximately one half of the slow acetylators developed evidence of Dilantin intoxication.[27] Kutt et al. then demonstrated a noncompetitive inhibition of Dilantin metabolism by isoniazid in liver microsomes; they also showed that genetically determined Dilantin toxicity was the result of a defect in hydroxylation, presumably due to an enzyme with low activity.[109,110]

As with hydralazine and procainamide, the appearance of a lupus syndrome occurs in a portion of the patients who are treated with this drug. Although the auto-immune manifestations generally subside after the Dilantin is discontinued, the authors have observed one young man in whom the clinical evidence of lupus has continued for over five years after the agent was stopped. The father of this young man has spontaneous lupus erythematosus. It appears likely that clinical manifestations of the immune phenomena after the administration of Dilantin may, as with procainamide and hydralazine, be determined by the immune capacities of the host.

Methyldopa

In the decade since alpha-methyldopa has become one of the most widely used antihypertensive agents, a variety of side effects of the agent have been described. A positive Coombs' test appears within 3 to 37 months, but usually within 18 months, in approximately one quarter of the patients to whom methyldopa is administered.[202] An auto-immune hemolytic anemia develops in a small percentage of these sensitized individuals but usually subsides promptly when the drug is discontinued. Antinuclear factors appear in the serum of 15 per cent of patients on prolonged methyldopa therapy; fever and abnormal liver-function tests have also been noted.[26,51,186] These unusual immunological manifestations may appear as isolated manifestations or in varying combinations.

At present no evidence has been presented to link the appearance of the auto-immune reactions of methyldopa to either an underlying rheumatic diathesis, as was discussed in relation to procainamide, or to any unusual metabolism of the drug, as may be true for hydralazine; however, another unusual genetic interaction has been noted. An IgG antibody, which is present in serum and can also be eluted from erythrocytes, is present in those patients who have positive Coombs' tests. Unlike the situation in the usual drug-related hemolytic anemia, this antibody also reacts against the red cells of patients who have not received the drug. Furthermore, Worlledge et al. noted an Rh specificity, leading these investigators to suggest the possibility that the drug or a metabolite may be incorporated into the red cells, causing alterations in the normal red-cell antigens.[202] Although these antibodies may persist for several weeks, neither they nor the antinuclear factors have remained evident for prolonged periods, as have some of the responses to other agents discussed in this section. Fortunately, the incidence of hemolytic anemia is low but the red-cell antibodies may cause difficulty in the crossmatching of blood.

THE GENETIC CONTRIBUTION TO COMMON CARDIOVASCULAR PROBLEMS

Hypertension

The importance of heredity as a determinant of blood pressure, including hypertension, has often been obscured in debates as to whether blood pressure is dictated by a number of genes, i.e. is polygenic, or if the idiopathic group of diseases called essential hypertension is due to effects of a single gene locus. This review will focus on evidence pertaining to the genetic role in hypertensive disease in human population groups regardless of mechanism and on pertinent animal experiments which help elucidate the degree to which hypertension and environmental influences on blood pressure, such as salt intake, are predicated on genes.

POPULATION SURVEYS

Studies in a number of countries have indicated that blood pressure among the various population groups is distributed in a unimodal or gaussian fashion. A recent report of this sort is that by Miall, who also pointed out that members within a given kinship tend to be clustered within the bell-shaped distribution curve rather than dispersed throughout it.[131] From a recalculation of some of Miall's earlier data and a comparison with polygenically determined stature, Acheson and Fowler concluded that the role of heredity in the regulation of blood pressure was even more important than previously thought.[1]

Strong additional support for the importance of heredity in essential hypertension is found in the study of VanderMolen and co-workers.[191] These investigators compared the degree of concordance for hypertension in identical and nonidentical twins. Although the sample was relatively small and should be extended, the incidence of hypertension in both members of the identical pairs was significantly greater than in the fraternal twins. Even so, in one quarter of the fraternal twins, if one member was hypertensive the other had elevated blood pressure; this is a significantly greater incidence than would be expected in a random sample of the population. These twin data are the most compelling evidence in support of the role of heredity in the etiology of hypertension. It is doubtful if further population surveys of blood pressure will lend much to the understanding of hypertension unless some pertinent correlative parameters are identified. In other words, it seems clearly established that hypertension is the result of many genes as well as of environmental influences. However, in certain individuals or groups, a single determinant may far outweigh all other factors, and methods need to be developed to evaluate these. Experimental animals with genetically determined hypertension are being used to evaluate specific physiological mechanisms with the hope that specific molecular determinations of their elevated blood pressure will be found.

ETHNIC DIFFERENCES

The incidence of hypertension varies considerably among different ethnic groups. Evaluation of epidemiological studies in different countries and among different racial groups has been extremely difficult because of methodological problems, so that comments will be limited primarily to studies of hypertension in black and white populations of the United States. The frequency and early age of onset of hypertension in the black patient has been emphasized by the report of Finnerty,[60] who found a history of hypertension in 48 per cent of the young black women attending a birth-control clinic, and by the mortality statistics accumulated by Berkson and Stamler.[13] It has been difficult to distinguish if this ethnic difference in incidence is due to environmental features, such as diet, adequacy of medical care, and psychological stresses, or to genetic factors. In a very detailed analysis, with controls for as many socioeconomic factors as possible, Howard and Holman clearly demonstrated that the increased incidence of hypertension in the American black could not be related in any primary sense to these factors alone.[87] Finnerty has rightly pointed out that the high incidence of hypertension in this population indicates a need for concerted efforts at detection and control. It is not clear, however, if response to the current therapeutic

armamentarium is as adequate in this group as in other ethnic groups. Indeed, the authors agree with an earlier observation by Finnerty that retinal vascular changes are sometimes present at an early age in the black in the absence of hypertension or other predisposing disorders, such as diabetes or a hemoglobinopathy.[61]

HYPERTENSIVE ANIMALS

Selection within inbred animal strains has demonstrated the rapidity with which the genes controlling blood pressure can be concentrated and has at the same time provided fascinating tools for the study of experimental hypertension. Dahl, Heine, and Tassinari chose rats from both ends of the unimodal distribution curve for blood pressure, which is similar to the usual human blood-pressure distribution.[41] Using these animals for selective breeding for three generations allowed them to develop two populations of rats which were dissimilar in blood pressure, with the disparity between the two groups being sharpened even more by the environmental adjunct of increased salt intake. Uninephrectomy produced mild hypertension in the sensitive rats but none in the resistant rats, while unilateral renal-artery constriction produced mild hypertension in the resistant rats and severe blood-pressure elevation in the sensitive rats.[93] This observation may be pertinent to the fact that many human subjects with renal-artery constriction do not develop hypertension. Both the sensitive and resistant strains developed severe hypertension following the classical Goldblatt procedure of renal-artery constriction and contralateral nephrectomy; if this procedure was performed on one of a parabiotic pair, however, it induced hypertension in the partner only if the operated rat was of the sensitive strain. In corollary studies it was demonstrated that renoprival hypertension in a nephrectomized sensitive rat did not induce hypertension in a parabiosed intact resistant rat.[102] On the basis of these studies, the investigators suggested that two pressor substances could be released from the kidneys of the sensitive strain, one of which was transmissible by parabiosis while the other was not. The resistant strain was thought to have the capacity to make only the nontransferable pressor.

Variation in pharmacological responsiveness in rats with unlimited hypertension is another approach which has been utilized by McGregor and Smirk.[119] In their colony of hypertensive rats, 5-hydroxytryptamine (serotonin) induced a much greater blood-pressure response than in either control or renal-hypertensive animals. It would be of considerable interest to know if strains of hypertensive rats developed by these two groups behave in comparable fashions to a variety of stimuli or if they may have selectively bred animals with different etiologies for this hypertension.

Other groups have demonstrated the same types of unimodal distribution curves for blood pressure in strains of mice and rats and, either by comparing strains[169] or by selective crossbreeding,[153] have demonstrated marked genetic influences, probably related to only a few genes. These animals can now be used in further experiments of the sort described above in the hopes of identifying physiological or biochemical defects which may be applicable to the human hypertensive patient.

Atherosclerosis

In few areas of medicine has more controversy raged than in the debates regarding the relative contributions of heredity and environment to the causation of atherosclerosis. In part, this is due to the fact that many environmental contributors to the disorder, such as cigarette smoking and dietary habits, have major economic backing and are deeply ingrained in the culture of the western world. In fairness, however, it is clear that genetic factors are important in the production of atherosclerosis, since virtually all surveys of white population groups have demonstrated a familial aggregation of atherosclerotic heart disease and of many of the

metabolic parameters known to be associated with an increased incidence of the disease.[46,47,172] Representative of such studies is that by Slack and Evans, in which first-degree relatives of patients with coronary heart disease were found to have dramatic increases in the rate of coronary disease, ranging from $2\frac{1}{2}$ to 7 times that of a control group, depending on the age and sex of the individual.[177]

A genetic susceptibility to atherosclerosis may be related to an intrinsic defect in the arterial wall, as in pseudoxanthoma elasticum,[122] to hypertension, to diabetes, or to a defect in lipid metabolism. In ethnic groups such as blacks and the Japanese in whom hypertension is common, the elevated blood pressure has seemed to contribute more to a high incidence of strokes than to coronary-artery disease. Accordingly, epidemiological studies of atherosclerosis in various parts of the world have generally been concerned primarily with correlations of serum cholesterols and the incidence of atherosclerosis. As emphasized by Keys, when the adoption of western dietary habits by a particular ethnic group leads to serum-cholesterol levels similar to those of western whites, the incidence of coronary-artery disease also approaches that of Europe and the United States.[101] A dramatic example of the importance of serum constituents, presumably lipids for the most part, and of the rapidity with which severe atheromatous disease can develop is found in recent cardiac transplant history. The coronary arteries of the previously healthy heart from a 24-year-old black donor were markedly narrowed by extensive coronary atherosclerosis after slightly more than $1\frac{1}{2}$ years of post-transplant life in a 58-year-old white hypercholesterolemic man.[189]

In view of the multiplicity of biochemical reactions and interrelated feedback-control systems which are involved in the absorption of exogenous cholesterol, the synthesis of endogenous cholesterol, and its excretion from the body, it is not surprising that the serum-cholesterol concentrations in most populations have a polygenic distribution.[46] (For an excellent review of cholesterol metabolism, see Dietschy and Wilson.[48]) Still, it is clear that a single gene can be a sufficiently powerful determinant of cholesterol level to dictate the dominant inheritance of coronary-artery disease in those individuals with familial hypercholesterolemia (type-II hyperlipoproteinemia).[66,157] Elevation of serum triglyceride levels is also a potent predicator of coronary-artery disease and is more strikingly abnormal in some of the hyperlipoproteinemic states than is the cholesterol concentration.[100] Regulation of serum triglycerides, which to date has not been tied to any single gene in any disease entity, was reviewed in detail recently by Havel.[83]

Currently considerable interest has been stimulated by reports that members of an African tribe with a low frequency of atherosclerosis have low serum-cholesterol concentrations while on a diet with two thirds of its calories furnished from fat.[85] The Masai are nomadic people who consume, almost exclusively, milk with some blood and meat; 50 per cent more calories come from fat than in the usual American or European diet. Although most studies in man have shown that feedback inhibition of cholesterol synthesis is limited,[48] it appears that the Masai have a very efficient negative feedback control of endogenous cholesterol synthesis, as well as an increased capacity to absorb dietary cholesterol. This combination produces a mean serum cholesterol of 135 mg/100 ml, which is only slightly lower than that found in another nomadic tribe of northern Kenya, the Samburu, which also eats a high-fat diet.[174] In contrast, the Rendille, a neighboring group with a similar life style and dietary habits, has much higher serum-cholesterol values.

A lessened incidence of atherosclerosis has been reported for a number of other population groups, such as the Bantu,[171] the Indians of the southwestern United States,[176] the Nigerians,[200] and others; often this has appeared to be due to nutritional inadequacies,

as reported from India,[167] or to cultural dietary habits.[154] Hopefully, and probably, the reports of the unique cholesterol metabolism of the Masai will stimulate more detailed analysis of lipid pathways in some of these groups rather than estimates of the balance of input, synthesis, and degradation reflected in serum values.

Evaluations of possible ethnic difference in atherosclerosis in one country have scarcely been less difficult than have been the comparisons among countries. In the United States, most studies have indicated that the incidence of atherosclerosis is significantly lower in blacks than in whites.[16,34,108,154] The most convincing studies have been those in which pathological confirmation of coronary-artery disease and infarction was present.[127,203] Interestingly, it appears that the sex difference in mortality from coronary-artery disease, which is striking in whites until relatively late in life, is not as marked in blacks.[108] Since hypertension, an accepted accelerator of atherosclerosis, is more common in blacks than in whites, a number of other coronary-proneness factors have been examined by a variety of investigators. Serum-cholesterol and triglyceride levels are approximately the same in blacks and whites in the younger age ranges but, with increasing age, remain stationary in the blacks while rising in the whites.[11,42] In a prospective study from Evans County, Georgia—in which a large number of socioeconomic factors and physiological and biochemical determinants were evaluated—it was suggested that the major cause for a lower incidence of coronary-artery disease in black men was a higher exercise level.[35]

The divergence of atherosclerosis appears early in life, at a time when exercise patterns may not be so dissimilar as they are later in life. In a study of autopsies on American soldiers who were killed in Vietnam, McNamara reported a high incidence of coronary-artery disease in asymptomatic young men between the ages of 18 and 37 years, generally comparably to a similar study from the Korean war by Enos.[53,126] Analysis of the Vietnam casualties by race revealed that 45 of the 91 white soldiers had significant coronary atherosclerosis while only 2 of the 14 black soldiers had comparable disease.[125]

It seems likely that some other racial, i.e. genetic, trait grants the black man relative immunity to coronary-artery disease without, of course, removing all liability to the stresses of elevated cholesterol, blood pressure, and cigarette smoking. Population enclaves which are isolated by geography or custom have relatively constricted gene pools, just as do animal strains which have been collectively bred to produce hypertension or resistance to warfarin. It is hardly surprising that racial differences in vascular disease occur. Exploration of these differences and the mechanisms behind them will contribute greatly to our understanding of the pathogenesis of the disorders and selective modes of treatment.

Chronic Lung Disease

Alpha₁-antitrypsin Deficiency

Recognition of genetic determinants of responses in drug influences provides the situation which is most amenable to corrective measures. However, delineation of genetically determined high-risk groups in the population may provide an opportunity to apply selectively prophylactic measures— abstinence from cigarette smoking, reduction in dietary intake, or avoidance of other environmental hazards. An excellent articulation by Haldane of this general thesis was quoted in a review by Keuppers:[105]

"I should be interested to know whether, to take a single example, the death rate among potters from bronchitis is still eight times that of the general population. If so, it would not be unreasonable if a certain proportion of the funds devoted to pottery research at Stoke-On-Trent were spent on research on potters rather than on pots. But while I am sure that our standards of industrial hygiene are shamefully low, it is important to realize that there is a side to this question which has so far been completely ignored. The majority of potters do not die of bronchitis. It is quite possible that, if we really understood the causation of this disease, we should find that only a fraction of potters are of a constitution which renders them liable to it. If so, we could eliminate potter's bronchitis by rejecting entrants into the pottery industry who are congenitally disposed to it. We are already making the attempt to exclude accident-prone workers from certain trades. The principle could perhaps be carried a good deal further. There are two sides to most of these questions involving unfavorable environments. Not only could the environment be improved, but susceptible individuals could be excluded."[79]

The above quotation from Kuepper's excellent review of alpha₁-antitrypsin deficiency introduces the question of the role of heredity in the production of chronic lung disease. The increasing prevalence of cor pulmonale secondary to chronic lung disease makes the inclusion of this topic pertinent to a volume on cardiovascular problems.

Recognition in the past decade that deficiency of one of the four electrophoretically identifiable serum proteinases is associated with parenchymal lung disease has stimulated great interest in the genetic variants of this protein. The clinical picture of individuals with very low levels (approximately 10 per cent of normal) of alpha₁-antitrypsin consists of the onset of symptoms in the fourth decade with rapidly progressive loss of lung tissue, particularly in the lower lobes. As would be anticipated, dyspnea is a major symptom which accompanies hyperlucency of the involved areas on x-ray, diminished perfusion on lung scans, and evidence of ventilation defects in pulmonary function. Symptoms of bronchitis are prominent in some patients as well.

Fortunately, separation of clinically recognizable phenotypes was virtually absolute in the initial studies and recognition of a simple mendelian mode of inheritance of alpha₁-antitrypsin was relatively simple.[55] In a comparison within a population group, individuals were found with high (approximately 200 mg/100 ml), intermediate (approximately 120 mg/100 ml), and low (approximately 25 mg/100 ml) levels of the glycoprotein, and family studies demonstrated that the intermediate levels represented the heterozygous state for genes, which, in homozygous individuals, produced either normal or low levels. More sophisticated electrophoretic techniques have subsequently allowed the definition of other phenotypes which appear to be the result of a number of alleles at a single gene locus, referred to as the Pi (for proteinase inhibitor) locus.[58] The more recently recognized Pi phenotypes have varying but, for the most part, lesser degrees of depression of alpha$_1$-antitrypsin than does the first variant described.

The alpha$_1$-antitrypsin deficiency is important not only because of the production of disease in the relatively infrequent homozygotes but also because of potential susceptibility of the more numerous heterozygotes to environmental stress. Evaluation of risk to the heterozygote cannot be determined from prospective data at present, but attempts have been made to study the problem by statistical comparisons of the frequency of the antitrypsin deficiency in patients with chronic lung disease versus a control population. In a study of 146 patients, Welch et al. reported a depression of antitrypsin levels in 12 per cent; however, this was not considered to be significantly greater than the incidence of 6 per cent (which approximates the heterozygote frequency in the population at large) in their control groups.[198] On the other hand, both Lieberman and Kueppers and Larson reported a significantly higher frequency of the deficiency in their series of patients with emphysema than in controls.[107,117] Stevens and co-workers have reexamined the data of Welch and added more, including pathological material, which demonstrate that heterozygotes develop lung disease more frequently than the population at large, albeit at a later age.[182] It appears prudent to consider that the probability is high that these heterozygotes constitute an at-risk group, perhaps the susceptible potters to whom Haldane referred.

In view of the activity of antitrypsin as an inhibitor of a number of proteolytic enzymes, hypotheses regarding the mode by which a deficiency produces pulmonary disease have naturally centered around this function. The major alternate hypotheses suggest that, in the deficient individual, uninhibited proteolytic enzymes, which have been released from peribronchial leukocytes, macrophages, or bacteria, destroy lung tissue or that the normal rate of breakdown of connective tissues of the lung parenchyma is accelerated.[91,106]

Cystic Fibrosis of the Pancreas

Cystic fibrosis is another entity in which the homozygous state is associated with severe pulmonary disease, as well as pancreatic and intestinal abnormality. As has been known for many years, the disorder becomes manifest in infancy or early childhood, but, in contrast to alpha$_1$-antitrypsin deficiency, the pulmonary disorder (secondary to repeated pulmonary infections in areas obstructed by viscous secretions) is dominantly in the upper lungs. The familial aggregation within one generation, gastrointestinal and pulmonary manifestations, and a reliable laboratory aid in the high-sweat sodium concentrations make the diagnosis relatively simple in childhood. Recognition may be more difficult in adults in whom the sweat sodium values are less reliable, except that low values virtually exclude the disorder. This is particularly true of those individuals in whom manifestations have been less pronounced in childhood or in whom pulmonary manifestations have predominated or where a familial aggregation is not present. Obviously, cor pulmonale can be the eventual result of the severe pulmonary disease and is becoming more frequent as survival is prolonged with antibiotic and pancreatic replacement therapy.[30,173]

Until recently it has not been possible to identify the heterozygous carriers of the gene for cystic fibrosis except as they became parents of diseased children. Careful studies of these heterozygotes demonstrate no deleterious effects of the gene, although earlier suggestions of marginal increases in sweat sodium levels or even of increased suscepti-bility to chronic pulmonary disease had been made.[150,201] A method for identifying hetero-zygotes and possibly for dividing the clinical entity of cystic fibrosis into two or more geno-types was reported by Bearn and Danes and promises new insights.[8] In cultured fibro-blasts and monocytes from both heterozygotes and homozygotes, these investigators found metachromatic staining in two distinct pat-terns, one of which could possibly be sub-divided. The method lacks specificity, since metachromasis can be detected in cell cul-tures from a small number of "normal" indi-viduals as well as from patients with one of the mucopolysaccharidoses. Nonetheless, it provides a tool for the objective classification of individuals by genotype.

CARDIOVASCULAR DISORDERS WITH MAJOR GENETIC INPUT

While the previous discussion emphasized the intricate relationship between the environ-ment and the genetic makeup of an individ-ual, it is also recognized that some cardio-vascular disorders are due primarily to inheritance, sometimes via a single gene. McKusick[120,121,123] and Taylor[187] have re-viewed these in the past, and only pertinent information regarding selective entities that are of interest will be updated.

Billowing or Ballooning Mitral Valves

Only in the last decade has it become clear that late systolic clicks and murmurs (or pre-cordial honks) are not extracardiac but indic-ative of a prolapsed or billowing mitral valve which may, at times, be associated with arrhythmias, significant mitral regurgitation, and T-wave electrocardiographic alterations. Complications, such as ruptured chorda tendineae or bacterial endocarditis, may be superimposed and the entity, although a rela-tively benign form of mitral-valve disease, is not always innocuous. While several studies have reported this condition to be familial and to transmit dominantly, it may also be sporadic.[90,159,175] A billowing valve also

occurs as part of the Marfan syndrome, a dom-inant disorder, and tends to be more common in tall, thin individuals.[14] It will probably be observed in other connective-tissue dis-orders as well, e.g. Ehlers-Danlos syndrome or homocystinuria, since the underlying ab-normality appears to be mucoid degeneration of the valve.[159] The case has been made that the billowing valve without the associated stigmata of Marfan's syndrome is a forme fruste of the latter disease, but the argument is weak and no families with Marfan's syn-drome have been reported in which some individuals have a prolapsing mitral valve as the only manifestation.

Congenital Heart Diseases

The theory that genetic factors play a role in certain cardiovascular anomalies is based on the following kinds of evidence: cardio-vascular defects of a specific nature occur in several members of a family; an increased incidence of congenital cardiac malforma-tions is seen in close relatives of patients with congenital heart defects; cardiovascular de-fects are noted as part of a larger constellation with a known genetic mode of transmission; twin studies, while indicating a low con-cordance rate, are compatible with a signifi-cant role being played by the genome of the individual; consanguinity increases the inci-dence of malformations in families with genetic disorders; and chromosomal derange-ments of known types are associated with spe-cific cardiac defects. Reports during the last decade have offered fairly compelling sup-port for all these points.

Data from these reports can be briefly sum-marized. It is probable that specific defects can be inherited within families, since most common congenital heart defects have been reported to cluster in families; however, it is often difficult to be certain that this is not by chance.[98,142,143] Examination of sibs and parents of probands with known heart de-fects reveals that 3 to 10 per cent of sibs and about 2 per cent of parents may be affected with similar defects.[50,143] On the other hand, when the children of parents with atrial or ventricular septal defects, for example, are evaluated, 37 and 21 times the estimated frequency of the respective anomaly in these individuals are found.[140] Rarely has it been possible to demonstrate a simple mendelian type of inheritance, and polygenic influences interacting with environmental stimuli are responsible for most congenital malformations.

The familial interatrial septal defect represents the best example of a congenital heart defect in which an autosomal dominant gene is responsible for the defect in many families, although, for most individuals with the disease, such a mechanism is not operative.[142] Dominantly inherited atrial septal defects have been described in association with other identifying features. Perhaps the best known of these entities is that which is combined with anomalies of the upper extremity.[86] More recently, Bizarro and colleagues have emphasized the association of atrial septal defects with prolonged A–V conduction.[15] The importance of this is that genetic prognosis in a patient with an atrial septal defect and one of these associated syndromes may be a risk of 50 per cent to the offspring.

In examining patients with known heart defects, a high incidence of associated extracardiac defects has been noted, varying from 11 to 41 per cent depending on the study;[19, 50,52] the high percentages indicate that clusters of defects tend to occur in the same individuals. While this relationship does not prove a genetic origin, and many classical teratogens produce multiple malformations, it is important to note them since they may permit easier recognition of a genetic syndrome. Multiple entities of this sort have been described,[187] but a few new ones merit comment. Deafness, congenital mitral regurgitation, short stature, and skeletal abnormalities were reported, in varying combinations, in six members of three generations of one family. An autosomal dominant inheritance with variable penetrance was considered to be the mode of transmission.[64] A dif-

ferent constellation of skeletal defects, deaf-mutism, and congenital heart disease was attributed to a dominant gene since children from the same mother by two fathers had identical defects.[103]

Since identical twins tend to have a concordancy rate of 30 to 46 per cent for major cardiac malformations, it has been said that such a rate indicates that strong genetic factors do not play a dominant role in these defects.[121] Others have taken issue with this, and pointed out that a strong genetic role is still prominent in these individuals.[141,187] Environmental factors superimposed on a genetic predisposition provide the most logical explanation for the concordancy rate in identical twins.

Idiopathic Hypertrophic Subaortic Stenosis (IHSS)

Since 1960, when Brent and colleagues demonstrated the autosomal dominant inheritance of muscular subaortic stenosis in three generations of two families, a large volume of literature on this entity has accumulated.[28] It appears that familial cases occur about one third of the time; the rest are sporadic. The entity is common enough that it should be suspected in patients with aortic stenosis and a family history of cardiac disease. Patients with familial IHSS or hypertrophic obstructive cardiomyopathy are usually diagnosed earlier, and more females are observed in this group than in the sporadic form. Although it has been suggested that various clinical manifestations and the prognosis may be different in the familial and sporadic cases, the course of the disease is so variable that this is questionable.[65] Furthermore, the familial incidence is probably underestimated since the disease may become manifest at any age from childhood to the seventh decade and, unless a careful survey of other family members is made, it may be erroneously assumed to be a sporadic case.

Numerous studies which present features distinguishing IHSS from valvular aortic stenosis have been published.[63,65,74,137] Characteristic findings include a decreased or unchanged pulse pressure in a postextrasystolic beat, an arterial pulse with a brisk upstroke and subsequent decline and rebound (which gives a spike-and-dome contour), a bifid left ventricular apical impulse, and, frequently, mitral regurgitation. Electrocardiographic evidence of septal hypertrophy and lack of evidence of aortic-root dilatation on x-ray are also commonly associated with IHSS.

It is generally accepted that the obstructive component is only one feature of the diffuse ventricular hypertrophy which characterizes this disease. This is clearly demonstrated in those families in which members with nonobstructive and obstructive varieties coexist.[65,137] Still, the muscular outflow obstruction produces many of the dramatic features which are accentuated by inotrophic agents and maneuvers which decrease ventricular volume.

Other Familial Cardiomyopathies

Although IHSS has been in the limelight in recent years, other types of familial cardiomyopathy have been described.[7,24,74] These include glycogen-storage disease, cardiomyopathy associated with Friedreich's ataxia, amyloidosis, endocardial fibroelastosis, myocardial hypertrophy, and familial cardiomegaly. Certain of these will be discussed in other sections. In autopsied patients with familial cardiomegaly (or cardiomyopathy), generalized cardiomegaly with nonspecific, patchy fibrosis and hypertrophy of surviving fibers has been described. In certain instances a PAS-positive material has also been noted.[24] Severe arrhythmias and heart block have occurred commonly. The mode of inheritance has usually followed a dominant pattern. Little is known regarding the real pathogenesis of this disorder, nor have biochemical or electron-microscopic studies helped our understanding thus far. A recently reported animal model for this disease will hopefully shed some light.[6]

Endocardial fibroelastosis in certain instances might also be considered as genetically determined, since several sibships and families have been reported with this disease.[62] Little understanding has occurred over the last ten years other than better clinical descriptions of the disorder, which appears to be transmitted as an autosomal recessive disorder.

It is pertinent to digress regarding the possible role in the cardiomyopathies of racial factors as they may reflect a particular gene pool. In an extensive review of cardiovascular diseases in the white and black races, Phillips and Burch concluded that heart failure in the absence of coronary-artery disease, hemodynamic overload, or specific myocardial defects, such as amyloid, is more common in blacks than whites.[155] Most writers agree with this conclusion, but at this point the consensus ends. Confusion and conflict abound in the writings on post- or peripartum heart failure, idiopathic cardiomegaly, and endomyocardial fibrosis—all entities accepted as being more common in black patients than in white.

Endomyocardial fibrosis has been described primarily in Rwanda immigrants in Uganda but is seen in some of the nearby areas of western Africa as well. It is characterized by heart failure of acute onset in individuals of all ages; signs of valvular insufficiency may appear. Davies collated the major features of the disease after some initial brief reports.[43,44] Distinguishing features are endocardial and subendocardial fibrosis of the ventricular inflow tracts which often leads to impairment of A–V valve function in a dilated but not hypertrophic heart.[39] This is clearly a separate entity from the other types of myocardial disease in which hypertrophy of the heart is a dominant feature.

Reports of myocardial disease from other areas of Africa and other regions of the world emphasize myocardial hypertrophy by the use of such terms as idiopathic myocardial hypertrophy and idiopathic cardiomegaly, which are well substantiated in postmortem reports in which heart sizes have ranged from

400 to 900 gm. Many authors have emphasized that nutritional inadequacies, alcoholism, and poverty have been frequent concomitants of this primary myocardial disease, as they were in the 50 patients described by Massumi and colleagues.[128] The clinical presentation of heart failure interspersed with mural thrombi and both systemic and pulmonary emboli but with no evidence of a hemodynamic stress is characteristic.

Most series of patients with postpartum heart failure have been drawn from the same population groups which provide most of the examples of primary myocardial disease; not surprisingly, the pathological picture from these groups is identical, also.[29,89,129] Unfortunately, neither prospective nor adequate long-term follow-up studies are available; however, Pierce, Price, and Joyce have pointed out a familial incidence of myocardial disease in patients with postpartum heart failure.[156] It seems likely that it represents merely one type of presentation of the idiopathic primary myocardial disease of blacks. Pregnancy, nutritional deficiency, or alcohol may serve only to unmask or exaggerate a genetically determined underlying metabolic defect. Hopefully, in the coming decade, some of the puzzles about these points will be unraveled.

Neuromuscular Disorders

Several neuromuscular diseases involve the cardiovascular system by effects on contractility or in the conduction system, or by ventilatory effects from impaired chest movement. Most of these are transmitted as single gene defects and are of special interest because this mode of inheritance makes it virtually certain that the identical biochemical defect is present in both cardiac and skeletal muscle. The greater accessibility of peripheral muscle for investigation of metabolic or structural biochemical defects may well provide an entree to the solution of the associated myocardial defect which may also be applicable to other problems of cardiac muscle in which a peripheral myopathy is not present.

Recent studies which demonstrate this approach have suggested abnormalities of myoglobin and the cytochrome system, but the data are not conclusive.[132,164,166,181]

Muscular Dystrophy

The classical form, Duchenne's pseudohypertrophic muscular dystrophy, is sex linked, and the heart is involved in most patients. The changes include cardiomegaly, congestive heart failure, arrhythmias, and occasionally sudden death. Tall right precordial R waves and deep limb-lead and lateral precordial Q waves constitute distinctive electrocardiographic abnormalities in this disorder, possibly related to a loss of posteriorly directed forces due to fibrosis in the posterobasal portion of the left ventricle.[151] The pathological changes are similar to those in skeletal-muscle diseases, namely, muscle-cell atrophy and replacement with fat and connective tissue. In addition to having different genetic patterns, the other types of muscular dystrophy are less rapidly progressive than the Duchenne type,[204] perhaps accounting for the fact that cardiac manifestations have been less prominent, although clearly present.[151]

Myotonic Dystrophy

This unique disorder is characterized by skeletal atrophy, myotonia, cataracts, frontal baldness, gonadal atrophy, and autosomal dominant inheritance. Cardiac symptoms, such as heart failure or arrhythmias, are rare, yet significant electrocardiographic abnormalities occur in about two thirds of the patients.[37] In contrast to the other muscular dystrophies, the changes are disturbances of both A–V and bundle branch conduction.

Friedreich's Ataxia

This is a rare and peculiar disorder which is usually inherited in an autosomal recessive pattern, although an occasional family with a dominant mode is seen. Features of both myopathy and neuropathy are present. Peripheral muscle wasting and weakness accompany evidence of spinocerebellar-tract degeneration. Cardiac abnormalities have been noted in about half of the living patients, including cardiomegaly, murmurs, pericardial effusion, and electrocardiographic abnormalities. In one sixth of the patients, the cardiac involvement results in death. At autopsy, virtually all patients have obvious changes, including hypertrophy and extensive diffuse interstitial fibrosis with degeneration and infiltration with lymphocytes. The conduction system and pericardium may also be involved.[69,84]

Familial Rhythm Disturbances

Various congenital arrhythmias, ranging from heart blocks to ectopic rhythm disturbances, have been ascribed to a genetic etiology since they cluster within family groups. Some of these appear to have a dominant mode of inheritance because of their appearance in successive generations; however, others have been noted in multiple siblings from apparently healthy parents, suggesting either a recessive mode of transmission or the continuing influence of an unidentified environmental factor.[70,170,194,195] Of particular interest are newly recognized entities which, like muscular subaortic stenosis, may not be exceedingly rare despite their recent discovery.

Sudden death has lent an uneasy fascination to the syndrome of Q–T interval prolongation, which was described by Jervell and Lange-Nielsen in 1957.[97] Its occurrence in deaf-mute children aided in its recognition and family studies suggested an autosomal recessive mode of inheritance. Subsequent detailed clinical and pathological investigations by James have demonstrated variable combinations of deafness, arrhythmias, syncope, and electrocardiographic changes in multiple family members in successive generations.[95] In addition, James has presented evidence for infarction in the vicinity of the sinus and A–V nodes due to marked narrowing of the nutrient arteries.

The work of Romano and colleagues removed deafness as a necessary concomitant of Q–T interval prolongation and sudden death and established that an autosomal dominant mode of transmission may be present;[163] however, it remains unclear if these are separate entities with differing physiological mechanisms. Recently, Garza et al. evaluated a number of pharmacological maneuvers in an affected family and suggested that propranolol was effective in decreasing the incidence of ventricular arrhythmias in its members.[68] The fact that sudden death due to disease in the vicinity of the A–V node may be a family trait, without either deafness or preceding electrocardiographic changes, was established by Green et al.[76]

Walther and co-workers were assisted in the recognition of another new cardiovascular syndrome involving the conduction system by the unusual degree of freckling which was present in involved members of a family.[196] Since their original report in 1966, other observers have noted the same association. Smith and colleagues summarized these articles, as well as properly classifying the electrocardiograms, from their cases and from the literature as varying types of fascicular block, including complete heart block with its expected prognostic implications.[179] Their publication also includes an excellent illustration of the lentigo which is a hallmark of the syndrome.

SYSTEMIC DISEASES OF GENETIC ORIGIN WITH MAJOR CARDIOVASCULAR INVOLVEMENT

Tissue-culture Techniques in Diagnosis

The importance of these methods in making diagnoses, not only of involved patients but also of genetic carriers, and in helping to elucidate biochemical defects makes it highly appropriate to introduce this section with a brief discussion of tissue-culture techniques as they are now applied to cardiovascular diseases. Although tissue cultures have been utilized for many years, it is mostly since 1956, with the finding that man had 46 and not 48 chromosomes, that culture techniques began to be applied extensively for clinical purposes. The most exciting frontier in this regard at the present time evolves around the use of these methods in preventive medicine, either by prenatal diagnosis or by heterozygote recognition.

CHROMOSOMAL DISORDERS AND CARDIOVASCULAR DEFECTS

Screening patients with congenital heart disease for chromosomal abnormalities has not been particularly rewarding.[71] Although minor chromosomal aberrations which are familial have been noted, these also occur in normal families. On the other hand, known chromosomal trisomy syndromes and certain sex chromosome anomalies have revealed a remarkable array of cardiovascular defects. Warkany and colleagues have reported that cardiac defects are frequent in the three common trisomies 21, 19, and D_1 (or 13–15).[197] In trisomy 21 (mongolism), 272 necropsies revealed 140 cardiac malformations (52 per cent), with ventricular septal defects in 68 (25 per cent), atrial septal defects in 61 (22 per cent), patent ductus arteriosus in 35 (13 per cent), endocardial cushion defects in 27 (10 per cent), and, less frequently, a variety of other defects. Of the 140 children with mongolism and heart defects, 64 (45 per cent) had only single lesions, whereas 76 (55 per cent) had combinations. In patients with trisomy 18, 84 necropsies revealed cardiac anomalies virtually in toto, with ventricular septal defects in 64 (74 per cent), patent ductus arteriosus in 47 (56 per cent), pulmonic stenosis in 18 (21 per cent), and many other defects in smaller percentages. Trisomy 13–15 (D_1) patients were autopsied in 32 instances and 27 (84 per cent) had cardiac malformations consisting of ventricular septal defects in 15 (47 per cent), patent ductus arteriosus in 12 (38 per cent), atrial septal defects in 8 (25 per cent), dextroposi-

tion in 7 (22 per cent), pulmonic stenosis in 4 (13 per cent), and atrial bicuspid valves in 3 (12 per cent); other lesions were uncommon. In both trisomy 18 and trisomy 13–15 (D_1), approximately three quarters of the children had multiple cardiac defects.

The sex chromosome abnormalities are quite different from the autosomal trisomies in regard to cardiac malformations. Klinefelter's syndrome (XXY), for example, has not usually been associated with cardiac anomalies. Thorough examinations of 50 patients with typical Klinefelter's syndrome (eunuchoid habitus, gynecomastia, small testes, aspermia, and increased urinary gonadotropins) did not detect any notable cardiac abnormality.[9] A few case reports of sporadic malformations in Klinefelter's syndrome have not indicated any patterns of cardiac anomalies.[161] Turner's syndrome (XO), with 45 chromosomes, on the other hand, is associated with a significant incidence of cardiovascular anomalies. Furthermore, it is apparent that Turner's syndrome, with its XO constitution, is associated with different cardiac defects than are Turner's phenotype, with XX or XY chromosomes, and mosaics, such as XO/XX. Nora and colleagues have observed two clusters of cardiovascular lesions which distinguish the XO syndrome from the other phenotypes.[144] Coarctation of the aorta occurred in 11 of 16 (70 per cent) patients with XO constitution, but not in others which had a Turner appearance but with the XX or XY chromosomes or mosaics, whereas pulmonic stenosis was noted in 21 of 24 (88 per cent) patients with XX, XY, or mosaic constitutions. Chaver-Carbello and Hayles have elaborated on males with the Turner's phenotype and normal XY chromosomes in a review of 86 patients in which, of 79 individuals whose cardiovascular status was evaluated, 38 had abnormalities including septal defects, either singly or in combination with a truncus or valvular stenosis, tetralogy, pure pulmonic or aortic stenosis, and others, but rarely coarctation.[36] Goldberg et al. have further commented on the Turner syn-

2

drome in females and also noted that, while coarctation was common in patients with XO, other cardiovascular lesions, including aortic stenosis and anomalous vessels, occurred.[72] Thus it appears that Turner's XO phenotype is associated with coarctation and, rarely, aortic stenosis or anomalous vessels, whereas the others show a wide variation in defects but favor the right side of the heart, as in pulmonic stenosis.

DETECTION OF HETEROZYGOTES AND PRENATALLY DETERMINED INBORN ERRORS

During the past decade, the development of several diagnostic procedures, including amniocentesis during certain phases of pregnancy, various enzymatic determinations, and several staining procedures, has made possible the experimental detection and sometimes clinical management of certain genetic defects. Detection as early as possible is important in considering therapeutic abortion but equally important is the management of some disorders by supplying the missing protein (as in agammaglobulinemia), limiting precursor intake (as in galactosemia), or depleting stored substances (as in Wilson's disease). Amniocentesis can be done at 12 weeks (transvaginally) to 15 weeks (transabdominally) of pregnancy.[12]

A continually growing number of familial metabolic disorders are now demonstrable by tissue culture and many of these can be detected prenatally.[12,136] Of interest to the cardiologist are cystic fibrosis, Marfan's syndrome, and the mucopolysaccharidoses, which can be suspected on the basis of metachromatic granules in amniotic cells; specific enzymatic deficiencies which can be demonstrated in glycogen-storage disease, homocystinuria, and Fabry's disease; and the presence of abnormal hormones which can be detected in the amniotic fluid, such as elevated pregnanetriol in the adrenogenital syndrome. Examination of karyotypes can be useful in sex-linked disorders or where a high risk for chromosomal aberration exists.

Connective-tissue Disorders

Little has been learned about the connective-tissue disorders since the excellent review of Marfan's syndrome, pseudoxanthoma elasticum, and Ehlers-Danlos syndrome by McKusick.[122] A few new emphases are worthy of note, however.

MARFAN'S SYNDROME

This disorder remains an enigma in regard to the question of whether the underlying defect is in the ground substance (collagen), connective tissue, or a combination of these. With the recent advances in knowledge regarding the crosslinking of collagen and elastin, it is tempting to hypothesize a defect similar to that produced by lathyrogenic agents, which inhibit crosslinking of these substances.[21] Dilatation of the aortic root and dissecting aneurysm are the most devastating cardiovascular manifestations in the Marfan's syndrome.[77,184] This has led to speculation that the use of agents which reduce the left ventricular ejection velocity may be of prophylactic value in patients with Marfan's syndrome, just as they have been reported to be in patients with active dissecting aneurysms.[199] The billowing mitral valve is the other frequent cardiovascular finding in Marfan's syndrome and, because of current interest in this entity, it has been attracting comment.[23]

EHLERS-DANLOS SYNDROME

Over 400 cases of this interesting autosomal dominant disorder have been described, with fragile, hyperextensible skin, hernias, easy bruising, subcutaneous nodules or spheroids (molluscoid pseudotumors), which may be calcified, and severe "cigarette-paper" scarring after trauma. The joints are unstable and extremely hyperextensible so that deformities due to trauma, easy spraining, and kyphoscoliosis may occur.

The cardiovascular manifestations are not yet as well defined nor as common as those in Marfan's syndrome, yet are quite distinct.

Dissecting aneurysms, aneurysms of the sinus of Valsalva, and abnormal or floppy mitral valves with mitral regurgitation have been described as in Marfan's; however, in addition, varicose veins, spontaneous rupture of arteries, and rupture after minor trauma have also been noted, as have fistulas of the aortic-inferior vena cava and carotid-cavernous sinus.[10,20,75,92] Several different congenital heart defects have been reported in association with the syndrome, but no striking correlation exists and these are probably coincidental.[20]

OSTEOGENESIS IMPERFECTA

This is also a generalized disorder of connective tissue, although it has often been thought of primarily as a bone disease. The cardiovascular manifestations are rare and only recently have been recognized as part of the disorder.[40] Aortic root dilatation with aortic insufficiency, mitral-valve abnormalities, and premature peripheral-artery calcification have been noted.

Abiotrophies

Several conditions classified as abiotrophies have now been described in the literature. Werner's syndrome, the most common of these rare disorders, consists of short stature, cataracts, tight skin (scleroderma-like) with hyperkeratosis, ulceration and calcification, premature loss of hair, atrophy of muscle, subcutaneous tissue and bones, diabetes mellitus, hypogonadism, severe premature vascular disease with medial calcification of arteries, and generalized atherosclerosis.[54] This last problem may lead to the usual complications, including death due to infarction. Occasionally, mitral- or aortic-valve calcification has been described. The etiology for this syndrome is unclear and the inheritance is recessive. Progeria, another recessive disorder, is characterized by precocious senility of striking degree. Death from coronary-artery disease may occur before age ten and severe atherosclerosis has been noted at autopsy.[185] Cockayne's syndrome,

also recessive, is the third of this group. Patients are dwarfed, have a precociously senile appearance, and develop retinal atrophy and pigmentation, deafness, excessive sensitivity, mental retardation, and intracranial calcifications.[67]

These three abiotrophies, or conditions in which life begins in a relatively normal fashion and then tissues deteriorate, are mentioned not because the cardiologist will probably see such patients in practice but because such conditions and pseudoxanthoma elasticum may hold clues to the pathogenesis and control of atherosclerosis and aging in general.

Hamartoses or Phakomatoses

Disorders of this group are characterized by an organizational defect leading to an abnormal admixture of tissues, such as hemangiomas, fibromas, adenomas, lipomas, etc. A variety of these exist, but only selected ones pertinent to cardiology will be presented here.

NEUROFIBROMATOSIS

Neurofibromas and café-au-lait spots are associated with tumors, benign and malignant, of the central nervous system, fibromas of internal organs, scoliosis, cystic lung disease, and giant nevi. Neurofibromatosis may also be associated with gigantism of the extremities without A–V malformations. Vascular lesions occur and appear to predominate in the kidneys, endocrine glands, heart, and gastrointestinal tract; this may lead to arterial obliteration or obstruction and, at times, to renal hypertension.[80] Abdominal coarctation has likewise been associated with neurofibromatosis. The analyzed obstructive tissue reveals intimal hypertrophy, fragmentation of the elastic tissue of the media, and fibrous adventitial reaction and is considered to be vascular neurofibromatosis.[80,178] These vascular lesions of neurofibromatosis occur as a pure intimal form of endothelial proliferation; a second form involves intimal and aneurysmal changes with atrophy of the muscular vessel wall; a third type is a nodular form located within the vessel wall.

Hypertension may also occur in neuro-fibromatosis because 4 to 23 per cent of these patients may have associated chromaffin tumors of the adrenal gland. Familial pheochromocytoma may well be a forme fruste of neurofibromatosis since café-au-lait spots and frank neurofibromas are observed in other family members.[168] While pheochromocytoma is the most common, other endocrine aberrations also occur, including diabetes insipidus, hyperparathyroidism, acromegaly, goiter, and myxedema.[190] About 50 per cent of individuals with neurofibromatosis have affected relatives and a dominant gene has been proposed as the inheritance pattern in these families.[122]

von Hippel-Lindau Syndrome

Another dominant disorder in this category is the von Hippel-Lindau syndrome for which the cardinal features are retinal angiomas and cerebellar hemangioblastoma.[130] A wide spectrum of hemangiomatous tumors of many organs also occurs. Hypertension and pheochromocytoma have been reported several times; however, renal cysts and tumors may also produce hypertension in this condition. Cardiac disease of uncertain etiology was also present in the cases described by Melmar and Rosen.[130] Whereas neurofibromatosis may present its symptomatology ranging from birth to adulthood, von Hippel-Lindau syndrome usually appears in middle life with symptoms of headache, polycythemia, or hypertension.

Tuberous Sclerosis

Still another dominant condition, tuberous sclerosis, occurs sporadically in a high proportion of cases (at least 75 per cent).[112,139] It is suggested by the triad of epilepsy (93 per cent), mental retardation (62 per cent), and adenoma sebaceum (62 to 83 per cent), with papular excrescences of the nasolabial folds. In addition, brain tumors (6 per cent), shagreen patches (peculiar, flat, large, macu-lar, truncal lesions), gingival and periungual fibromas (39 per cent), and phakomas or fundal tumors (76 per cent) occur, and intracranial calcification is frequent (51 per cent). Hamartomas, involving the kidneys, heart, lungs, and spleen, occur with a significant frequency (50 to 80 per cent) and, specifically, rhabdomyoma of the heart has been reported several times; of patients with rhabdomyomas of the heart, 50 per cent will have tuberous sclerosis.[73]

Inborn Errors of Metabolism

Generally, the inborn errors are recessive disorders and involve various enzyme deficiencies. The number of these which are recognized increase every year and not infrequently explain the underlying pathogenesis of a previously poorly understood genetic disorder. Several are of interest in cardiology.

Amino-acid Disorders

Many amino-acid disorders have been described, but homocystinuria is of special interest because it may mimic Marfan's syndrome. It has been only nine years since the first clinical descriptions of this disorder,[33] yet over 100 cases have now been reported, and it is predicted that the defect may be nearly as prevalent as phenylketonuria. The inheritance, as predicted, is as a recessive disorder with a defect in cystathionine synthetase, the enzyme which catalyzes the condensation of homocystine and serine to form cystathionine. Methionine and homocystine are involved in biochemical steps prior to this block, and these two substances accumulate in plasma and urine while endogenous cystine is deficient.[114]

The clinical manifestations mimic Marfan's syndrome in that arachnodactyly, pectus excavatum or carinatum, and ectopic lens are found in both and some 20 per cent of patients with Marfan's and 5 per cent of all patients with ectopic lens have homocystinuria.[32] The resemblance ends with the marfanoid habitus and ectopic lens, however, for, whereas patients with Marfan's syndrome have aortic dilatation and insufficiency or mitral-valve disease, patients with homocystinuria have not been shown, at least as yet, to suffer from these infirmities. In addition, loose-jointedness is not prevalent in homocystinurics while osteoporosis, flushed skin, malar flush, livedo reticularis, fine light hair, and fatty changes in the liver are. More important, thrombosis of large arteries, such as the carotids, coronaries, and femorals, and of veins, such as the inferior vena cava, occurs commonly in homocystinuria and frequently leads to death at an early age or to cor pulmonale.[32]

GLYCOGEN-STORAGE DISEASES

These recessive disorders consist of various enzymatic defects involved in glycogen metabolism in several organs. Three of some eleven forms have significant cardiac pathology: (1) Type II (Pompe's disease) results in an acid alpha$_1$, 4-glucosidase deficiency and is a generalized form, producing prostration, hypotonia, large failing hearts, and, frequently, death within the first year. In the past, some cases have been diagnosed as idiopathic myocardiopathy in infants because of the striking cardiac abnormality with heavy glycogen deposits. Severe left ventricular hypertrophy and strain, marked cardiomegaly on examination, and a short P–R interval on the electrocardiogram, as well as macroglossia in an infant, should alert one to Pompe's disease. (2) Type III (Forbes' disease) concerns a defect in the "debrancher" enzyme, amylo-1,6-glucosidase, and, in addition to the kidneys and liver, skeletal and heart muscle may be involved; the liver and heart show the predominant pathological effects. (3) Type V (McArdle's disease) predominantly involves the skeletal muscle, with exercise intolerance and intermittent myoglobinuria, striking serum creatine phosphokinase activity and electrocardiographic abnormalities which are observed after exercise.[162] In addition to these forms, McKusick[123] has classified as type X a form which appears to be limited to the heart, without generalized involvement.[5]

MUCOPOLYSACCHARIDOSES

These recessive disorders, like glycogen-storage disease, appear to exist as a number of variants. Some have profound cardiovascular effects, in addition to the usual corneal clouding, coarse features, and joint stiffness. Some 70 per cent of patients with Type I (Hurler's syndrome, or gargoylism) show evidence of cardiovascular disease. The disorder is characterized by deposits of complex glycoproteins in the connective tissue of most organs and excessive secretion of chondroitin sulfate B and heparitin sulfate. Generalized cardiomegaly and valvular deformities with mitral insufficiency occur and congestive heart failure results in death in about two thirds of patients. Type II (Hunter's syndrome) is a milder, more generalized form but genetically is also a sex-linked recessive and not autosomal. Type IV (Morquio's syndrome), a disorder of keratosulfate metabolism, and type V (Scheie's syndrome), abnormal chondroitin-B metabolism, may result in significant aortic insufficiency. These disorders and clinical descriptions have been reviewed by McKusick and hemodynamic studies have been carried out in some patients.[104,124]

OTHER INHERITED METABOLIC DISEASES

Another inherited metabolic disorder of interest is angiokeratoma corporis diffusum universale (Fabry's disease), a sex-linked recessive disorder with deposits of a glycolipid, ceramidetrihexoside, in the skin, kidneys, heart, nerve tissue, and muscle, secondary to deficiency of ceramidetrihexosidase which cleaves galactose from the moiety.[25] Signs and symptoms which develop during childhood consist of small, dark lesions of the skin of the trunk, febrile episodes, renal failure with proteinuria, bouts of abdominal pain, and neuropathy. Glycolipid deposits are seen in vascular smooth muscle and cardiac muscle and in the valves, and may lead to cardiomegaly, hypertension, heart failure, or symptoms suggesting ischemic heart disease.[59]

REFERENCES

1. Acheson, R. M., and Fowler, G. B.: On the inheritance of stature and blood pressure. J. Chronic Dis., 20:731, 1967.
2. Alarcón-Segovia, D., Wakim, K. G., Worthington, J. W., and Ward, L. E.: Clinical and experimental studies on the hydralazine syndrome and its relationship to systemic lupus erythematosus. Medicine, 46:1, 1967.
3. Alarcón-Segovia, D., Worthington, J. W., Ward, L. E., and Wakim, K. G.: Lupus diathesis and the hydralazine syndrome. New Eng. J. Med., 272:462, 1965.
4. Allott, E. N., and Thompson, J. C.: The familial incidence of low pseudocholinesterase levels. Lancet, 2:517, 1956.
5. Antopol, W., Boas, E. P., Levison, W., and Tuchman, L. R.: Cardiac hypertrophy caused by glycogen storage disease in a 15-year-old boy. Amer. Heart J., 20:546, 1940.
6. Bajusz, E.: Hereditary cardiomyopathy: A new disease model. Amer. Heart J., 77:686, 1969.
7. Barold, S. S., et al.: Familial cardiomyopathy: A clinical, hemodynamic and angiographic study in one family. Chest, 57:141, 1970.
8. Bearn, A. G., and Danes, B. S.: A genetic study of cystic fibrosis of the pancreas in cell culture. Trans. Assoc. Amer. Physicians, 82:248, 1969.
9. Becker, K. L., et al.: Klinefelter's syndrome: Laboratory findings in 50 patients. Arch. Intern. Med., 118:314, 1966.
10. Beighton, P.: Lethal complications of the Ehlers-Danlos syndrome. Brit. Med. J., 3:656, 1968.
11. Benedek, T. G., and Sunder, J. H.: Comparisons of serum lipid and uric acid content in white and Negro men. Amer. J. Med. Sci., 260:331, 1970.
12. Bergsma, D. (Ed.): Symposium on intrauterine diagnosis: Birth Defects. Original Articles Series, 7:1, 1971.
13. Berkson, D. M., and Stamler, J.: Epidemiological findings on cerebrovascular diseases and their implications. J. Atheroscler. Res., 5:189, 1965.
14. Bittar, N., and Sosa, J. A.: The billowing mitral valve leaflet. Circulation, 38:763, 1968.
15. Bizarro, R. O., et al.: Familial atrial septal defect with prolonged atrioventricular condition. Circulation, 41:677, 1970.
16. Blache, J. O., and Handler, F. P.: Coronary artery disease: A comparison of the rates and patterns of development of coronary arteriosclerosis in the Negro and white races with its relation to clinical coronary artery disease. Arch. Path., 50:189, 1950.
17. Blomgren, S. E., Condemi, J. J., Bignall, M. C., and Vaughn, J. H.: Antinuclear antibody induced by procainamide. A prospective study. New Eng. J. Med., 281:64, 1969.
18. Blunt, M. H., and Evans, J. V.: Changes in the concentration of potassium in the erythrocytes and in haemoglobin type in Merino sheep under a severe anaemic stress. Nature, 200:1215, 1963.
19. Boesen, I., Melchior, J. C., Terslev, E., and Vendel, S.: Extracardiac congenital malformations in children with congenital heart diseases. Acta Paediat., 146(Suppl.):28, 1963.
20. Bopp, P., et al.: Cardiovascular aspects of Ehlers-Danlos syndrome. Circulation, 32:602, 1965.
21. Bornstein, P.: The cross-linking of collagen and elastin and its inhibition in osteolathyrism. Amer. J. Med., 49:429, 1970.
22. Bourne, J. G., Collier, H. O. J., and Somers, G. F.: Succinylcholine (succinoylcholine): Muscle relaxant of short action. Lancet, 1:1225, 1952.
23. Bowers, D.: Pathogenesis of primary abnormalities of the mitral valve in Marfan's syndrome. Brit. Heart J., 6:679, 1969.
24. Boyd, D. L., Mishkin, M. E., Feigenbaum, H., and Genovese, P. D.: Three families with familial cardiomyopathy. Ann. Intern. Med., 63:386, 1965.
25. Brady, R. O., et al.: Enzymatic defect in Fabry's disease. Ceramidetrihexosidase deficiency. New Eng. J. Med., 276:1163, 1967.
26. Breckenridge, A., et al.: Positive direct Coombs' tests and antinuclear factor in patients with methyldopa. Lancet, 2:1265, 1967.
27. Brennan, R. W., Dehejia, H., Kutt, H., and McDowell, F.: Diphenylhydantoin intoxication attendant to slow inactivation of isoniazid. Neurology, 18:283, 1968.
28. Brent, L. B., et al.: Familial muscular subaortic stenosis. Circulation, 21:167, 1960.
29. Brockington, I. F.: Postpartum hypertensive heart failure. Amer. J. Cardiol., 27:650, 1971.
30. Brusilow, S. W.: Cystic fibrosis in adults. Ann. Rev. Med., 21:99, 1970.
31. Callan, H. G.: The organization of genetic units in chromosomes. J. Cell Sci., 2:1, 1967.
32. Carey, M. C., Donovan, D. E., Fitzgerald, O., and McAuley, F. D.: Homocystinuria. I. A clinical and pathological study of nine subjects in six families. Amer. J. Med., 45:7, 1968.
33. Carson, N. A. J., et al.: Homocystinuria. A new inborn error of metabolism associated with mental deficiency. Arch. Dis. Child., 38:425, 1963.
34. Cassel, J. C.: Review of 1960 through 1962 cardiovascular disease prevalence study. Arch. Intern. Med., 128:890, 1971.
35. Cassel, J. C., et al.: Occupation and physical activity and coronary heart disease. Arch. Intern. Med., 128:920, 1971.
36. Chaves-Carballo, E., and Hayles, A. B.: Ullrich-Turner syndrome in the male. Mayo Clin. Proc., 41:843, 1966.
37. Church, S.: The heart in myotonia atrophica. Arch. Intern. Med., 119:176, 1967.

38. Conney, A. H.: Pharmacological implications of microsomal enzyme induction. Pharmacol. Rev., *19*:317, 1967.

39. Connor, D. H., et al.: Endomyocardial fibrosis in Uganda (Davies' disease). Amer. Heart J., *74*:687, 1967; *75*:107, 1968.

40. Criscitello, M. G., Ronan, J. A., Besterman, M. M., and Schoenwelter, W.: Cardiovascular abnormalities in osteogenesis imperfecta. Circulation, *31*:255, 1965.

41. Dahl, L. K., Heine, M., and Tassinari, L.: Role of genetic factors in susceptibility to experimental hypertension due to chronic excess salt ingestion. Nature, *194*:480, 1962.

42. Danowski, T. S., Tinsman, C. A., and Moses, C.: Hydrocortisone and/or desiccated thyroid in physiologic dosage. VIII. Lipid and body fluid patterns in North American Negro and white prisoners. Metabolism, *12*:117, 1963.

43. Davies, J. N. P.: Endocardial fibrosis in Uganda. E. Afr. Med. J., *25*:10, 1948.

44. Davies, J. N. P.: Some considerations regarding obscure diseases affecting the mural endocardium. Amer. Heart J., *59*:600, 1960.

45. Davies, R. O., Marton, A. V., and Kalow, W.: The action of normal and atypical cholinesterase of human serum upon a series of esters of choline. Canad. J. Biochem., *38*:545, 1960.

46. Deutscher, S., Epstein, F. H., and Kjelsberg, M. O.: Familial aggregation of factors associated with coronary heart disease. Circulation, *33*:911, 1966.

47. Deutscher, S., Ostrander, O. D., and Epstein, F. H.: Familial factors in premature coronary heart disease. A preliminary report from the Tecumseh community health study. Amer. J. Epidem., *91*:233, 1970.

48. Dietschy, J. M., and Wilson, J. D.: Regulation of cholesterol metabolism. New Eng. J. Med., *282*:1128, 1179, 1241, 1970.

49. Dubois, E. L.: Procainamide induction of a systemic lupus erythematosus-like syndrome. Medicine, *48*:217, 1969.

50. Ehlers, K. H., and Engle, M. A.: Familial congenital heart disease. I. Genetic and environmental factors. Circulation, *34*:503, 1966.

51. Elkington, S. G., Schreiber, W. M., and Conn, H. O.: Hepatic injury caused by L-alpha methyldopa. Circulation, *40*:589, 1969.

52. Emerit, I., Vernant, P., Corone, P., and Grouchy, J. de: Extracardiac malformations associated with congenital cardiopathies. Acta Genet. Med., *16*:27, 1967.

53. Enos, W. F., Holmes, R. H., and Beyer, J.: Coronary disease among United States soldiers killed in action in Korea: Preliminary report. JAMA, *152*:1090, 1953.

54. Epstein, C. J., Martin, G. M., Schultz, A. L., and Motulsky, A.: Werner's syndrome. Medicine, *45*:177, 1966.

55. Eriksson, S.: Pulmonary emphysema and alpha₁-antitrypsin deficiency. Acta Med. Scand., *175*:197, 1964.

56. Evans, D. A. P., and White, T. A.: Human acetylation polymorphism. J. Lab. Clin. Med., *63*:394, 1964.

57. Evans, F. T., Gray, P. W. S., Lehmann, H., and Silk, E.: Sensitivity to succinylcholine in relation to serum-cholinesterase. Lancet, *1*:1229, 1952.

58. Fagerhol, M. K., and Braend, M.: Serum prealbumia: Polymorphism in man. Science, *149*:986, 1965.

59. Ferrans, V. J., Hibbs, R. G., and Burda, C. D.: The heart in Fabry's disease. A histochemical and electronmicroscopic study. Amer. J. Cardiol., *24*:95, 1969.

60. Finnerty, F. A., Jr.: Hypertension is different in blacks. JAMA, *216*:1634, 1971.

61. Finnerty, F. A., Jr.: Toxemia of pregnancy as seen by an internist: An analysis of 1,081 patients. Ann. Intern. Med., *44*:358, 1956.

62. Fixler, D. E., et al.: Familial occurrence of the contracted form of endocardial fibroelastosis. Amer. J. Cardiol., *26*:208, 1970.

63. Flamm, M. D., Harrison, D. C., and Hancock, E. W.: Muscular subaortic stenosis. Circulation, *38*:846, 1968.

64. Forney, W. R., Robinson, S. J., and Pascoe, D. J.: Congenital heart disease, deafness, and skeletal malformations: A new syndrome? J. Pediat., *68*:14, 1966.

65. Frank S., and Braunwald, E.: Idiopathic hypertrophic subaortic stenosis. Circulation, *37*:759, 1968.

66. Fredrickson, D. S., Levy, R. I., and Lees, R. S.: Fat transport in lipoproteins—an integrated approach to mechanisms and disorders. New Eng. J. Med., *276*:34, 94, 148, 215, 273, 1967.

67. Fujimoto, W. Y., Greene, M. L., and Seegmiller, J. E.: Cockayne's syndrome. J. Pediat., *75*:881, 1969.

68. Garza, L. A., Vick, R. L., Nora, J. J., and McNamara, D. G.: Heritable Q–T prolongation without deafness. Circulation, *41*:39, 1970.

69. Gauthier, E. J.: Cardiac disease in Friedreich's ataxia. Ann. Intern. Med., *60*:892, 1964.

70. Gazes, P. C., Culler, R. M., Taber, E., and Kelly, T. E.: Congenital familial cardiac conduction defects. Circulation, *32*:32, 1965.

71. German, J., Ehlers, K. H., and Engle, M. A.: Familial congenital heart disease. II. Chromosomal studies. Circulation, *34*:517, 1966.

72. Goldberg, M. B., Scully, A. L., Solomon, I. L., and Steinbach, H. L.: Gonadal dysgenesis in phenotypic female subjects. Amer. J. Med., *45*:529, 1968.

73. Golding, R., and Reed, G.: Rhabdomyoma of the heart. New Eng. J. Med., *276*:957, 1967.

74. Goodwin, J. F.: Congestive and hypertrophic cardiomyopathies. Lancet, *1*:731, 1970.

75. Green, G. J., Schuman, B. M., and Barrow, J.: Ehlers-Danlos syndrome complicated by acute hemorrhagic sigmoid diverticulitis, with an unusual mitral valve abnormality. Amer. J. Med., *41*:622, 1966.

76. Green, J. R., Jr., et al.: Sudden unexpected death in three generations. Arch. Intern. Med., *124*:359, 1969.

77. Grondin, C. M., Steinberg, C. L., and Edwards, J. E.: Dissecting aneurysm complicating Marfan's syndrome (arachnodactyly) in a mother and son. Amer. Heart J., *77*:301, 1969.

78. Gutsche, B. B., Scott, E. M., and Wright, R. C.: Hereditary deficiency of pseudocholinesterase in Eskimos. Nature, *215*:322, 1967.

79. Haldane, J. B. S.: *Heredity and Politics*. London, Allen and Unwin, 1938. (Quoted with permission of the publisher.)

80. Halperin, M., and Currarino, G.: Vascular lesions causing hypertension in neurofibromatosis. New Eng. J. Med., *273*:248, 1965.

81. Harris, H., Robson, E. B., Glen-Bott, A. M., and Thornton, J. A.: Evidence for non-allelism between genes affecting human serum cholinesterase. Nature, *200*:1185, 1963.

82. Harris, H., and Whittaker, M.: Differential inhibitions of human serum cholinesterase with fluoride: Recognition of two new phenotypes. Nature, *191*:496, 1961.

83. Havel, R. J.: Pathogenesis, differentiation and management of hypertriglyceridemia. Advances Intern. Med., *15*:117, 1969.

84. Hewer, R. L.: The heart in Friedreich's ataxia. Brit. Heart J., *31*:5, 1969.

85. Ho, K-J., et al.: The Masai of East Africa: Some unique biological characteristics. Arch. Path., *91*:387, 1971.

86. Holt, M., and Oram, S.: Familial heart disease with skeletal malformations. Brit. Heart J., *22*:236, 1960.

87. Howard, J., and Holman, B. L.: The effects of race and occupation on hypertension mortality. Milbank Mem. Fund Quart., *48*:263, 1970.

88. Hughes, H. B., Biehl, J. P., Jones, A. P., and Schmidt, L. H.: Metabolism of isoniazid in man as related to occurrence of peripheral neuritis. Amer. Rev. Tuberc., *70*:266, 1954.

89. Hull, E., and Hidden, E.: Postpartal heart failure. Southern Med. J., *31*:265, 1938.

90. Hunt, D., and Sloman, G.: Prolapse of the posterior leaflet of the mitral valve occurring in eleven members of a family. Amer. Heart J., *78*:149, 1969.

91. Hunter, C. C., Jr., Pierce, J. A., and LaBorde, J. B.: Alpha₁-antitrypsin deficiency. A family study. JAMA, *205*:93, 1968.

92. Imahori, S., Bannerman, R. M., Graf, C. J., and Brennan, J. C.: Ehlers-Danlos syndrome with multiple arterial lesions. Amer. J. Med., *47*:967, 1969.

93. Iwai, J., et al.: Genetic influence on the development of renal hypertension in parabiotic rats. J. Exp. Med., *129*:507, 1969.

94. Jacob, F., and Monod, J.: Genetic regulatory mechanisms in the synthesis of proteins. J. Molec. Biol., *3*:318, 1961.

95. James, T. N.: Congenital deafness and cardiac arrhythmias. Amer. J. Cardiol., *19*:627, 1967.

96. Jelliffe, R. W., and Blankenhorn, D. H.: Effect of phenobarbital on digitoxin metabolism. Clin. Res., *14*:160, 1966.

97. Jervell, A., and Lange-Nielson, F.: Congenital deaf-mutism, functional heart disease, with prolongation of the Q–T interval and sudden death. Amer. Heart J., *54*:59, 1957.

98. Kahler, R. L., Braunwald, E., Plauth, W. H., Jr., and Morrow, A. G.: Familial congenital heart disease. Amer. J. Med., *40*:384, 1966.

99. Kalow, W., and Genest, K.: A method for the detection of atypical forms of human serum cholinesterase. Determination of dibucaine numbers. Canad. J. Biochem., *35*:339, 1957.

100. Kennel, W. B., Castelli, W. P., Gordon, T., and McNamara, P. M.: Serum cholesterol, lipoproteins, and the risk of coronary heart disease. The Framingham study. Ann. Intern. Med., *74*:1, 1971.

101. Keys, A., et al.: Lessons from serum cholesterol studies in Japan, Hawaii, and Los Angeles. Ann. Intern. Med., *48*:83, 1958.

102. Knudsen, K. D., et al.: Genetic influence on the development of renoprival hypertension in parabiotic rats. J. Exp. Med., *310*:1353, 1969.

103. Koroxendis, G. T., Webb, N. C., Jr., Moschos, C. B., and Lehan, P. H.: Congenital heart disease, deaf-mutism and associated somatic malformations occurring in several members of one family. Amer. J. Med., *40*:149, 1966.

104. Krovetz, L. J., Lorinez, A. E., and Schiebler, G. L.: Cardiovascular manifestations of the Hurler syndrome. Circulation, *31*:132, 1965.

105. Kueppers, F.: Alpha₁-antitrypsin: Physiology, genetics and pathology. Humangenetik, *11*: 177, 1971.

106. Kueppers, F., and Bearn, A. G.: A possible experimental approach to the association of hereditary alpha₁-antitrypsin deficiency and pulmonary emphysema. Proc. Soc. Exp. Biol. Med., *121*: 1207, 1966.

107. Kueppers, F., and Larson, R. K.: Obstructive lung disease and alpha₁-antitrypsin deficiency gene heterozygosity. Science, *165*:899, 1969.

108. Kuller, L.: Sudden deaths in arteriosclerotic heart disease. Amer. J. Cardiol., *24*:617, 1969.

109. Kutt, H., Verebely, K., and McDowell, F.: Inhibition of diphenylhydantoin metabolism in rats and in rat liver microsomes by antitubercular drugs. Neurology, *18*:706, 1968.

110. Kutt, H., Wolk, M., Scherman, R., and McDowell, F.: Insufficient parahydroxylation as a cause of diphenylhydantoin toxicity. Neurology, *14*:542, 1964.

111. Ladd, A. T.: Procainamide-induced lupus erythematosus. New Eng. J. Med., *267*:1357 1962.

112. Lagos, J. C., and Gomez, M. R.: Tuberous sclerosis: Reappraisal of a clinical entity. Mayo Clin. Proc., *42*:26, 1967.

113. Lappat, E. J., and Cawein, M. J.: A familial study of procainamide-induced systemic lupus erythematosus. Amer. J. Med., *45*:846, 1968.

114. Laster, L., Spaeth, G. L., Mudd, S. H., and Finkelstein, J. D.: Homocystinuria due to cystathionine synthase deficiency. Ann. Intern. Med., *63*:1117, 1965.

115. Lewis, R. J., Spivack, M., and Spaet, T. H.: Warfarin resistance. Amer. J. Med., *42*: 620, 1967.

116. Lewis, R. J., and Trager, W. F.: Warfarin metabolism in man: Identification of metabolites in urine. J. Clin. Invest., *49*:907, 1970.

117. Lieberman, J.: Heterozygous and homozygous alpha₁-antitrypsin deficiency in patients with pulmonary emphysema. New Eng. J. Med., *281*:279, 1969.

118. Link, K. P., Berg, D., and Barker, W. M.: Partial fate of warfarin in the rat. Science, *150*:378, 1965.

119. McGregor, D. D., and Smirk, F. H.: Vascular responses to 5-hydroxytryptamine in genetic and renal hypertensive rats. Amer. J. Physiol., *219*:687, 1970.

120. McKusick, V. A.: Genetic factors in cardiovascular diseases. J. Amer. Geriat. Soc., *9*: 465, 1961.

121. McKusick, V. A.: A genetical view of cardiovascular disease. Circulation, *30*:326, 1964.

122. McKusick, V. A.: *Heritable Disorders of Connective Tissue*, 3rd ed. St. Louis, C. V. Mosby Co., 1966.

123. McKusick, V. A.: *Mendelian Inheritance in Man: Catalogs of Autosomal Dominant, Autosomal Recessive, and X-Linked Phenotypes*, 2nd ed. Baltimore, Johns Hopkins Press, 1968.

124. McKusick, V. A., et al.: The genetic mucopolysaccharidoses. Medicine, *44*:445, 1965.

125. McNamara, J. J.: Personal communication, 1971.

126. McNamara, J. J., Molot, M. A., Stremple, J. F., and Cutting, R. T.: Coronary artery disease in combat casualties in Vietnam. JAMA, *216*:1185, 1971.

127. McVay, L. V., Jr., and Keil, P. G.: Myocardial infarction with special reference to the Negro. Arch. Intern. Med., *96*:762, 1955.

128. Massumi, R. A., et al.: Primary myocardial disease: Report of 50 cases and review of the subject. Circulation, *31*:19, 1965.

129. Meadows, W. R.: Postpartum heart disease. Amer. J. Cardiol., *6*:788, 1960.

130. Melmon, K. L., and Rosen, S. W.: Lindau's disease. Amer. J. Med., *36*:595, 1964.

131. Maill, W. E.: Heredity and hypertension. Practitioner, *207*:20, 1971.

132. Miyoshi, K., et al.: Myoglobin subfractions: Abnormality in Duchenne type of progressive muscular dystrophy. Science, *159*:736, 1968.

133. Molina, J., et al.: Procainamide-induced serologic changes in asymptomatic patients. Arthritis Rheum., *12*:608, 1969.

134. Moore, S. L., et al.: The production of hemoglobin C in sheep carrying the gene for hemoglobin A: Hematologic aspects. Blood, *28*: 314, 1966.

135. Motulsky, A. G.: Pharmacogenetics. Progr. Med. Genet., *3*:49, 1964.

136. Nadler, H. L.: Prenatal detection of genetic defects. J. Pediat., *74*:132, 1969.

137. Nasser, W. K., et al.: Familial myocardial disease with and without obstruction to left ventricular outflow. Circulation, *35*:638, 1967.

138. Neitlich, H. W.: Increased plasma cholinesterase activity and succinylcholine resistance: A genetic variant. J. Clin. Invest., *45*:380, 1966.

139. Nevin, N. C., and Pearce, W. G.: Diagnostic and genetical aspects of tuberous sclerosis. J. Med. Genet., *5*:273, 1968.

140. Nora, J. J., et al.: Risk to offspring of parents with congenital heart defects. JAMA, *209*: 2052, 1969.

141. Nora, J. J., Gilliland, J. C., Sommerville, R. J., and McNamara, D. G.: Congenital heart disease in twins. New Eng. J. Med., *277*:568, 1967.

142. Nora, J. J., McNamara, D. G., and Fraser, F. C.: Hereditary factors in atrial septal defect. Circulation, *35*:448, 1967.

143. Nora, J. J., and Meyer, T. C.: Familial nature of congenital heart diseases. Pediatrics, *37*: 329, 1966.

144. Nora, J. J., Torres, F. G., Sinha, A. K., and McNamara, D. G.: Characteristic cardiovascular anomalies of XO Turner syndrome, XX and XY phenotype and XO/XX Turner mosaic. Amer. J. Cardiol., *25*:639, 1970.

145. O'Reilly, R. A.: The second reported kindred with hereditary resistance to oral anticoagulant drugs. New Eng. J. Med., *282*:1448, 1970.

146. O'Reilly, R. A., and Aggeler, P. M.: Determinants of the response to oral anticoagulant drugs in man. Pharmacol. Rev., *22*:35, 1970.

147. O'Reilly, R. A., et al.: Hereditary transmission of exceptional resistance to coumarin anticoagulant drugs: The first reported kindred. New Eng. J. Med., *271*:809, 1964.

148. O'Reilly, R. A., Aggeler, P. M., and Leong, L. S.: Studies on the coumarin anticoagulant drugs: The pharmacodynamics of warfarin in man. J. Clin. Invest., *42*:1542, 1963.

149. O'Reilly, R. A., Pool, J. G., and Aggeler, P. M.: Hereditary resistance to coumarin anticoagulant drugs in man and rat. Ann. N.Y. Acad. Sci., *151*:913, 1968.

150. Orzalesi, M. M., Kohner, D., Cook, C. D., and Shwachman, H.: Anamnesis, sweat electrolyte and pulmonary function studies in parents of patients with cystic fibrosis of the pancreas. Acta Paediat., *52*:267, 1963.

151. Perloff, J. K., DeLeon, A. C., Jr., and O'Doherty, D.: The cardiomyopathy of progressive muscular dystrophy. Circulation, *33*:625, 1966.

152. Perry, H. M., Jr., Sakamoto, A., and Tan, E. M.: Relationship of acetylating enzyme to

hydralazine toxicity. J. Lab. Clin. Med., 70: 1020, 1967.

153. Phelan, E. L.: Genetic and autonomic factors in inherited hypertension. Circ. Res., 27 (Suppl. II):65, 1970.

154. Phillips, J. H., Jr., and Burch, G. E.: Cardiovascular disease in the white and Negro races. Amer. J. Med. Sci., 238:97, 1959.

155. Phillips, J. H., Jr., and Burch, G. E.: A review of cardiovascular diseases in the white and Negro races. Medicine, 39:241, 1960.

156. Pierce, J. A., Price, B. O., and Joyce, J. W.: Familial occurrence of postpartal heart failure. Arch. Intern. Med., 111:651, 1963.

157. Piper, J., and Orrild, L.: Essential familial hypercholesterolemia and xanthomatosus: Follow-up study of twelve Danish families. Amer. J. Med., 21:34, 1956.

158. Pollak, V. E.: Antinuclear antibodies in families of patients with systemic lupus erythematosus. New Eng. J. Med., 271:165, 1964.

159. Pomerance, A.: Ballooning deformity (mucoid degeneration) of atrioventricular valves. Brit. Heart J., 31:343, 1969.

160. Pyörälä, K., and Nevanlinna, H. R.: The effect of selective and nonselective inbreeding on the rate of warfarin metabolism in the rat. Ann. Med. Exp. Fenn., 46:35, 1968.

161. Rao, V. S., and Mooring, P. K.: Ebstein's anomaly in XXY Klinefelter's syndrome. Amer. J. Dis. Child., 120:164, 1970.

162. Ratinov, G., Baker, W. P., and Swaiman, K. F.: McArdle's syndrome with previously unreported electrocardiographic and serum enzyme abnormalities. Ann. Intern. Med., 62: 328, 1965.

163. Romano, C., Gemme, G., and Pongiglione, R.: Aritmie cardiache rare dell'eta' pediatrica. II. Accessi sincopali per fibrillazione ventricolare parossistica. (Presentazione del primo case della letteratura pediatrica italiana.) Clin. Pediat., 45:656, 1963.

164. Rowland, L. P., Dunne, P. B., Penn, A. S., and Maher, E.: Myoglobin and muscular dystrophy. Arch. Neurol., 18:141, 1968.

165. Rubinstein, H. M., et al.: Silent cholinesterase gene: Variations in the properties of serum enzyme in apparent homozygotes. J. Clin. Invest., 49:479, 1970.

166. Samaha, F. J., and Gergely, J.: Biochemical abnormalities of the sarcoplasmic reticulum in muscular dystrophy. New Eng. J. Med., 280:184, 1969.

167. Sarvothan, S. G., and Berg, J. N.: Prevalence of coronary heart disease in an urban population in northern India. Circulation, 37:939, 1968.

168. Saxena, K. M.: Endocrine manifestations of neurofibromatosis in children. Amer. J. Dis. Child., 120:265, 1970.

169. Schlager, G., and Weibust, R. S.: Genetic control of blood pressure in mice. Genetics, 55: 497, 1967.

170. Schneider, R. G.: Familial occurrence of Wolff-Parkinson-White syndrome. Amer. Heart J., 78:34, 1969.

171. Schrire, V., and Uys, C. J.: Cardiac infarction in the Bantu. Amer. J. Cardiol., 2:453, 1958.

172. Schweitzer, M. D., Clark, E. G., Gearing, F. R., and Perera, G. A.: Genetic factors in primary hypertension and coronary disease—a reappraisal. J. Chronic Dis., 15:1093, 1962.

173. Shwachman, H., Kulczycki, L. L., and Khaw, K. T.: Studies in cystic fibrosis. A report of 65 patients over 17 years of age. Pediatrics, 36:689, 1965.

174. Shaper, A. G., and Jones, K. W.: Serum cholesterol in camel-herding nomads. Lancet, 2:1305, 1962.

175. Shell, W. E., Walton, J. A., Clifford, M. E., and Willis, P. W.: The familial occurrence of the syndrome of mid-late systolic click and late systolic murmur. Circulation, 39:327, 1969.

176. Sievers, M. L.: Myocardial infarction among southwestern American Indians. Ann. Intern. Med., 67:800, 1967.

177. Slack, J., and Evans, K. A.: The increased risk of death from ischaemic heart disease in first degree relatives of 121 men and 96 women with ischaemic heart disease. J. Med. Genet., 3:239, 1966.

178. Smith, C. J., Hatch, F. E., Johnson, J. G., and Kelly, B. J.: Renal artery dysplasia as a cause of hypertension in neurofibromatosis. Arch. Intern. Med., 125:1022, 1970.

179. Smith, R. F., Pulicicchio, L. U., and Holmes, A. V.: Generalized lentigo: Electrocardiographic abnormalities, conduction disorders and arrhythmias in three cases. Amer. J. Cardiol., 25:501, 1970.

180. Solomon, H. M.: Variations in metabolism of coumarin anticoagulant drugs. Ann. N.Y. Acad. Sci., 151:932, 1968.

181. Spiro, A. J., et al.: A cytochrome-related inherited disorder of the nervous system and muscle. Arch. Neurol., 23:103, 1970.

182. Stevens, P. M., Hnilica, V. S., Johnson, P. C., and Bell, R. L.: Pathophysiology of hereditary emphysema. Ann. Intern. Med., 74:672, 1971.

183. Sunahara, S., Urano, M., and Ogawa, M.: Genetical and geographic studies on isoniazid inactivation. Science, 134:1530, 1961.

184. Synbar, P. N., Baldwin, B. J., Silverman, M. E., and Galumbos, J. T.: Marfan's syndrome with aneurysm of ascending aorta and aortic regurgitation. Amer. J. Cardiol., 25:483, 1970.

185. Talbot, N. B., et al.: Progeria: Clinical, metabolic, and pathologic studies on a patient. Amer. J. Dis. Child., 69:267, 1945.

186. Tallgren, L. G., and Servo, C.: Hyperpyrexia in association with administration of L-alpha methyldopa. Acta Med. Scand., 186:223, 1969.

187. Taylor, W. J.: Genetics and the cardiovascular system. In: *The Heart: Arteries and Veins*, 2nd ed. (Hurst, J. W., and Logue, R. B., Eds.). New York, McGraw-Hill, 1970.

188. Thomas, C. A., Jr., Hamkalo, B. A., Misra, D. N., and Lee, C. S.: Cyclization of eucaryotic deoxyribonucleic acid fragments. J. Molec. Biol., 51:621, 1970.

189. Thomason, J. G.: Production of severe atheroma in a transplanted human heart. Lancet, 2:1088, 1969.

190. Tisherman, S. E., Gregg, F. J., and Danowski, T. J.: Familial pheochromocytoma. JAMA, 182:150, 1962.

191. VanderMolen, R., et al.: A study of hypertension in twins. Amer. Heart J., 79:454, 1970.

192. Vesell, E. S., and Page, J. G.: Genetic control of Dicumarol levels in man. J. Clin. Invest., 47:2657, 1968.

193. Vesell, E. S., and Page, J. G.: Genetic control of the phenobarbital-induced shortening of plasma antipyrine half-lives in man. J. Clin. Invest., 48:2202, 1969.

194. Wagner, C. W., and Hall, R. J.: Congenital familial atrioventricular dissociation. Amer. J. Cardiol., 19:593, 1967.

195. Wallgren, G., and Agorio, E.: Congenital complete A–V block in three siblings. Acta Paediat., 49:49, 1960.

196. Walther, R. J., Polansky, B. J., and Grots, I. A.: Electrocardiographic abnormalities in a family with generalized lentigo. New Eng. J. Med., 275:1220, 1966.

197. Warkany, J., Passarge, E., and Smith, L. B.: Congenital malformations in autosomal trisomy syndrome. Amer. J. Dis. Child., 112:502, 1966.

198. Welch, M. H., Reinecke, M. E., Hammarsten, J. F., and Guenter, C. A.: Antitrypsin deficiency in pulmonary disease: The significance of intermediate levels. Ann. Intern. Med., 71:533, 1969.

199. Wheat, M. W., Jr., Palmer, R. F., Bartley, T. D., and Sealman, R. C.: Treatment of dissecting aneurysms of the aorta without surgery. J. Thorac. Cardiov. Surg., 50:364, 1965.

200. Williams, A. O.: Atherosclerosis in the Nigerian. J. Path., 99:219, 1969.

201. Wood, J. A., et al.: A comparison of sweat chlorides and intestinal fat absorption in chronic obstructive pulmonary emphysema and fibrocystic disease of the pancreas. New Eng. J. Med., 260:951, 1959.

202. Worledge, S. M., Carstairs, K. C., and Dacie, J. V.: Autoimmune haemolytic anemia associated with α-methyldopa therapy. Lancet, 2:135, 1966.

203. Yater, W. M., et al.: Coronary artery disease in men eighteen to thirty-nine years of age. Amer. Heart J., 36:334, 481, 683, 1948.

204. Zundel, W. S., and Tyler, F. H.: The muscular dystrophies. New Eng. J. Med., 273:537, 596, 1965.

Chapter 2

IMMUNOLOGICAL ASPECTS OF
CARDIOVASCULAR DISORDERS

C. I. Roberts, B.M., M.R.C.P., and M. H. Lessof, M.D., F.R.C.P.

Immune reactions involve the production of antibody proteins and sensitized cells which are directed against foreign antigens. In the recovery from infection, and possibly in the elimination of neoplastic cells, such reactions can be beneficial. However, undesirable effects of antibodies and sensitized cells occur, leading to diseases which have been broadly grouped as having an "auto-immune" etiology. In addition, the surgeon engaged in organ transplantation has learned to regard the immune response to a foreign graft as a major postoperative problem.

The great interest in auto-immunity in recent years has led to problems in separating fact from speculation. For example, the finding of an autoantibody, that is, an antibody reacting with an appropriate tissue antigen, is no longer sufficient to establish an auto-immune etiology for any disease process which may be present. It is necessary to show how the antibody could be related to one of the recognized immunopathological mechanisms and, ideally, to isolate the antigen and use it experimentally to reproduce the disease. These considerations make it

necessary to analyze the techniques used by investigators, as they often have important limitations.

A concise summary of immunopathological mechanisms is that of Gell and Coombs,[48] which describes four types of mechanism. Type I concerns the reaction of free antigen with antibody passively sensitizing the cell surface. This leads to the release of a number of pharmacologically active agents, such as histamine, heparin, bradykinin and slow-reacting substance. This is the mechanism thought to be responsible for various atopic and allergic reactions, including allergic lung diseases such as asthma, and for anaphylactic reactions.

Type II concerns an antibody reaction with either an antigenic component of a cell surface or an antigen or hapten attached to a cell surface. With the mediation of complement cell lysis can occur, as in hemolytic anemia and blood-transfusion reactions.

Type III involves antigen and antibody reacting in antigen excess, forming soluble complexes which are deposited in blood-vessel walls. With binding of some comple-

31

ment components polymorphs accumulate, with release of lysosomal enzymes. Various forms of nephritis are of this type, and a similar mechanism may sometimes be demonstrable in polyarteritis nodosa or in the vasculitis which may accompany rheumatoid arthritis.

Type IV concerns specifically modified mononuclear cells reacting with an antigen at local sites. The reaction seen in certain infected tissues is of this type, as in the lung in pulmonary tuberculosis. A round cell infiltrate is a feature of the histology in many auto-immune or autoallergic diseases. More than one of these mechanisms may be evident in the same disorder.

Most techniques used to study possible auto-immune reactions depend on the demonstration of serum factors reacting with various types of antigen. The type of antigen used and its mode of preparation can modify the results, and in general only free antibody will be demonstrated. That attached to cell surfaces or complexed with antigen will not, unless special techniques are used. In order to identify cellular reactions, an in vitro model must be devised to allow the measurement of changes produced when lymphocytes react with their antigen, e.g. lymphocyte transformation or the inhibition of leukocyte migration.

IMMUNOLOGICAL ASPECTS OF INFECTION AND AUTO-IMMUNE REACTIONS

The clinical pattern of an infectious disease is greatly influenced by the host's response and, more specifically, by the host's immune reactions. It is well known that there are virus infections which may themselves be harmless but which can be rapidly fatal if a brisk immune reaction occurs. A classical example is lymphocytic choriomeningitis in mice. Animals infected with the virus in the neonatal period may develop an extensive viremia, and the virus is disseminated throughout the body. At this age, in the absence of an immune response, most animals show no evidence of disease in the first few months of life.[87] When adult mice are infected, however, a brisk and widespread lymphocytic reaction occurs (type IV), with a major lymphocytic infiltration of the meninges very similar to that seen in human lymphocytic choriomeningitis. Neonatal thymectomy, irradiation, or the use of antilymphocytic globulin may prevent this reaction,[54] but when the immune response is abrogated by these methods the virus persists in the circulation. In that case the outcome may be influenced by any form of immune reaction which can still occur. While the cellular reaction remains depressed, circulating antibody frequently develops; in this case complexes of virus and antibody are deposited in the kidney (type III reaction) and in the ensuing months fatal renal disease develops in an increasing proportion of the animals. In this relatively benign infection the immune reaction can thus be fatal. The development of a lymphocytic reaction may be followed by extensive tissue damage and death, and even if this is suppressed the formation of immune complexes may also lead to death by causing capillary damage and renal failure.

These are not the only disease patterns seen in association with infection. In animals a number of infections cause disease manifestations which are reminiscent of the various clinical syndromes seen in man. New Zealand black (NZB) mice frequently develop a hemolytic anemia with a positive Coombs' test, and virtually all mice of this strain are affected by the age of nine months. About half of them have antinuclear factor in their blood and there is a high incidence of renal disease and of reticuloendothelial neoplasms.[57] In this disease, with its auto-immune manifestations, an immune complex nephritis (type III reaction) is often the immediate cause of death, and Dixon et al.[33] have shown that DNA and antibody against DNA may both be deposited in the affected glomeruli, together with complement. Although the significance of autoantibody formation is far from clear, in this case antibodies are present which are capable of reacting with DNA from a variety of sources and which appear to be of pathogenetic importance in causing immune complex disease.

The tendency to produce reactions of an auto-immune nature was at first thought to be due to an inherited defect of the immune response. However, electron-microscopic evidence of a virus of the murine leukemia group has suggested that this is basically an infective condition, in which, as in lymphocytic choriomeningitis, the type of immune response determines the clinical pattern of the disease. Virus has been found not only in adult animals but also in the fetus, and it appears to be transmitted from one generation to the next. Antigens from viruses in this leukemia group have been found in NZB mice at about the age when a positive Coombs' test develops. By the age of nine months the mouse begins to eliminate this antigen, and antibody then appears in the circulation. As in serum sickness, the stage of antigen-antibody balance may follow, and there is progressive renal damage. Deposits of a virus of this group have been seen in the mesangium of the glomerulus in a few cases.[83]

In man there are now numerous examples of the immunological disorders provoked by infection. In leprosy, for example, a whole spectrum of clinical manifestations ranges from an illness resembling serum sickness, seen in lepromatous leprosy, to the tuberculoid forms accompanied by local lymphocytic infiltration. Autoantibodies, including antiheart factors, may be seen in leprosy,[105] and antinuclear and other autoantibodies are seen in syphilis,[131] glandular fever,[69] infective hepatitis,[43] and other noninfective types of tissue injury such as burns. The Wassermann reaction itself is an auto-immune response, and Waldenström has pointed out that if the spirochete had never been discovered syphilis would provide an ideal model of an "auto-immune" disease: lymphocytic infiltration, vasculitis and abnormal autoantibodies are all prominent features of this condition. In systemic lupus erythematosus the findings in

mice have raised the possibility that the disease might be due to a similar reaction to viral infection. A number of groups have described myxovirus-like inclusions in various tissues.[47,51,72,86] Antibodies to the Epstein-Barr virus have also been reported.[41] However, similar syndromes have been seen in patients given procainamide,[75] hydralazine and methyldopa.[15,25] This makes it likely that the lupus reaction is not the result of a specific infection but rather the result of a particular type of immune response in which immune complex deposition and lymphocytic reactions both play an important part. In the abnormal immune response seen in polyarteritis nodosa, an overt or latent virus infection has also been suggested as a cause in some cases.[127]

Auto-immune reactions are by no means confined to infections, and the manner in which they arise may not be constant in different situations. Their transient appearance after various types of tissue damage, including the infarction of brain or cardiac muscle, suggests that a "mopping-up" response to tissue destruction or to the release of sequestered antigen may be a frequent occurrence which leads to disease only in special circumstances.

There are other ways in which auto-immune reactions may arise, and it is possible that various modifications of the surface of living host cells by viruses, drugs, or other agents may render the living cells antigenic. Although this might lead to autoallergic cell damage, it has been postulated that such a mechanism may also be capable of a protective role, by destroying deviant cells in early cancer.

IMMUNE MECHANISMS IN CARDIOVASCULAR DISEASE

Subacute Bacterial Endocarditis

In bacterial endocarditis the adverse immune response to an infection is well known. In this disease death may occur long after the eradication of the infective agent. One third of the deaths are due to renal disease and uremia, but this is not embolic in most cases. Renal involvement is equally common in left- and right-sided heart infections, and the appearance is that of a diffuse glomerulonephritis. The "lumpy-bumpy" appearance of immune complex deposition may be seen on electron microscopy. In association with this, autoantibodies may develop as the disease progresses and rheumatoid (antiglobulin) factors are common, as are positive Kahn reactions. Cryoglobulins are found in most cases at one time or another,[37] and this is usually taken as further evidence of an abnormal antibody response. Hopes of improving the results of treatment of this disease must depend on improved control of the complications as well as of the infection itself.

The Collagen Diseases

Austen[2] has pointed out that this term was originally introduced to describe a group of diseases with common or overlapping clinical and histological features. In all of them there is widespread damage to connective tissue and blood vessels, and a necrotizing angiitis is suggested as the basic pathological feature. The clinical manifestations of a particular disease will be caused by partial or complete occlusion of vessels, the size and type of vessel involved determining the pattern of the disease. The diseases usually included in the collagen group include rheumatoid arthritis, systemic lupus erythematosus, scleroderma and polymyositis. They share a high incidence of nonorgan-specific antibodies such as antinuclear factor and rheumatoid factor. Related to this group, but without the high incidence of circulating antibodies, are polyarteritis nodosa and a variety of more or less well-defined inflammatory diseases of blood vessels—giant-cell arteritis, the aortic arteritis of Takayashu, and allergic granulomatous angiitis. A role in the etiology of these diseases is given to immune mechanisms, particularly type-III reactions with immune complex deposi-

tion[126,127] and probably type-IV cell-mediated reactions.

All these diseases affect more than one organ system, and the cardiovascular system is often involved. When a generalized vasculitis occurs, the myocardium can be diffusely affected or can show areas of infarction from coronary-artery occlusions. Pericarditis occurs often, although it may not dominate the clinical picture. Endocarditis and valve lesions are also described.

Barker[6] has recently reviewed rheumatoid arthritis and heart disease. Two main types of heart lesion are described: (1) Granulomas, similar in pattern to the subcutaneous nodules, can occur in the myocardium, endocardium, pericardium and all four valves. Although the valve lesions do not often affect valve function, a case is recorded of aortic regurgitation leading to valve replacement. (2) Nonspecific inflammations can affect myocardium, endocardium and pericardium. Kirk and Cosh[73] have stressed the pericarditis, finding a 30 per cent incidence of healed lesions in eight series of patients coming to necropsy. They went on to demonstrate clinical signs of pericarditis in 31 out of 100 consecutive patients admitted to the hospital with active rheumatoid arthritis. They concluded that the pericardial involvement was usually benign and self-limiting. Liss and Bachmann[80] described a case going on to constrictive pericarditis requiring surgery, and reviewed a further 25 cases in the literature. Despite these examples of lesions requiring surgery, Hart's conclusion[52] remains accurate: that clinically significant rheumatoid heart disease is rare.

Brigden et al.[16] concluded that heart lesions develop in nearly all patients with systemic lupus erythematosus at some time. The most common manifestation is pericarditis, often painless and often accompanied by an effusion. Endocarditis, first recorded by Libman and Sacks in 1924,[79] is present in half of the cases studied at necropsy, but it rarely results in significant valvular obstruction or regurgitation. Myocarditis is less common but may be associated with arrhythmias and conduction disturbances. A coronary-artery vasculitis, with generalized subendothelial fibrinoid necrosis and proliferation of fibroblasts, can lead to narrowing of the vessel lumen with occasional thrombosis and possible infarction.

Sclerodermal heart disease, with patchy replacement of heart muscle by fibrous tissue, was first described by Weiss et al. in 1943;[125] it is relatively rare. The most common type of cardiac involvement is right and left ventricular failure secondary to pulmonary and systemic hypertension. Pulmonary hypertension in scleroderma was recently reviewed by Trell and Lindström,[117] who describe both lung fibrosis and hyperplastic changes in the pulmonary arteries with medial hypertrophy and intimal proliferation. As in the other collagen diseases, asymptomatic pericarditis is common.[89]

In polymyositis and dermatomyositis, changes are seen in heart muscle similar to, but less severe than, those seen in skeletal muscle.[88] Some muscle fibers show fragmentation, loss of striation and vacuolization while between them cellular infiltrates may occur. Clinically, tachycardia is most often seen, with occasional conduction disturbances and, rarely, congestive failure.

In polyarteritis nodosa and the related vasculitis syndromes variable clinical features occur depending on the site of vascular involvement, the rapidity and intensity with which the process develops and the presence of associated conditions. Holsinger et al.[55] made a special study of the heart in 66 cases of polyarteritis nodosa coming to necropsy. They related death to congestive cardiac failure in 44 per cent of the cases, with hypertension contributing to this. Myocardial infarction was more often due to arteritis of small vessels than to a major coronary occlusion. While immune complex deposition is usually thought of as the most likely underlying mechanism in these diseases, Ueda et al.[120] have recently described a variety of antibodies to vascular tissues in aortitis,

raising the possibility that these antibodies may themselves initiate the tissue damage (type II).

A number of other diseases often included in the collagen group may have important cardiac complications. The aortic-valve lesions of ankylosing spondylitis are well known.[1,118] Carditis with conduction disturbances and aortic incompetence can also occur in Reiter's disease.[23] A rarer condition, seen in some cases in association with rheumatoid arthritis or systemic lupus erythematosus, is relapsing polychondritis;[90] here, too, aortic regurgitation may occur.[58]

Postcardiotomy and Postinfarction Syndromes

In an early report on the effects of mitral-valve surgery[107] it was noted that illness sometimes occurred weeks or months after the operation. This was associated with pericarditis and pleurisy, sometimes with effusions, and with pneumonia, occasional hemoptysis and arthralgia. The erythrocyte sedimentation rate was raised. This complication was first called the postcommissurotomy syndrome, but in 1958 Ito et al.[59] showed that it could occur after surgery for congenital heart disease. It has also been described after penetrating stab wounds to the chest[104] and after implantation of pacemakers.[35] Dressler[34] drew attention in 1956 to a similar set of symptoms occurring in the weeks following myocardial infarction. All reports agree that attacks after both cardiotomy and infarction can recur, and Soloff et al.[107] describe one patient who had 14 episodes at monthly intervals after mitral valvotomy.

The incidence of the syndrome varies in different reports. Soloff et al.[107] found it in 24 per cent of their patients, and Larson[77] in 1957 reported it in 51 of 137 patients after mitral valvotomy (37 per cent). A uniform set of criteria for making the diagnosis would be needed for a true estimate, but with modern techniques the incidence of a postcardiotomy syndrome is probably closer to the 10 per cent of Paul Wood[128] than to the higher estimates.

Theories as to the etiology of the postcardiotomy syndrome have included reactivation of rheumatic disease,[107] a traumatic or hemorrhagic pericarditis,[91,128] and, more recently, an auto-immune response. Increasing awareness that similar symptoms could follow myocardial infarction, and surgery in patients who had not had rheumatic fever, seemed to discredit the original idea of rheumatic reactivation. However, it remained difficult to explain the delayed and sometimes recurrent appearance of the syndrome on the basis of a traumatic or hemorrhagic pericarditis. In 1960 Kaplan[63] suggested that autoantibodies might be involved in both rheumatic fever and the postcommissurotomy state. In 1969 he and Frengley[70] pointed out that in both the postcardiotomy and postinfarction syndromes participation of an immune mechanism is suggested by the latent period and the prompt response to steroid treatment. The clinical manifestations of pericarditis, pleurisy and arthralgia are also common in "collagen" diseases, and systemic lupus erythematosus is mentioned in the differential diagnosis of the postcardiotomy syndrome by some authors.

These considerations have stimulated a search for autoantibodies and three sensitive but relatively nonspecific serological tests have been used. Most frequently used has been the immunofluorescent technique, in which a patient's serum is applied to frozen sections of heart muscle and the fluorescent anti-globulin staining method is used to detect attached globulin molecules. The second test (used by one group) is the antiglobulin consumption test, which uses an antiglobulin assay method to detect the globulin from a patient's serum absorbed by a homogenate of heart tissue. Both these techniques include all the antigens of heart tissue in the test substrate, but only with the fluorescent test is some localization of the reacting antigen possible. The third test involves coating saline-soluble antigens of heart muscle onto tanned sheep red-blood cells. The sensitized cells will then agglutinate when exposed to serum containing an appropriate antibody.

Espinosa, Kushner and Kaplan[40] reviewed the antigenicity of heart tissue. They refer to one group of heart-specific antigens, including a particulate one localized to sites between the myofibrils and two or three saline-soluble antigens. A second group of insoluble antigens is shared by heart and skeletal muscle, and a third group by smooth muscle as well. In such a complex system it is difficult to isolate one antigen which might have stimulated the appearance of an antibody, and the techniques referred to above will have limited ability to localize the source of a reacting antigen. The literature contains many references to the appearance of heart-reactive antibodies in patients who have undergone cardiotomy, or who have suffered a myocardial infarct, but the varying methods and substrates used make comparison difficult.

Table 1.   Summary of Antiheart Antibody Tests

Condition Studied	Positive Results with Various Tests		
	Immunofluorescence[1]	Antiglobulin Consumption[2]	Tanned Red Cell[3]
Postinfarction (all cases)	10–32%	3%	23–27%
Postinfarction syndrome	55%	43%	75–100%
Postcardiotomy (all cases)	60–100%	16%	10–17%
Postcardiotomy syndrome	82%	73%	86–100%

[1] Data from Kaplan et al.,[66] Hess et al.,[53] Van der Geld,[122] and Zabriskie et al.[132]
[2] Data from Van der Geld.[122]
[3] Data from Ehrenfeld et al.,[38] Robinson and Brigden,[96,97] and Itoh et al.[60]

None of the techniques can demonstrate whether a cell-mediated reaction might also be occurring.

Table 1 summarizes the results of studies on the appearance of antiheart antibodies in patients with and without symptoms of the postinfarction and postcardiotomy syndromes. These data are derived from papers published by the groups listed below the table. It is worth noting that the total numbers studied are small, e.g. the results of the immunofluorescent test refer to only 9 patients with the postinfarction syndrome and 11 patients with the postcardiotomy syndrome. In general, while antibodies have been detected in varying numbers of patients after uncomplicated infarction or cardiotomy, more patients have been found to have antibodies when symptoms are present. It has been suggested[38,60] that these antibodies are a result of cardiac damage and do not have a pathogenetic effect. However, Robinson and Brigden[96] noted that the symptoms of a postcardiotomy syndrome may wax and wane parallel with the appearance and disappearance of antibody, and suggested that the antibodies might cause the syndrome. Itoh et al.[60] noted that, when infarcted heart muscle was used as a source of antigen, their test gave a higher number of positive results in the postinfarction syndrome. The possibility that infarction might change an antigen, rendering it more immunogenic, arises. Further progress in our understanding of these syndromes must await further analysis of antigens and antibodies, together with further immunopathological studies of the heart, pericardium and pleura.

The suggestion of Burch and Colcolough[18] that these syndromes might be caused by reactivation of a latent virus infection deserves mention. They quote the work of Pearce[94] with rabbits in 1942, showing that needling or handling of the heart can increase tissue damage caused by a subsequent viral infection. Having found Coxsackie antigens in heart tissue at routine autopsy,[17] they suggest that similar viruses might lie latent

to be reactivated by the trauma of surgery and the tissue damage of myocardial infarction. The delayed appearance of symptoms might be difficult to explain on this basis, but the hypothesis is well worth further study.

Rheumatic Fever

The immunological techniques referred to above have been extensively used in studies on rheumatic fever.[70] Immunofluorescent studies from Kaplan et al.,[66] Hess et al.,[53] and Zitnan and Bosmansky[133] report positive reactions between serum factors and heart muscle in 25 to 63 per cent of patients with rheumatic fever, 12 to 21 per cent of patients with inactive rheumatic heart disease, and 0 to 4 per cent of normal controls. Antiglobulin consumption tests, complement-fixation tests and the tanned red-cell hemagglutination techniques also show a high frequency of autoantibodies to heart tissue in rheumatic fever. Several different types of heart antigen were used in these tests, suggesting that multiple autoantibodies may be present. It has been claimed that the appearance of some of these antibodies, particularly those directed to particulate cardiac antigens, correlates with the clinical course of rheumatic fever.[20,53]

The work of Kaplan and Meyeserian[65] has suggested a cross-reacting immune response, provoked by group A beta-hemolytic streptococci but leading to the formation of antibodies which also react with heart muscle cells. Antibodies to streptococcal cells may be shown by immunofluorescent methods to have an affinity for the sarcolemma and subsarcolemmal sarcoplasm of heart muscle fibers, and this affinity is lost when the serum is absorbed with streptococcal cell walls or cell membranes.[71] In the cell wall, the responsible antigen appears to be present in a molecular complex with M protein, the factor associated with virulence in group A streptococcus.[70] A cross reaction has also been reported between streptococcal group A carbohydrate and a structural glycoprotein of heart valves.[50]

Kaplan and Svec[67] have demonstrated a cross-reactive antibody in the sera of more than 50 per cent of patients with rheumatic fever, inactive rheumatic heart disease or acute glomerulonephritis, and in 24 per cent of patients with a recent streptococcal infection. In those with uncomplicated streptococcal infection or glomerulonephritis the antibody was present without evidence of cardiac involvement. Zabriskie et al.[132] have attempted quantitative immunofluorescent studies, and conclude that sera of patients with acute rheumatic fever have about four times as much of this antibody as is found in sera of patients without cardiac symptoms after streptococcal infection.

It has been suggested that similar cross reactions may be responsible for other immunological disorders, including Crohn's disease and ulcerative colitis.[32,92] However, the finding of autoantibodies in other situations may have a different significance. As suggested above, they could represent a response to the breakdown of infected cells or might also represent an immune reaction provoked by cells which have virus, drugs or other foreign substances on their surface. In clinical situations in which they provide useful markers of disease, it sometimes appears that the presence of autoantibodies relates to the duration and other features of the disease rather than to its activity. Even when their presence is established, therefore, their significance remains to be established.

In rheumatic fever, immunopathological observations lend some support to the idea that the antibodies demonstrated might be more than "markers" of the disease. Kaplan and Dallenbach[64] showed bound gamma globulin in scattered deposits in 18 per cent of atrial biopsy specimens from patients with clinically inactive rheumatic heart disease. In studies on hearts of children dying of acute rheumatic fever, the myocardium of all chambers was massively infiltrated by bound globulin and the Blc component of complement.[68] The deposits were concentrated in the sarcolemma and subsarcolemma, in smooth muscle in the walls of arteries and veins, and in interstitial connective tissue. Gamma G was present in largest amounts, with variable amounts of gamma A and gamma M. In Aschoff lesions and in cellular elements globulins were virtually absent. The valves showed intense staining for gamma G only, with no evidence of complement binding.

The significance of these observations is not yet certain. The possibility exists that antibody to streptococcal antigen cross reacts with heart antigen and causes direct damage, or that the antibody reaction is against decapsulated streptococcal L-forms which have invaded the myocardium.[76] It is also possible that damage may arise from the deposition of immune complexes. The cellular lesions could result from a coincidental lymphocytic immune reaction. These speculations must be tempered by the knowledge that attempts to induce typical rheumatic lesions by injecting streptococcal antigens into experimental animals have not been successful.[114] When live streptococci are used some successes have been claimed.[22,27]

While the streptococcus has become established as important in the etiology of rheumatic fever, the fact remains that only 3 per cent of patients with streptococcal infections develop carditis and, of these, 50 to 60 per cent do not have a recurrence of rheumatic fever with the second streptococcal infection.[24] Burch et al.[19] have suggested that preoccupation with the streptococcus has prevented other agents from being studied. They point out that Coxsackie virus B4 can produce cardiac lesions resembling rheumatic fever in experimental animals[113] and argue that acute and chronic heart disease in man might be caused by similar agents. As noted above in relation to the postcardiotomy and postinfarction syndromes, a variety of factors might predispose to viral infection or to reactivation of a latent infection. The immune events after streptococcal infection would then be regarded as "conditioning" the heart for viral attack. Some support for the hypothesis comes from demonstration by immunofluorescence of viral antigens in valvular tissue examined at routine autopsy.[17]

TRANSPLANTATION AND THE HEART

Lower et al.[81] have recently reviewed the results of heart transplantation to September 1970. A study of the transplant registry supplemented by direct communication with transplant teams showed a total of 165 transplants in 162 patients. There were 22 survivors (13.3 per cent). The operation had been performed by 59 different teams in 20 countries. Approximately two thirds of the patients had died within three months of the operation from rejection or infection, and some lessening in enthusiasm for the procedure was suggested by the comparison between the 27 operations performed in the single month of November 1968 and only 14 between January and September 1970.

The group at Stanford University[109] have reported on 25 patients operated on between January 1968 and September 1970. Donor and recipient were matched for major blood groups, but in only two cases was there good matching of histocompatibility antigens. Five patients in the series had survived for more than one year, and four of these were still alive, one patient having reached 22 months. Calculating survival on life-table methods they showed a 40 per cent survival at six months, with 34 per cent for 12 and 18 months. In an analysis of causes of death they ascribe three deaths to preexisting disease of the pulmonary vessels, one to a cerebrovascular accident, five to rejection and eight to infection. In an earlier report from another center, Cooley et al.[26] reviewed 9 deaths in 17 patients. One was ascribed to preexisting disease, five to rejection and three to infection. These sets of figures illustrate that the main problem in heart transplantation is that of rejection and its management.

There have been some excellent recent reviews of the background to graft rejec-

tion.[42,101] An individual's tissues carry a unique complement of histocompatibility antigens, probably on the cell surface. After transplantation into another individual, recognition of the "foreign" nature of the graft occurs. This depends either on release of antigenic material into the host's bloodstream[85] or on migration of host antigen-recognizing cells into the graft.[111] A sequence of events follows[119] whereby the host's immune system produces a population of specifically sensitized lymphocytes and humoral antibodies. Graft rejection then occurs at a rate determined by the intensity of the immune response and by the anatomy of the graft. A combination of immunopathological processes is responsible, including the direct effect of antibody, a lymphocytic reaction, and possibly immune complex deposition.[9]

Further analysis of this problem for a particular organ involves discussion of its antigen content, and of the ways in which rejection processes impair its function and can be recognized clinically.

Antigenicity of the Heart

It is usually stated that the full spectrum of histocompatibility antigens is present on all living nucleated cells. However, quantitative differences among various cell types can occur, and there may be some qualitative differences.[8]

Organ-specific antigens may also be of importance in transplantation, and the presence of antiheart antibodies in the serum of patients with chronic rheumatic heart disease or ischemic heart disease has already been noted. It has been suggested by Watts[26] that some cases of hyperacute rejection may occur because of the existence of preformed antiheart antibodies and that all potential recipients should be screened for these antibodies. Ellis and Zabriskie[39] have looked for heart antibodies by immunofluorescence before and after transplantation in nine patients, and found them to be present initially in two patients. Rossen et al.,[99] also using immunofluorescence, found antibodies to heart muscle in 15 out of 17 patients before heart transplantation. Neither group comments on any particularly adverse course for these patients. This aspect of heart antigenicity and its effect on transplantation need further study.

In view of the heart's antigenicity and susceptibility to rejection, a number of attempts have been made to determine the degree to which donor and recipient must be matched before prolonged function is possible. Working with rats, Freeman and Steinmuller[45] found heart homografts to be as rapidly rejected as skin. Barker and Billingham[7] confirmed this observation, but went on to study the fate of skin and heart grafts in rats across a wider range of genetic disparities. They concluded that in the absence of major histocompatibility barriers heart grafts usually survive longer than skin grafts. Boyd et al.[14] worked with a closed colony of beagles in which a possible histocompatibility system (DL-A) had been isolated. When heterotopic heart transplants were carried out between litter mates with DL-A compatibility they survived for a mean time of 53.2 days. This compares with a figure of 28.6 days for renal homograft survival in similar exchanges.[95] Bos et al.[13] also used beagles and showed that identity between donor and recipient for the major histocompatibility locus DL-A resulted in prolonged heart-graft survival, but did not prevent ultimate rejection.

These experimental observations suggest that a close similarity between donor and recipient antigens is desirable to reduce the rejection reaction to manageable proportions. It is doubtful if the minor variations in survival of different organs in the same situation will prove to have any clinical significance.

Patterns of Rejection

Thomson[115] has pointed out that interpretation of the histology of a rejected heart graft in man must take several factors other than immunological ones into account. Some lesions may have been present before transplantation; ischemic damage could occur between removal of the donor heart and reestablishment of a coronary circulation; secondary effects on the heart of events leading to the death of the recipient might be present; and some of the immunosuppressive measures might cause cardiac damage.

In the experimental animal both acute and chronic patterns of rejection have been distinguished.[29,30] Acute rejection is characterized by cellular invasion of the vessels and myocardium, with considerable edema. Foci of muscle necrosis develop, and the endocardial and subendocardial cellular infiltrates may lead to endocardial damage and overlying thrombi. Macroscopically, punctate hemorrhages are seen in a thickened, stiff ventricular wall. Similar changes have been described in man.[26] Involvement of the atrioventricular conduction tissue has been commented on[108] and, while the mononuclear cell infiltrates dominate the picture, serum antibodies may also play a part. Goldman et al.[49] have studied heterotopic heart transplants in mongrel dogs matched only for blood group. Frozen sections of rejected hearts showed globulin deposits along the sarcolemmal sheath of the muscle fibers. Immunoglobulin G was demonstrated in eluates from rejected hearts and was shown to react with lymphocytes, erythrocytes and heart muscle. Antibody activity detected in the heart eluate was usually also present in the animal's serum. When hearts were transplanted into animals with serum containing antibodies, sarcolemmal immunoglobulin G deposits appeared as early as 10 minutes after transplantation. Polymorphs could be seen to form margins on the endothelium of small blood vessels within 15 minutes. Surprisingly, fibrin and platelet thrombi and hyperacute rejection did not occur, in contrast to some reports on kidney transplants in similar circumstances.[82] Rossen et al.[99] have studied 15 human hearts that had been rejected. All of them showed immunoglobulins G, A and M in varying quantities in the sarcolemma, muscle fibers and coronary arteries. Relatively more immunoglobulin was found in hearts of patients who died of rejection soon after transplantation.

Chronic rejection involves the coronary arteries at all levels. Lower et al.[81] have pointed out that of 17 patients dying beyond six months after transplantation most have shown intimal hyperplasia in coronary vessels resulting in arrhythmias and heart failure. Dempster[30] has reviewed the development of these obliterative lesions. The vessel wall becomes edematous, and endothelial cells are damaged and displaced. Fibrin and platelet thrombi are deposited on the damaged intima and organization of these can lead to complete occlusion of the vessel. Thomson[116] recorded gross atheroma in a heart transplanted from a 24-year-old donor to a 58-year-old recipient. This was in position for only $19\frac{1}{2}$ months, but showed extensive atheroma at necropsy, including severe involvement of the mitral valve. Kosek et al.[74] have carried out further investigations into heart-graft arteriosclerosis and atheroma, and relate their development to endothelial damage and hypoxia of the arterial wall. The pathogenesis of these changes may have an immunological basis, although it is not clear whether individual or organ-specific antigens are involved. It has been established that any sort of damage to blood vessels—enzymatic, hormonal or mechanical—predisposes them to atheroma. Van Winkle and Levy[123,124] have induced an illness similar to serum sickness in rabbits, and have shown that this potentiates the atherogenic effect of a high-cholesterol diet. Further support for an immune mechanism comes from a demonstration in man of laminar deposits of immunoglobulin in arteries showing intimal thickening.[99]

If rejection is to be controlled, some way of diagnosing it short of cardiac biopsy must be found. In acute rejection the clinical features are malaise, weakness, fever, dyspnea, anorexia and progressive signs of cardiac failure. A pericardial friction rub and triple gallop rhythm may appear. Unfortunately most of these features could occur with other complications of recent cardiac surgery. Changes in the blood, such as increases in levels of cardiac enzymes and leukocytosis, may be noted but are again nonspecific. Stinson et al.[108] have reviewed the clinical diagnosis of cardiac rejection. The electrocardiogram has proved of greatest assistance. The features noted include decreased voltage, atrial arrhythmias, rightward deviation of the mean electrical axis and ischemic S-T segment changes. Ultrasound cardiography has also been used.[102] An increase in heart size, thickening of the left ventricular wall and variable decreases in the transverse diameter of the left ventricular cavity have been recorded.

The diagnosis of chronic rejection may be made only after vascular lesions have led to severe myocardial dysfunction. It has been claimed by Kahn et al.[62] that scintiscanning with [131]cesium may reveal areas of decreased myocardial blood flow and function some weeks before other clinical manifestations of rejection appear, and this correlates with histological evidence of chronic rejection in two of their patients.

Ellis and Zabriskie[39] have suggested that the severity of a rejection episode might be judged by the appearance and titer of a heart-reactive antibody. They use an immunofluorescent method and find that antibodies to heart muscle appear in the serum soon after cardiac transplantation. In one case high titers were present during each clinical and laboratory episode of rejection, while in a second the suspicion of rejection was not supported either by antibody titers or necropsy findings. The problem in accepting this technique as a precise monitor of cardiac rejection lies in the observations recorded above on the appearance of antibodies after various surgical and ischemic insults to the heart. In addition, while Ellis and Zabriskie found antibodies before transplantation in only 2 out of 9 patients, Rossen et al.[99] reported them (also by immunofluorescence) in 15 out of 17 patients. Problems may thus arise in interpreting results after transplantation.

While the end-results of rejection can be described, their pathogenesis is less clear. Most groups work on the assumption that histocompatibility differences initiate the reaction, although Dempster[31] has criticized this view. Further progress in transplantation may depend on bypassing or safely suppressing both sensitized cells and the antibody response.

Prospects for the Control of Rejection

HISTOCOMPATIBILITY TESTING

After the ABO red-cell antigen system, the most important histocompatibility system in man is known as the HL-A system.[10,28,56] This consists of a large number of antigenic factors. Collaborative experiments among different laboratories have led to the serological definition of a number of antigens. Most of these are "strong" antigens, in that grafts exchanged across them are subject to rapid rejection. Recently a multicenter collaborative report on the result of 162 tissue-typed renal transplants[44] has shown that when donor and recipient are matched for three or four major HL-A antigens the results are much better than when only two antigens are shared. A record of 25 per cent of well-matched transplants in this series was made possible by the agreement to fly appropriate kidneys to suitable recipients at other centers. In heart transplantation the problems of obtaining suitable grafts and of preserving them for transport have yet to be solved, and similar evidence on the importance of histocompatibility testing has not been produced except in animals.[13]

All the evidence suggests that histocompatibility matching will prove just as important in heart transplantation as it has in renal transplantation, despite the recent claim[110] that survival beyond two years is possible even with several HL-A incompatibilities. However, leukocyte typing and other techniques, such as mixed leukocyte culture,[3] can be fully utilized only when the problems of supply and storage of donor organs have been solved.

IMMUNOSUPPRESSION

Agents used in controlling rejection include antilymphocyte globulins, antimetabolites, alkylating agents, and corticosteroids. In addition to suppressing immune responses, some of them have a less specific effect as anti-inflammatory agents. Several recent reviews have appeared.[4,11,103] Antilymphocyte serum[61,129] appears to have its main action against long-lived lymphocytes, the function of which is to recognize antigen and initiate the immune response. Some problems have arisen in using this type of serum in man, and the spectacular prolongation of graft survival seen in experimental animals has not been realized in many hands. Some impure preparations have been used, and difficulties have arisen over rapid removal of the foreign protein from the circulation,[21] leading, in the case of the kidney, to damage to the transplanted organ. These problems have recently been reviewed.[5,130] In heart transplantation the failure of two thirds of the recorded human grafts because of rejection or infection[81] reveals that much remains to be learned.

The infective complications are due to the nonspecific action of conventional immunosuppressive agents. Stinson et al.[109] record a total of 47 separate infections (i.e. attributable to a single organism) in 15 patients, and in 8 cases infection led to death. The agents involved included gram-negative bacteria in 19, gram-positive bacteria in 6, viruses in 11 (9 of these cytomegalovirus), fungi in 7 and protozoa in 4. In several patients, several organisms were present simultaneously, especially in 6 cases with fatal pulmonary infection. The combination of agents used, interfering with both cellular and humoral responses and with the normal process of inflammation, allows normally nonpathogenic organisms to flourish. The reduced tissue responses make the diagnosis of infection more difficult.

A more insidious problem with immuno-suppression is the possible increase in incidence of malignant tumors after long-term therapy. Penn et al.[93] describe 11 patients out of Starzl's series of 236 renal-homograft recipients with various forms of malignant disease. When this number is expressed as a percentage of those surviving beyond four months from operation, the figure is 6 per cent. An estimate of the incidence of neoplasia in a comparable healthy group (with an age range of $3\frac{1}{2}$ to 49 years) produces a figure of 0.058 per cent. When the 11 cases from Denver are added to 28 from other renal-transplant centers and one case from South Africa in a heart-transplant recipient, the total number reported comes to 40. Of these, 23 were varieties of epithelial carcinoma, some of which were treatable, and 17 were mesenchymal (15 being various types of lympho-recticular tumor). It has been proposed that some of the malignancies result from loss of the immune surveillance system by which mutant cells are normally detected and destroyed. Until better control of immuno-suppressive dosage is possible, or until there are new ways of avoiding rejection, the risk of malignancy appears likely to continue.

The importance of finding less empirical ways of arriving at the dosage of immuno-suppressive agents is illustrated by one of Starzl's patients who developed an intra-cranial lymphoma. This was successfully irradiated, and her immunosuppression was drastically reduced without rejection of her homograft. In 1970 she had survived three years from transplantation and two and a half years from diagnosis of the tumor.[93] It could be argued that she was at first given more immunosuppressive therapy than she really needed, and had the dose been optimal the tumor might not have developed. In most centers, the therapy is adjusted in relation to signs and symptoms of rejection, and high doses of drugs are given both at the time of transplantation and during rejection episodes. Munro et al.[84] have developed an in vitro technique which they hope will provide a measure of the effectiveness of a given drug regimen in controlling a patient's ability to reject his graft. Their test, which depends on inhibition of the tendency of human lymphocytes to form rosette-like clusters with sheep red cells, enabled them to predict rejection crises in their patients and to deal with them by controlled increases in immunosuppression. While much work remains to be done on the theoretical basis of the technique, further results will be awaited with interest.

ENHANCEMENT AND TOLERANCE

The problems of immunosuppression have been outlined above. These would be less serious if there were adequate means of organ storage to allow full tissue matching to be carried out, but progress in this direction has been slow. This has led to an interest in finding other ways of avoiding rejection.

Enhancement refers to the prolongation of graft survival by the induction or administration of antibodies to graft antigens. Provided that these antibodies are not themselves cytotoxic, they have been shown to interfere with the immune response in a number of situations. Much of the early work on the phenomenon was done with tumors,[106,121] but Stuart et al.[112] and French and Batchelor[46] have shown that incompatible rat-kidney transplants could be made to survive long periods after treatment of recipients by passive transfer of enhancing antiserum. In a thoughtful review on enhancement Russell[100] concludes that caution is needed in applying the technique in man. In inducing enhancement the balance between cytotoxic and protective effects of humoral antibody is critical. He argues that the appearance of antibody spontaneously in patients is usually associated with advancing damage to the transplant, and suggests that some form of passive treatment may be necessary, involving the administration of antiserum against histocompatibility antigens. The production of such an antiserum will depend on progress in the purification of these antigens and in the separation of cytotoxic and enhancing antibodies. In heart transplants the problem of chronic rejection might still arise despite avoidance of the early acute attack.

Tolerance is a term introduced by Billingham et al.[12] in 1956 to refer to a central failure of the immunological response to specific antigens "brought about by exposure of animals to antigenic stimuli before the maturation of the faculty of immunological response." Since that time various ways of rendering mature animals tolerant to different antigens have been discovered.[36] Theories to explain tolerance have become more complex with the discovery of the interaction of two populations of lymphocytes in the immune response.[98] It now seems probable from in vitro studies on the H antigens of Salmonella adelaide that antibody is involved in the process also. The balance between induction of tolerance or immunity by a given antigen may depend on a particular combination of antigen dose, reacting cell population and avidity of induced antibody.[78] Different antigens will demand different combinations. Before the principle can be applied in human transplantation, progress in isolating and purifying histocompatibility antigens will have to be made.

SUMMARY AND CONCLUSIONS

In the recent past, the significance of autoantibodies in cardiovascular disorders and other diseases may have been over-emphasized. The techniques used to detect such antibodies have notable limitations and in many cases detect only free antibody. Such antibodies are not always cytotoxic and there is a need for further study of the cellular reactions which may also be present.

In infections of various kinds, including bacterial endocarditis, immunological reactions may be a direct cause of tissue damage. Auto-immune reactions may also result from tissue damage of various types, including tissue damage caused by infection. The basic pathogenesis of various connective-tissue disorders remains unknown, but in virtually all of these conditions there may be a widespread vasculitis with diffuse myocarditis, areas of myocardial infarction, pericarditis or endocarditis.

After cardiotomy or myocardial infarction a variety of antiheart antibodies may be found even in the absence of symptoms, and there does not appear to be any reliable test which can distinguish among a normal reaction to tissue damage, an exaggerated immune response, or the activation of a virus infection. Activation of a virus infection could also, conceivably, have a contributory role in some cases of rheumatic fever, although here the most notable immunological observations concern the well-established evidence of a cross-reacting immune response to the streptococcus, which may itself explain the cardiac damage seen in this condition.

An analysis of immunological mechanisms in disease has a particular relevance to the problems of heart transplantation. Rejection has been a major problem, and even when it is controlled there may be rapid deterioration of function and death due to a chronic obliterative attack on blood vessels. Immunosuppression has reversed some crises, but at the cost of high mortality from toxicity and infection. Antilymphocyte globulin may be of value and is still under trial. Progress in tissue typing cannot easily be applied until methods of storing the heart can be improved. The prospects for enhancement in heart transplantation also seem doubtful, and significant progress may depend on the development of specific ways of rendering a recipient tolerant to the foreign antigens on his graft.

REFERENCES

1. Ansell, B. M., Bywaters, E. G. L., and Doniach, I.: The aortic lesion of ankylosing spondylitis. Brit. Heart J., *20*:507, 1958.
2. Austen, K. F.: Connective tissue diseases ("collagen diseases") other than rheumatoid arthritis. In: *Cecil-Loeb Textbook of Medicine.* Philadelphia, W. B. Saunders, 1971.

3. Bach, F. H., and Bach, M. L.: Mixed leukocyte cultures in transplantation immunology. Transplantation Proc., 3:942, 1971.

4. Bach, J. F.: Immunosuppression by chemical agents. Transplantation Proc., 3:27, 1971.

5. Balner, H.: Perspectives of immunosuppression. Transplantation Proc., 3:949, 1971.

6. Barker, A.: Rheumatoid arthritis and rheumatoid heart disease. New Zeal. Med. J., 73:14, 1971.

7. Barker, C. F., and Billingham, R. E.: Histocompatibility requirements of heart and skin grafts in rats. Transplantation Proc., 3:172, 1971.

8. Barker, C. F., Lubaroff, D. M., and Silvers, W. K.: Lymph node cells. Their differential capacity to induce tolerance of heart and skin homografts in rats. Science, 172:1050, 1971.

9. Batchelor, J. R.: Mechanism of graft rejection. Proc. Roy. Soc. Med., 62:953, 1969.

10. Batchelor, J. R.: Tissue typing. Brit. J. Hosp. Med., 2:1199, 1969.

11. Berenbaum, M. C.: Immunosuppressive agents and allogeneic transplantation. J. Clin. Path., 20 (Suppl.):471, 1967.

12. Billingham, R. E., Brent, L., and Medawar, P. B.: Quantitative studies on tissue transplantation immunity. III. Actively acquired tolerance. Philos. Trans. Roy. Soc. B., 239: 357, 1956.

13. Bos, E., et al.: Histocompatibility in orthotopic heart transplantation in dogs. Transplantation Proc., 3:155, 1971.

14. Boyd, A. D., et al.: Role of the DL-A system of canine histocompatibility in cardiac transplantation. Transplantation Proc., 3:152, 1971.

15. Breckenridge, A., et al.: Positive direct Coombs test and antinuclear factor in patients treated with methyl dopa. Lancet, 2:1265, 1967.

16. Brigden, W., Bywaters, E. G. L., Lessof, M. H., and Ross, I. P.: The heart in systemic lupus erythematosus. Brit. Heart J., 22:1, 1960.

17. Burch, G. E., et al.: Coxsackie B viral myocarditis and valvulitis identified in routine autopsy specimens by immunofluorescent techniques. Amer. Heart J., 74:13, 1967.

18. Burch, G. E., and Colcolough, H. L.: Postcardiotomy and postinfarction syndromes. A theory. Amer. Heart J., 80:290, 1970.

19. Burch, G. E., Giles, T. D., and Colcolough, H. L.: Pathogenesis of rheumatic heart disease: Critique and theory. Amer. Heart J., 80:556, 1970.

20. Burgio, G. R., Severi, F., Vaccaro, R., and Rossini, R.: Antibodies reacting with heart tissue in the course of rheumatic fever in children. Schweiz. Med. Wschr., 96:431, 1966.

21. Butler, W. T., et al.: Antilymphocyte globulin turnover rates in heart transplant patients. Clin. Res., 17:72, 1969.

22. Cayeux, P., Panizel, J., Cluzan, R., and

Levillain, R.: Streptococcal arthritis and cardiopathy experimentally induced in white mice. Nature, 212:688, 1966.

23. Cliff, J. M.: Spinal bony bridging and carditis in Reiter's disease. Ann. Rheum. Dis., 30: 171, 1971.

24. Coburn, A. F., and Moore, L. V.: Salicylate prophylaxis in rheumatic fever. J. Paediat., 21:180, 1942.

25. Condemi, J. J., Moore-Jones, D., Vaughan, J. H., and Mitchell, P. H.: Antinuclear antibodies following hydralazine toxicity. New Eng. J. Med., 276:586, 1967.

26. Cooley, D. A., et al.: Cardiac transplantation: general considerations and results. Ann. Surg., 169:892, 1969.

27. Cromartie, W. J., and Craddock, J. G.: Rheumatic like cardiac lesions in mice. Science, 154:285, 1966.

28. Dausset, J.: The genetics of transplantation antigens. Transplantation Proc., 3:8, 1971.

29. Dempster, W. J.: Human heart transplantation. Brit. Med. J., 1:695, 1968.

30. Dempster, W. J.: An assessment of allotransplanted hearts. Brit. J. Hosp. Med., 2:1243, 1969.

31. Dempster, W. J.: HL-A histocompatibility. Lancet, 1:495, 1971.

32. Deodhar, S. D., Mickener, W. M., and Farmer, R. G.: A study of the immunological aspects of chronic ulcerative colitis and transmural colitis. Amer. J. Clin. Path., 51:591, 1969.

33. Dixon, F. J., Edgington, T. S., and Lambert, P. H.: Non-glomerular antigen-antibody complex nephritis. In: Immunopathology V, International Symposium. Basel, Schwake, 1967.

34. Dressler, W.: A post myocardial infarction syndrome. A preliminary report of a complication resembling idiopathic recurrent benign pericarditis. JAMA, 160:1379, 1956.

35. Dressler, W.: Postcardiotomy syndrome after implantation of a pacemaker. Amer. Heart J., 63:757, 1962.

36. Dresser, D. W., and Mitchison, N. A.: The mechanism of immunological paralysis. Advances Immun., 8:129, 1968.

37. Dreyfuss, F., and Librach, G.: Gold precipitable serum globulins ("cold fractions," "cryoglobulins") in subacute bacterial endocarditis. J. Lab. Clin. Med., 40:489, 1952.

38. Ehrenfeld, E. N., Gery, I., and Davies, A. M.: Specific antibodies in heart disease. Lancet, 1:1138, 1961.

39. Ellis, R. J., and Zabriskie, J. B.: Heart reactive antibody: A monitor of cardiac rejection. Transplantation Proc., 3:905, 1971.

40. Espinosa, E., Kushner, I., and Kaplan, M. H.: Antigenic analysis of heart tissue. Amer. J. Cardiol., 24:508, 1969.

41. Evans, A. S., Rothfield, N. F., and Niederman, J. C.: Raised antibody titres to E. B. virus in systemic lupus erythematosus. Lancet, 1: 167, 1971.

42. Evans, D. B., and Sells, R. A.: Rejection: the immune reaction and its control. Brit. J. Hosp. Med., 2:1249, 1969.
43. Farrow, L. J., et al.: Autoantibodies and the hepatitis. Brit. Med. J., 2:693, 1970.
44. Festenstein, H., et al.: Multicentre collaboration in 162 tissue typed renal transplants. Lancet, 2:225, 1971.
45. Freeman, J. S., and Steinmuller, D.: Acute rejection of skin and heart allografts in rats matched at the major rat histocompatibility locus. Transplantation, 8:530, 1969.
46. French, M. E., and Batchelor, J. R.: Immunological enhancement of rat kidney grafts. Lancet, 2:1103, 1969.
47. Fresco, R.: Tubular (myxovirus like) structures in glomerular deposits from a case of lupus nephritis. Fed. Proc., 27:170, 1967.
48. Gell, P. G. H., and Coombs, R. R. A.: Classification of allergic reactions responsible for clinical hypersensitivity and disease. In: Clinical Aspects of Immunology. Oxford, Blackwell Scientific Publications, 1970.
49. Goldman, B. S., et al.: Antibodies in the serum and on the heart of dogs with cardiac allografts. Transplantation Proc., 3:515, 1971.
50. Goldstein, I., Halpern, B., and Robert, L.: Immunological relationship between streptococcus A polysaccharide and the structural glycoprotein of heart valve. Nature, 213:46, 1967.
51. Gyorkey, F., Min, K. W., Sincovics, J. G., and Gyorkey, P.: Systemic lupus erythematosus and myxovirus. New Eng. J. Med., 280:333, 1969.
52. Hart, F. D.: Rheumatoid arthritis: Extraarticular manifestations. Brit. Med. J., 2:131, 1969.
53. Hess, E. V., Finn, C. W., Taranta, A., and Ziff, M.: Heart muscle antibodies in rheumatic fever and other diseases. J. Clin. Invest., 43:886, 1964.
54. Hirsch, M. S., and Murphy, F. A.: Effects of antilymphoid sera on viral infections. Lancet, 2:37, 1968.
55. Holsinger, D. R., Osmundsen, P. J., and Edwards, J. E.: The heart in periarteritis nodosa. Circulation, 25:610, 1962.
56. Hors, J., Feingold, N., Fradelizi, D., and Dausset, J.: Critical evaluation of histocompatibility in 179 renal transplants. Lancet, 1:609, 1971.
57. Howie, J. B., and Hellyer, B. J.: The immunology and immunopathology of NZB mice. Advances Immun., 9:215, 1968.
58. Hughes, R. A. C., Berry, C. L., Seifer, M., and Lessof, M. H.: Relapsing polychondritis. Three cases with a clinicopathological study and literature review. Quart. J. Med., in press.
59. Ito, T., Engle, M. A., and Goldberg, H. P.: Post-pericardiotomy syndrome following surgery for non-rheumatic heart disease. Circulation, 17:549, 1958.
60. Itoh, K., Ohkun, I. H., Kimura, E., and Kimura, Y.: Immunoserological studies on myocardial infarction and post-myocardial infarction syndrome. Jap. Heart J., 10:485, 1969.
61. James, K.: The preparation and properties of antilymphocytic sera. Progr. Surg., 7:140, 1969.
62. Kahn, D. R., et al.: Diagnosis of chronic rejection after cardiac transplantation. Transplantation Proc., 3:380, 1971.
63. Kaplan, M. H.: The concept of autoantibodies in rheumatic fever and in the post commissurotomy state. Ann. N.Y. Acad. Sci., 86:974, 1960.
64. Kaplan, M. H., and Dallenbach, F. D.: Immunologic studies of heart tissue. III. Occurrence of bound gammaglobulin in auricular appendages from rheumatic hearts. Relationship to certain histopathologic features of rheumatic heart disease. J. Exp. Med., 113:1, 1961.
65. Kaplan, M. H., and Meyeserian, M.: An immunological cross reaction between group A streptococcal cells and human heart tissue. Lancet, 1:706, 1962.
66. Kaplan, M. H., Meyeserian, M., and Kushner, I.: Immunologic studies of heart tissue. IV. Serologic reactions with human heart tissue as revealed by immunofluorescent methods: isoimmune, Wassermann and autoimmune reactions. J. Exp. Med., 113:17, 1961.
67. Kaplan, M. H., and Svec, K. H.: Immunologic relation of streptococcal and tissue antigens. III. Presence in human sera of streptococcal antibody cross-reactive with heart tissue. Association with streptococcal infections, rheumatic fever and glomerulonephritis. J. Exp. Med., 119:651, 1964.
68. Kaplan, M. H., Bolande, R., Rakita, L., and Blair, J.: Presence of bound immunoglobulins and complement in the myocardium in acute rheumatic fever. New Eng. J. Med., 271:637, 1964.
69. Kaplan, M. H., and Tan, E. M.: Antinuclear antibodies in infectious mononucleosis. Lancet, 1:561, 1968.
70. Kaplan, M. H., and Frengley, J. D.: Autoimmunity to the heart in cardiac disease. Amer. J. Cardiol., 24:459, 1969.
71. Kaplan, M. H., and Rakita, L.: In: Immunological Diseases, Vol. 2 (Samter, M., Ed.). Little, Brown, & Co., Boston, 1971.
72. Kawano, K., Miller, L., and Kimmelstiel, P.: Virus like structures in lupus erythematosus. New Eng. J. Med., 281:1228, 1969.
73. Kirk, J., and Cosh, J.: The pericarditis of rheumatoid arthritis. Quart. J. Med., 38:397, 1969.
74. Kosek, J. C., Bieber, C., and Lower, R. R.: Heart graft arteriosclerosis. Transplantation Proc., 3:512, 1971.

75. Ladd, A. G.: Procainamide-induced lupus erythematosus. New Eng. J. Med., *267*:1357, 1962.
76. Lannigan, R., and Zaki, S. A.: Sub-microscopic particles in the lesions of rheumatic carditis. Lancet, *1*:1098, 1965.
77. Larson, D. L.: Relation of the post commissurotomy syndrome to the rheumatic state. Circulation, *15*:203, 1957.
78. Levey, R. H.: Immunological tolerance and enhancement: A common mechanism. Transplantation Proc., *3*:41, 1971.
79. Libman, E., and Sacks, B.: A hitherto undescribed form of valvular and mural endocarditis. Arch. Intern. Med., *33*:701, 1924.
80. Liss, J. P., and Bachmann, W. T.: Rheumatoid pericarditis treated by pericardiectomy. Arthritis Rheum., *13*:869, 1970.
81. Lower, R. R., et al.: Current state of clinical heart transplantation. Transplantation Proc., *3*:333, 1971.
82. MacDonald, A., et al.: Heparin and aspirin in the treatment of hyperacute rejection of renal allografts in presensitised dogs. Transplantation, *9*:1, 1970.
83. Mellors, R. C., Aoki, T., and Huebner, R. J.: Further implications of murine leukaemia virus in the disorders of NZB mice. J. Exp. Med., *129*:1045, 1969.
84. Munro, A., et al.: Clinical evaluation of a rosette inhibition test in renal allotransplantation. Brit. Med. J., *2*:271, 1971.
85. Najarian, J. S., May, J., and Cochrum, K. C.: Mechanism of antigen release from canine kidney homotransplants. Ann. N.Y. Acad. Sci., *129*:76, 1966.
86. Norton, W. L.: Endothelial inclusions in active lesions of S.L.E. J. Lab. Clin. Med., *74*:369, 1969.
87. Oldstone, M. G. A., and Dixon, F. J.: Lymphocytic choriomeningitis: Production of antibody by tolerant infected mice. Science, *158*: 1193, 1967.
88. O'Leary, P. A., and Waisman, M.: Dermatomyositis: study of 40 cases. Arch. Derm. Syph., *41*:1001, 1940.
89. Oram, S., and Stokes, W.: The heart in scleroderma. Brit. Heart J., *23*:243, 1961.
90. Owen, D. S., Irby, R., and Toome, E.: Relapsing polychondritis with aortic involvement. Arthritis Rheum., *13*:869, 1970.
91. Papp, C., and Zion, M. M.: The post commissurotomy syndrome. Brit. Heart J., *18*:153, 1956.
92. Perlmann, P., Hammarstrom, S., Lagercrantz, R., and Gustafsson, B. E.: Antigen from colon of germ free rats and antibodies in human ulcerative colitis. Ann. N.Y. Acad. Sci., *124*:377, 1965.
93. Penn, I., Halgrimson, C. G., and Starzl, T. E.: *De novo* malignant tumours in organ transplant recipients. Transplantation Proc. *3*: 773, 1971.
94. Pearce, J. M.: Susceptibility of the heart of the rabbit to specific infection in viral disease. Arch. Path., *34*:319, 1942.
95. Rapoport, F. T., et al.: Histocompatibility studies in a closely bred colony of dogs. I. Influence of leukocyte group antigens upon renal allograft survival in the unmodified host. J. Exp. Med., *131*:881, 1970.
96. Robinson, J., and Brigden, W.: Immunological studies in the post-cardiotomy syndrome. Brit. Med. J., *2*:706, 1963.
97. Robinson, J., and Brigden, W.: Recurrent pericarditis. Brit. Med. J., *2*:272, 1968.
98. Roitt, I. M., et al.: The cellular basis of immunological responsiveness. Lancet, *2*:367, 1969.
99. Rossen, R. D., Butler, W. T., Johnson, A. H., and Mittal, K. K.: Immunofluorescent and serologic studies of the humoral antibody response to cardiac allotransplantation in man. Transplantation Proc., *3*:445, 1971.
100. Russell, P. S.: Immunological enhancement. Transplantation Proc. *3*:960, 1971.
101. Russell, P. S., and Winn, H. J.: Transplantation I. New Eng. J. Med., *282*:786, 1970.
102. Schroeder, J. S., et al.: Acute rejection following cardiac transplantation. Phonocardiographic and ultra-sound observations. Circution, *40*:155, 1969.
103. Schwartz, R. S.: Immunosuppressive drug therapy. In: *Human Transplantation* (Rapoport, F. T., and Dausset, J., Eds.). New York, Grune and Stratton, 1968.
104. Segal, F., and Tabatznik, B.: Post-pericardiotomy syndrome following penetrating stab wounds of the chest: Comparison with post commissurotomy syndrome. Amer. Heart J., *59*:175, 1960.
105. Shaper, A. G., and Kaplan, M. H.: Malarial antibodies and autoantibodies to heart and other tissues in the immigrant and indigenous peoples of Uganda. Lancet, *1*:1342, 1968.
106. Snell, G. D.: Immunologic enhancement. Surg. Gynec. Obstet., *130*:1109, 1970.
107. Soloff, L. A., et al. Reactivation of rheumatic fever following mitral commissurotomy. Circulation, *8*:481, 1953.
108. Stinson, E. B., et al.: Cardiac transplantation in man. I. Early rejection. JAMA, *207*: 2233, 1969.
109. Stinson, E. B., Griepp, R. B., Dong, E., and Shumway, N. E.: Results of human heart transplantation at Stanford University. Transplantation Proc., *3*:337, 1971.
110. Stinson, E. B., et al.: Correlation of histocompatibility matching with graft rejection and survival after cardiac transplantation in man. Lancet, *2*:459, 1971.
111. Strober, S., and Gowans, J. L.: The role of lymphocytes in the sensitization of rats to renal homografts. J. Exp. Med., *122*:347, 1965.
112. Stuart, F. P., Saitoh, T., Fitch, F. W., and Spargo, B. H.: Immunological enhancement of renal allografts in the rat. Surgery, *64*:17, 1968.

113. Sun, S. C., et al.: Coxsackie B4 pancarditis in cynomologus monkeys resembling rheumatic fever. Brit. J. Exp. Path., *48*:655, 1967.
114. Taranta, A.: Of man's heart valves and strep's cell walls. Ann. Intern. Med., *66*:1287, 1967.
115. Thomson, J. G.: Heart transplantation in man —necropsy findings. Brit. Med. J., *1*:511, 1968.
116. Thomson, J. G.: Production of severe atheroma in a transplanted human heart. Lancet, 2: 1088, 1969.
117. Trell, E., and Lindström, C.: Pulmonary hypertension in systemic sclerosis. Ann. Rheum. Dis., *30*:390, 1971.
118. Toone, E. C., Pierce, E. L., and Hennigar, G. R.: Aortitis and aortic regurgitation associated with rheumatoid spondylitis. Amer. J. Med., *26*:255, 1959.
119. Turk, J. L.: Lymphocyte response to antigens A. Afferent side of sensitization arc. Response to lymphocytes to antigens. Transplantation, *5*:952, 1967.
120. Ueda, H., et al.: Further immunological studies of aortitis syndrome. Jap. Heart J., *12*:1, 1971.
121. Uhr, J. W., and Möller, G.: Regulatory effect of antibody on the immune response. Advances Immun., *8*:81, 1968.
122. Van der Geld, H.: Antiheart antibodies in the post pericardiotomy and the post myocardial infarction syndrome. Lancet, 2:617, 1964.
123. Van Winkle, M., and Levy, L.: Effect of removal of cholesterol diet upon serum sickness —cholesterol induced atherosclerosis. J. Exp. Med., *128*:497, 1968.
124. Van Winkle, M., and Levy, L.: Further studies on the reversibility of serum sickness—cholesterol induced atherosclerosis. J. Exp. Med., *132*:858, 1970.
125. Weiss S., Stead, E. A., Warren, J. V., and Bailey, O. T.: Scleroderma heart disease. Arch. Intern. Med., *71*:749, 1943.
126. Whaley, K., and Buchanan, W. W.: Immunological mechanisms in the pathogenesis of systemic lupus erythematosus. Scot. Med. J., *15*:261, 1970.
127. Wigley, R. D.: The aetiology of polyarteritis nodosa. A review. New Zeal. Med. J., *71*: 151, 1970.
128. Wood, P.: An appreciation of mitral stenosis. Brit. Med. J., *1*:1051, 1954.
129. Woodruff, M. F. A.: Antilymphocytic serum. Antibiot. Chemother., *15*:234, 1969.
130. Woodruff, M. F. A.: Antilymphocyte serum and its mode of action. Transplantation Proc., *3*:34, 1971.
131. Wright, D. M., et al.: New antibody in early syphilis. Lancet, *1*:740, 1970.
132. Zabriskie, J. B., Hsu, K. C., and Segal, B. C.: Heart-reactive antibody associated with rheumatic fever: characterization and diagnostic significance. Clin. Exp. Immun., 7:147, 1970.
133. Zitnan, D., and Bosmansky, K.: Antimyocardial serum factors in rheumatic fever detected by the immunofluorescence method. Acta Rheum. Scand., *12*:267, 1966.

Chapter 3

THE CURRENT STATUS OF CARDIAC GLYCOSIDE ASSAY TECHNIQUES*

Thomas W. Smith, M.D., and Edgar Haber, M.D.

"... It is much easier to write upon a disease than upon a remedy. The former is in the hands of nature, and a faithful observer, with an eye of tolerable judgement, cannot fail to delineate a likeness. The latter will ever be subject to the whims, the inaccuracies, and the blunders of mankind."   Withering, 1778

These words, penned nearly 200 years ago, find a sympathetic audience among contemporary investigators interested in the clinical pharmacology of digitalis glycosides. As was apparent to Withering,[134] the narrow margin between therapeutic and toxic effects of cardiac glycosides results in a relatively high incidence of toxicity in routine clinical use. An incidence ranging from about 8 to 20 per cent has been reported in most series of hospitalized patients receiving digitalis.[7,15,106] A recent prospective survey of 931 successive admissions to a single medical service at

* Portions of the work described herein were supported by U.S. Public Health Service Grant HEP-06664, National Heart and Lung Institute Grant IROI HE-14325, American Heart Association Grant-in-Aid #70718, and Grant-in-Aid #1068 from the Massachusetts Heart Association, Northeast Chapter. Dr. Smith is an Established Investigator of the American Heart Association.

Boston City Hospital revealed a 23 per cent incidence of digitalis intoxication in patients receiving maintenance doses of cardiac glycosides.[7] An additional 6 per cent of digitalized patients were judged possibly toxic at the time of admission. Another recent study of 1,080 consecutively monitored patients receiving digoxin revealed a 13.3 per cent incidence of toxic cardiac rhythm disturbances.[15]

Earlier studies have been largely retrospective in design and this may account, at least in part, for an apparently increasing incidence in toxicity in recent studies. Increased use of potent diuretics with consequent renal potassium losses and increased prevalence of advanced cardiac disease also have been suggested as possible contributing factors, but it seems likely that improved monitoring methods and increased awareness of the spectrum of rhythm disturbances caused by digitalis excess account for much of the increase.

At the other extreme, substantial numbers of patients have been found to be markedly underdigitalized. Eleven per cent of patients fell into this category in the series of hospital-ized patients reported by Beller et al.,[7] while as many as 36 per cent of patients presumed to be receiving appropriate maintenance doses of cardiac glycosides were found to be underdigitalized in a prospective outpatient study.[54] Reasons for the difficulty in selection of proper doses include patient variation in the correct maintenance dose, inability accu-rately to measure the therapeutic effect in clinical practice, and the nonspecificity of many symptoms of toxicity in addition to the notoriously narrow therapeutic:toxic ratio.[27]

Thus, it is clear from epidemiological studies of the sort discussed above that there is substantial room for improvement in the clinical management of individual digitalized patients. Recent advances in the measure-ment of serum or plasma* concentrations of cardiac glycosides have provided the clinician with additional information for the assessment of the individual problem patient, and the clinical investigator with new tools for the elucidation of various special problems in the clinical pharmacology of these drugs. The purpose of the present review is to discuss in detail current methods for the measurement of cardiac glycoside concentrations, and to summarize the results of a rapidly expanding number of studies employing these techniques.

RATIONALE

A number of lines of evidence have sug-gested that data on serum cardiac glycoside concentration might bear a meaningful rela-tionship to pharmacological or clinical effect. It has been apparent since the time of Withering that alterations in cardiac rhythm produced by digitalis are dose-related phe-nomena, as are most of the extracardiac mani-festations such as gastrointestinal or central nervous system toxicity.[68,86] Ample evidence is now available that serum digitalis concen-trations rise with increasing dosage,[9–11,19,28,]

* Serum and plasma cardiac glycoside concentra-tion measurements give essentially identical results, and the term "serum concentration" as used in the remainder of this review may be considered synony-mous with serum or plasma concentration.

[37,38,56,75,76,87,88,98,109] so that a correlation between serum digitalis concentration and clinical state would be expected to exist, at least statistically.

Data relating serum and myocardial digoxin concentrations provide an additional basis for the use of serum digitalis levels. The studies of Doherty and Perkins[31] estab-lished a relatively constant ratio of serum to myocardial digoxin concentration in dogs after the attainment of serum-tissue equilib-rium. In humans as well, Doherty et al.[32] observed a relatively constant ratio of serum to myocardial digoxin concentration, leading these authors to postulate the possible clinical usefulness of methods for the quantitation of serum digoxin levels. Nevertheless, total myocardial digoxin content undoubtedly includes nonspecific drug binding as well as binding to specific receptors,[62,84] so that even total myocardial digoxin concentration can-not a priori be assumed to bear a one-to-one relationship to effect.

Further rationale for the use of serum digitalis concentrations may be found in the growing body of evidence implicating Na^+, K^+-activated "transport" adenosine triphos-phatase in the mechanism of cardiac glycoside action upon the heart.[1,12,65,100,110] Direct evidence has been obtained in studies employ-ing the giant axon and red blood cells of the squid that this enzyme system, located within the plasma membrane, is inhibited by cardio-active steroids only when the latter are present at the external cell surface. Using a squid giant axon preparation in which ion and/or drug concentrations could be indepen-dently varied on both sides of the membrane, Caldwell and Keynes observed that Na^+ flux was inhibited only when ouabain was present at the outer surface.[26] Concentra-tions of ouabain 100-fold higher placed inside the axon were without demonstrable effect on Na^+ flux. Analogous results were obtained in experiments with human red blood cells by Hoffman.[58] After demonstrating sub-stantial reduction of active Na^+ flux when strophanthidin was present at the outer surface of intact cells, cells were exposed at the inner surface alone by lysis and resealing in the presence of strophanthidin, followed by washing to remove external traces of the agent. No inhibition of active Na^+ efflux was observed under the latter circumstances, yet the strophanthidin-containing lysate from these cells produced Na^+ efflux inhibition in normal cells exposed at the outer surface. Finally, the polarity of cellular response to cardiac glycosides has also been shown in the isolated toad bladder by Herrera.[55] In this structurally more complex model, active Na^+ transport was shown to be diminished by ouabain only when present at the basal (serosal) surface. Thus, it may be that an important mediator of digitalis effect lies in close proximity to the external cell surface, a site which would be maximally responsive to serum digitalis concentrations. (Although a convincing case can be made for Na^+, K^+ adenosine triphosphatase inhibition as an important mechanism of toxic electrophysiological effects of digitalis, it should be noted that the mechanism of inotropic effect, recently reviewed by Lee and Klaus,[67] is less certain.)

Recent animal experimental studies also support the concept of a potentially useful relationship between serum digoxin concentration and electrophysiological effects on the heart. Barr et al.[2] studied the relationships between serum digoxin concentration and drug-induced changes in cardiac automaticity in dogs given single and multiple doses of digoxin. The dominant serum half-time of digoxin was found to be 26.9 hours by radioimmunoassay, in good agreement with previous studies using tritium-labeled digoxin.[31] The rate of decline in serum digoxin concentration was not influenced by preexisting body stores of the drug within the range studied. Changes in automaticity were evaluated in two ways, using provocation of repetitive ventricular responses by low-energy endocardial stimuli[72] and by tolerance to infusion of the rapidly acting cardoi-active steroid acetyl strophanthidin. The electro-

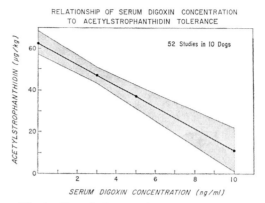

RELATIONSHIP OF SERUM DIGOXIN CONCENTRATION
TO ACETYLSTROPHANTHIDIN TOLERANCE

52 Studies in 10 Dogs

Fig. 1. The relationship of acetyl strophanthidin tolerance to serum digoxin concentration in dogs. Rising serum digoxin concentration results in decreasing doses of acetyl strophanthidin needed to precipitate ventricular tachycardia. The shaded area defines 95 per cent confidence limits. (From Barr et al.[2])

physiological effects of digoxin as judged by these criteria were significantly related to serum digoxin concentration. As shown in Figure 1, over a range of 0 to 10 ng/ml, serum digoxin concentration was inversely correlated with acetyl strophanthidin tolerance; for each 1.0 ng/ml increase in digoxin level, a mean value of 5.2 µg/kg less acetyl strophanthidin was needed to evoke ventricular tachycardia.

DIGITALIS ASSAY TECHNIQUES

The literature related to quantitation of digitalis glycoside concentrations has expanded rapidly in recent years. Table 1 lists the various approaches which have been employed, followed by the drug(s) to which each method has been applied and relevant references. Certain of the advantages and disadvantages of most of these methods have been discussed recently.[111]

No discussion of this sort would be complete without mention of the classical chemical methods used to measure relatively large quantities of cardiac glycosides (microgram to milligram range). The standard U.S.P. assay system for digitoxin involves measurement of the optical density at 495 mµ after reaction of digitoxin with alkaline picrate.[127]

Table 1. Approaches to Digitalis Concentration Determination

I. CHEMICAL METHODS OF LIMITED SENSITIVITY (MICROGRAM TO MILLIGRAM RANGE)*

  A. ALKALINE PICRATE: digitoxin[127]

  B. ALKALINE DINITROBENZENE: digoxin[127]

  C. XANTHYDROL: digitoxin and digoxin[59]

II. MICROMETHODS SUITABLE FOR MEASUREMENT OF NANOGRAM QUANTITIES

  A. DUCK EMBRYO BIOASSAY: lanatoside C;[43] digitoxin[44]

  B. RADIOISOTOPE LABELING: digitoxin;[33] digoxin;[33] ouabain;[33,78,85] acetyl digitoxigenin;[126] peruvoside;[63] lanatoside C;[17] digitoxigenin;[64] proscillardin;[36] dihydro-ouabain;[36] convallatoxol[36]

  C. PHYSICOCHEMICAL METHODS
    1. Double isotope dilution derivative: digitoxin[75,76]
    2. Gas-liquid chromatography: digoxin[130]

  D. NA+, K+–ACTIVATED ADENOSINE TRIPHOSPHATASE INHIBITION
    1. Red cell rubidium uptake inhibition
      a. [86]Rb radioactivity measurement: digitoxin;[46,70,71,98,101] digoxin[10,13,49,70,71,101]
      b. Atomic absorption spectrophotometry of nonradioactive rubidium:
         digitoxin;[16,97] lanatoside C[16,97]
    2. Microsomal Na+, K+–activated adenosine triphosphatase inhibition: digitoxin;[9,20] digoxin[21]

  E. COMPETITIVE PROTEIN BINDING
    1. Radioimmunoassay: digoxin;[28,38,56,66,94,109,112,113] digitoxin;[95,114] deslanoside;[115] ouabain[104,116]
    2. Adenosine triphosphatase enzymatic isotopic displacement: digoxin and digitoxin[18]

* An exhaustive review of these methods is beyond the scope of this discussion.

Sample preparation is tedious, and the sensitivity is such that the method is suitable only for samples in the milligram range. The U.S.P. assay for digoxin is also a colorimetric procedure in which digoxin is reacted with alkaline dinitrobenzene.[127] The presence of an activated methylene group in the lactone ring results in a colored product which is read at 620 mμ. Again, the method is exacting and relatively insensitive.

Jelliffe developed improved methods for the chemical determination of microgram quantities of digitoxin and digoxin which could be used for studies of urinary excretion of these drugs.[59] This procedure employs chloroform extraction, successive alkali and water washes, thin-layer chromatographic isolation, elution, and xanthydrol quantification. It lacks the requisite sensitivity for serum determinations.

The remainder of this review will be concerned with methods of high sensitivity which are capable of quantitating the minute concentrations of digitalis compounds present in the serum of patients receiving usual therapeutic doses. Much of the development of earlier techniques such as the various bioassay methods, including the duck embryo bioassay, has been ably reviewed by Friedman, St. George, and Bine.[44] The refinements introduced by these authors allowed the detection of concentrations of digitoxin and lanatoside C as low as 5 ng/ml.[44,45]

With the rapid growth of radioisotope technology in the 1950s, it became possible to label cardiac glycosides with ^{14}C and tritium (^{3}H). The development and application of isotope-labeling techniques to problems in the clinical pharmacology of digitalis glycosides have been extensively reviewed by Doherty.[33] A wealth of important information has been obtained by the direct administration of labeled cardiac glycosides to experimental animals and human volunteers, and this approach continues to yield highly useful data.[6,34,40,50,74,80,81,93,96,107] It should also be recognized that most of the remaining methods listed in Table 1 are dependent upon the availability of nuclides or radioactively labeled compounds of high specific activity.

Methods employing physicochemical techniques include the double isotope dilution derivative assay of digitoxin and a recently developed gas-liquid chromatographic assay for digoxin. Lukas and Peterson[75] devised the elegant but complex digitoxin method, which has been applied to quantitation of digitoxin in plasma, whole blood, urine, and stool. ^{3}H-digitoxin is used to monitor procedural losses of digitoxin, while acetic anhydride-1-^{14}C is used to convert digitoxin to the triacetate. The method is capable of detecting 10 ng of digitoxin, and has been employed in studies of various aspects of digitoxin pharmacodynamics.[75,76] Probably the greatest asset of this approach is its high degree of specificity, which suits it admirably to studies of the complex metabolic patterns of digitoxin. Although technically demanding, double isotope dilution derivative assay systems have been widely used in the measurement of aldosterone[60] and may logically find further application in the elucidation of cardiac glycoside metabolic pathways.

The gas-liquid chromatographic method for assay of digoxin recently described by Watson and Kalman,[130] like the double isotope derivative digitoxin assay discussed above, requires an initial extraction step. An internal ^{3}H-digoxin standard is added to the plasma sample to quantitate losses and methylene chloride extraction is carried out; this is followed by preliminary purification on a florisil column and thin-layer chromatography on silica gel G. The heptafluorobutyrate derivative is then formed and the extract chromatographed again on silica gel. Gas-liquid chromatography is then carried out with electron capture detection to enhance sensitivity. As does the double isotope derivative method for digitoxin, this method has a high degree of specificity which should prove useful in the study of metabolic patterns.

The discovery of Schatzmann[103] that cardiac glycosides are potent inhibitors of cellular monovalent cation transport laid the groundwork for the red blood cell ^{86}Rb uptake inhibition assay originally introduced by Lowenstein.[70] Initially modified by Lowenstein and Corrill,[71] the method has been further developed by other workers for both digoxin[10,13,49] and digitoxin[29,46,98] measurement. Serum or plasma samples are initially extracted with water-immiscible organic solvents and the extract is assayed for ability to inhibit red blood cell ^{86}Rb uptake. ^{86}Rubidium, a potassium analogue in this system, is actively pumped into red cells and is used because of its relatively convenient radioactive half-life. Unknown samples are estimated by comparison with a standard curve defined with known amounts of the glycoside to be measured. Several of the important variables in this type of assay system have been defined by Bertler and Redfors[10] and by Gjerdrum.[46] Although some investigators have reported values for plasma digoxin concentrations with this technique which tend to be somewhat higher than those obtained by other methods,[49] more recent reports[11] reflect good agreement with the methods to be discussed subsequently. As in other methods requiring an extraction step, particular care must be given to the details of the extraction procedure to insure uniform recovery of standards and unknown samples.

An interesting variant of the red cell ^{86}Rb uptake inhibition assay is the method described by Bourdon and Mercier.[16] Inhibition of red cell Rb$^+$ uptake by extracted cardiac glycosides forms the basis of this procedure, but quantitation of Rb$^+$ concentrations is accomplished by atomic absorption spectrophotometry rather than by counting gamma radiation from ^{86}Rb.

Conceptually similar to the ^{86}Rb uptake inhibition assay is the approach developed by Burnett and Conklin for the measurement of serum digitoxin and digoxin concentrations. This technique, as originally described for digitoxin,[20] again employs the inhibitory properties of cardiac glycosides toward Na^+, K^+-activated adenosine triphosphatase, in this case from brain cortex. Plasma samples are first extracted with methylene dichloride and the extracts are included in a buffer system containing ATP and partially purified microsomal Na^+, K^+-activated adenosine triphosphatase prepared from pork brain. Increasing amounts of digitoxin result in increasing inhibition of the cleavage of ATP; enzymatic activity is quantitated by a colorimetric assay of the inorganic phosphate liberated. The sensitivity of the method is adequate over the range of plasma digitoxin concentrations of clinical interest.

This method has recently been extended to the measurement of plasma digoxin concentrations.[21] The enhanced sensitivity necessary to measure clinically relevant plasma digoxin levels was obtained by incubating the plasma extract to be assayed with pork brain Na^+, K^+ adenosine triphosphatase in the absence of K^+. Binding of cardiac glycosides to the enzyme with consequent inhibition of adenosine triphosphatase activity is maximal when K^+ is absent during the incubation step, and this modification allowed a sensitivity of 0.3 ng/ml to be achieved. As the authors point out, although the procedure is less precise than radioimmunoassay and more time consuming, it has the advantage of applicability in the clinical laboratory without radioisotope counting equipment. This procedure and the method of Bourdon and Mercier[16] are the only techniques in current use which do not require isotope counting facilities of some kind.

The remaining methods for serum glycoside measurement are based upon competitive binding of radioactively labeled and unlabeled cardiac glycosides to a specific binding site provided by antibody or Na^+, K^+ adenosine triphosphatase. The general principles of competitive protein-binding assays have been discussed at length in a recent volume.[92]

Competitive binding of cardiac glycosides to Na^+, K^+ adenosine triphosphatase has been used by Brooker and Jelliffe for the measurement of both digoxin and digitoxin levels in an extensive clinical experience.[18] Serum (5 ml) is extracted with chloroform and the extract is allowed to compete with ^3H-ouabain for specific binding sites on guinea-pig brain Na^+, K^+ adenosine triphosphatase. ^3H-ouabain bound to the enzyme is separated by centrifugation, and the amount of unbound ^3H-ouabain displaced from the binding site by cardiac glycosides in the sample is subjected to liquid scintillation counting. Correction for extraction efficiency of various cardiac glycosides must be made, but was found to be relatively constant at 89.2 ± 4.9 per cent (1 S.D.) for digoxin and 46.9 ± 4.4 per cent for digitoxin. The method is potentially applicable to any cardiac glycoside which can be reproducibly extracted from serum. Although the method is not specific for any single cardiac glycoside, the authors feel that this may be an advantage in some situations where uncertainty exists as to the drug the patient is taking.

Our own experience has been based on a radioimmunoassay approach.[112] Butler and Chen[22] immunized rabbits with a protein-digoxin conjugate synthesized by periodate oxidation of vicinal hydroxyl groups on the terminal digitoxose moiety of digoxin, followed by Schiff-base coupling of the resulting aldehyde intermediate to ϵ-amino groups of lysine in the carrier protein. Antibodies were obtained which were shown to bind digoxin. Antisera obtained in this way have been characterized in detail[115] with results different in several important ways from previous studies of antibodies directed against steroid haptenes. Exceptionally high affinity and specificity for digoxin were found late in the immune response. Studies of antisera from an animal immunized over 97 weeks showed 5.8 mg/ml of digoxin-specific antibody with an average intrinsic association constant (Ko) of 1.7×10^{10} L/M. Sips analysis of equilibrium dialysis data also documented relative homogeneity of binding-site affinities. The Ko for digitoxin was found to be 32-fold lower despite the marked

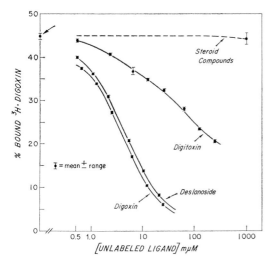

Fig. 2. Haptene inhibition curves for rabbit digoxin-specific antiserum, showing the extent to which digoxin, deslanoside, and digitoxin displace tritiated digoxin from the antibody binding site. The arrow on the vertical axis denotes control binding in the absence of unlabeled ligand.[115] Horizontal lines denote the range of duplicate determinations. (Reprinted with permission from Biochemistry.)

with ^{3}H-digoxin for antibody binding sites, despite the lack of any glycoside content at all. In contrast, endogenous steroid compounds produced measurable displacement only when present in more than 1,000-fold molar excess. This property of selected digoxin-specific antisera confers remarkable specificity on the radioimmunoassay procedure. It should be noted, however, that all antisera which bind digoxin cannot a priori be assumed to display this degree of specificity, and haptene displacement experiments of this sort should be carried out before use of new antisera for radioimmunoassay purposes.

A radioimmunoassay approach to the measurement of clinically relevant serum concentrations of a cardiac glycoside was first successfully employed in the measurement of serum digitoxin concentrations by Oliver et al.[95] Digitoxigenin was succinylated at the C-3 position and coupled to serum albumin for use as an antigen. Rabbit antisera were obtained which could be used

structural similarity between digoxin and digitoxin.

Specificity of digoxin binding was also assessed in haptene inhibition experiments with a number of cardiac glycoside analogues and endogenous steroid compounds. As shown in Figure 2, deslanoside, which differs from digoxin in the presence of an additional glucose sugar coupled to the terminal digitoxose residue, displaces ^{3}H-digoxin from the antibody binding site virtually as effectively as the homologous haptene digoxin. Digitoxin, on the other hand, competes much less effectively despite the difference of only a single hydroxyl group at the C-12 position of the steroid ring. Thus, the most important determinants of binding appear to reside toward the C-D ring end of the steroid moiety, most distal to the point where the haptene was coupled to the carrier protein of the antigen. Further support for the importance of antigenic determinants on the aglycone is found in Figure 3, in which it can be seen that digoxigenin also competes effectively

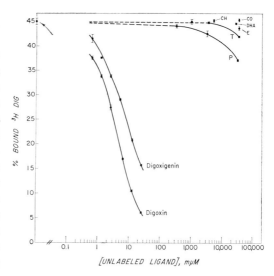

Fig. 3. Haptene inhibition curves for the same rabbit antidigoxin antiserum shown in Figure 2. Digoxigenin is shown in addition to the endogenous steroid compounds cholesterol (CH), cortisol (CO), dehydroepiandrosterone (DHA), 17-β-estradiol (E), testosterone (T), and progesterone (P). The arrow on the ordinate indicates binding in the absence of unlabeled ligand; horizontal lines denote ranges of duplicate determinations.[115] (Reprinted with permission from Biochemistry.)

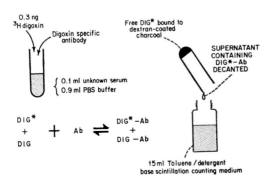

Fig. 4. General scheme for radioimmunoassay of serum cardiac glycoside concentrations.[113] In this example, unlabeled digoxin (DIG) in 0.1 ml of the unknown serum completes with tritiated digoxin (DIG*) for binding sites of digoxin-specific antibody (Ab). See text for further explanation. (Reprinted with permission from American Heart Journal.)

for quantitation of digitoxin by measurement of the extent to which it displaced ^{125}I-labeled tyrosine-digitoxigenin from antibody binding sites. Chloroform extraction of digitoxin from serum is required in this method, and antibody-bound and free tracer are separated by the use of a second antibody to rabbit gamma globulin.

The radioimmunoassay technique which has evolved in our laboratory[109,112–114,116] is briefly summarized in Figure 4. In this case an aliquot of serum containing unlabeled digoxin (without prior extraction) is brought to a convenient volume with buffer and an appropriate tracer quantity of ^{3}H-digoxin is added. The amount of tracer used is determined by the range of digoxin concentrations to be measured, and this in turn depends upon the size of the serum aliquot used. For resolution of digoxin concentrations over the clinically relevant range from 0.2 to 20 ng/ml, a tracer quantity of about 2 to 3 ng is suitable. Thus, for a 0.1 ml aliquot of serum 0.3 ng of tracer is used. The high specific activity of commercially available ^{3}H-digoxin insures adequate counting rates for these small amounts of tracer. After thorough mixing, an amount of digoxin-specific antiserum is added which will bind about 40 to 50 per

cent of tracer counts in the absence of unlabeled drug. This amount of antibody is selected to strike an optimum balance between sensitivity and precision. During a brief incubation, an equilibrium is established (Fig. 4) in which the amount of ^{3}H-digoxin bound to antibody combining sites depends upon the amount of unlabeled digoxin in the sample.

Dextran-coated charcoal is then added to separate antibody-bound from free ^{3}H-digoxin. Care should be taken to expose both the known samples used to construct the standard curve and the unknown samples to the charcoal for similar lengths of time, since the equilibrium shown in Figure 4 may be pulled toward the left as free digoxin is bound to the charcoal. This tendency proves to be of little consequence when high-affinity antibodies are used, but may become an increasing problem with antisera of lower affinity. After centrifugation to remove the charcoal, antibody-bound ^{3}H-digoxin remaining in the supernatant phase is quantitatively decanted into scintillation counting vials containing a toluene-detergent base counting fluid. Samples are then counted (usually for two minutes) in a liquid scintillation counter equipped with a ^{226}radium external standard for quenching correction. When results are urgently needed, a sample can be run in one hour without serious compromise of accuracy.

Figure 5 shows a typical standard curve obtained with known, gravimetrically determined amounts of crystalline digoxin. Because of the relatively large number of samples assayed daily in our laboratory, we have developed a simple computer program which corrects raw counts per minute for background and quenching and plots the reciprocal count rate against a linear scale of digoxin concentration. The limited heterogeneity of antibody binding-site affinities in the antisera used results in a rectilinear plot as shown in Figure 5B. The computer plots this line by least squares linear regression analysis, compares count rates for unknown samples, and prints out the concentration value. A

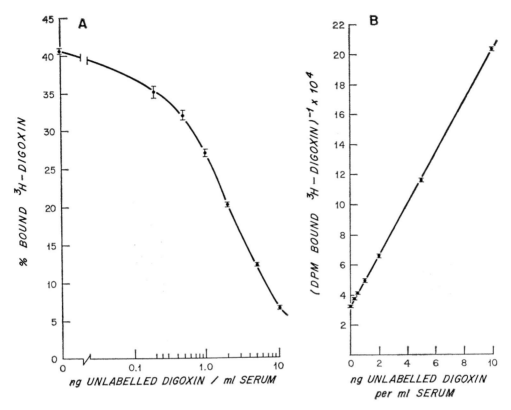

Fig. 5. Standard curves obtained by the procedures outlined in Figure 4. *A:* Per cent of ³H-digoxin tracer bound by the antibody is plotted against a logarithmic scale of unlabeled digoxin concentration in the sample. Horizontal lines indicate ranges of duplicate determinations. It is apparent that a 0.2 ng/ml concentration is readily measurable in the 0.1 ml sample. *B:* The same data are plotted as reciprocal antibody-bound counts (corrected for background and quenching) against a linear scale of unlabeled digoxin concentration. The rectilinear plot obtained is well suited to computer usage. (Reprinted with permission from American Heart Journal.)

single technician is able to assay up to 50 samples in duplicate in a normal working day.

The antiserum used in the above-described assay system can also be used for the determination of serum deslanoside concentrations because of the binding characteristics shown in Figure 2. Known amounts of deslanoside are used to construct the standard curve, and ³H-digoxin is used as tracer in the system.

An analogous system for the measurement of serum digitoxin concentrations also uses the same antiserum with ³H-digitoxin as the tracer.[114] Although the somewhat lower affinity of the antibody population of digitoxin would theoretically lower the sensitivity of the technique, this is not a problem since

the range of serum digitoxin concentrations encountered clinically is about tenfold higher than that of digoxin, presumably because of greater binding to serum albumin.[77]

While freedom from the necessity to perform preliminary extraction procedures on serum prior to assay is usually an advantage of the radioimmunoassay approach described above, there may be occasions where extraction is advantageous. Following radioisotope imaging procedures such as lung, brain, or thyroid scans, residual radioactivity in the blood of the patient may interfere for a time with the assay.[119] We routinely scan for the presence of gamma-emitting isotopes on an auxiliary channel of the scintillation counter to exclude the possibility of this source of error. If present, the problem can be dealt with by one of the various extraction techniques used in other assay systems, or by the method described by Butler.[23]

Radioimmunoassay procedures for digoxin employed in other laboratories[28,37,56,66,94,123] are basically similar to that described above—all using similar antigen synthesis, dextran-coated charcoal separation, and ^{3}H-digoxin tracer techniques. The commercial availability of radioimmunoassay kits with a choice of tritium or ^{125}I tracers has made both digoxin and digitoxin assay methods widely available to laboratories with the necessary counting equipment.

A radioimmunoassay technique has recently been developed for the rapidly acting cardiac glycoside ouabain.[116] Antibodies with high affinity and specificity for ouabain were raised in rabbits by challenge with an antigen consisting of a conjugate of ouabain linked through its rhamnose sugar to terminal α-amino groups of poly-D,L alanyl-human serum albumin. Serial determinations of antibody titer showed that ouabain-specific antibodies were present as early as 3 weeks and rose in titer over the initial 20 to 33 weeks of immunization. Specific immunoglobulin levels as high as 6.5 mg/ml antiserum were reached in one rabbit at the end of 45 weeks. Average intrinsic association constants for ouabain were 1.3×10^9 L/M and 1.6×10^9 L/M in antisera from two rabbits studied in detail. Restricted heterogeneity of binding-site affinities and high specificity were demonstrated, as in the digoxin-specific antibodies previously discussed. Significant cross reactivity was observed only with other cardio-active steroid compounds such as acetyl strophanthidin, digoxin, and digitoxin, while endogenous steroids showed no measurable cross reaction even when present in 1,000-fold excess. It is of interest that compounds which tend to cross react with both digoxin-specific and ouabain-specific antibodies all share the C-13 methyl and C-14 hydroxyl groups, the cis fusion of C and

D rings, and the α, β unsaturated lactone ring attached at C-17, characteristics lacking in endogenous steroids from mammalian species. Competition between ^{3}H-ouabain tracer and unlabeled ouabain allows the measurement of plasma or urine ouabain concentrations as low as 0.1 ng/ml without the need of extraction procedures.

The accuracy of all of the methods for cardiac glycoside assay discussed above ultimately depends upon the accuracy of the standard curve with which unknown samples are prepared. It is therefore of paramount importance that meticulously prepared standards of well-defined purity and stability be used with all assay systems.

CLINICAL EXPERIENCE: THE RELATIONSHIP BETWEEN SERUM CARDIAC GLYCOSIDE CONCENTRATIONS AND DIGITALIS TOXICITY

Studies in Patients without Toxicity

Recent publications reflect substantial agreement regarding serum digoxin and digitoxin levels encountered in clinical practice, despite the variety of assay methods used and the number of laboratories engaged in these studies. Table 2 summarizes data from a number of studies which included groups of patients receiving usual maintenance digoxin doses without clinical or electrocardiographic evidence of toxicity. As noted, larger doses of digoxin were associated with higher serum concentrations of the drug in all studies in which this relationship was specifically examined.[10,28,38,56,88,109,112] As expected in the light of earlier studies,[14,35,82] impairment of renal function was also associated with higher serum digoxin concentrations.[7,38,109] In comparing data from the various studies listed, the times at which blood samples were obtained for assay must be carefully noted. For example, the relatively low mean serum digoxin concentration of 1.0 ng/ml in nontoxic patients observed by Beller et al.[7] is probably due in large part to

Table 2. Serum or Plasma Digoxin Concentrations: Nontoxic Patients

Authors (ref.)	Method	Dose (mg/day)	Mean Conc. (ng/ml)	Mean Conc. All Doses (ng/ml)
Beller et al.[7]	Radioimmunoassay			1.0
Bertler and Redfors[10]	[86]Rb uptake	0.25	0.8	
		0.5	1.3	
Bertler and Redfors[11]	[86]Rb uptake			0.9
Brooker and Jelliffe[18]	Enzymatic displacement			1.4
Burnett and Conklin[21]	ATPase inhibition			1.2
Chamberlain et al.[28]	Radioimmunoassay	0.125	0.5	1.4
		0.25–0.375	0.9	
		0.5	1.5	
		0.625–0.75	2.1	
Evered and Chapman[38]	Radioimmunoassay	0.25 on alt. days	0.9	1.38
		0.25	1.2	
		0.5	1.42	
		0.75	1.85	
Fogelman et al.[42]	Radioimmunoassay			1.4
Grahame-Smith and Everest[49]	[86]Rb uptake			2.4
Hoeschen and Proveda[56]	Radioimmunoassay	0.25	0.8	
		0.5	1.3	
Morrison, Killip and Stason[88]	Radioimmunoassay	0.25	0.76	
		0.5	1.25	
Smith, Butler and Haber[112]	Radioimmunoassay	0.25	1.1	
		0.5	1.4	
Smith and Haber[109]	Radioimmunoassay	0.25	1.2	1.4
		0.5	1.7	
		0.75 + above	2.3	
Oliver, Parker and Parker[94]	Radioimmunoassay			1.6

the fact that some patients had had no digoxin for up to 48 hours prior to the time of serum sampling.

The red cell ^{86}Rb uptake inhibition results reported by Grahame-Smith and Everest[49] yielded somewhat higher values than those obtained by other workers. The time of plasma sampling was not stated, and an earlier time relative to the last digoxin dose may explain this result, since Bertler and Redfors (also using a red cell ^{86}Rb uptake inhibition method) reported results closely similar to those obtained in the other studies listed.[10] Comparable values have also been reported by Ritzmann et al.[101] The mean values for nontoxic patients, then, can be seen

to cluster around 0.8 to 1.6 ng/ml. It is of interest to note that Marcus et al., studying normal volunteers by the direct oral administration of 0.5 mg of tritiated digoxin per day, obtained a mean steady-state blood level of 1.4 ± 0.3 (S.D.) ng/ml 8 hours after the last dose.[83]

Data summarizing serum or plasma digitoxin concentrations in nontoxic patients on usual therapeutic regimens are summarized in Table 3. As in the case of digoxin, increasing doses of digitoxin are associated with increasing serum concentrations of the drug.[9,87,98] In contradistinction, however, the general experience has been that serum digitoxin concentrations on any given dose

Table 3. Serum or Plasma Digitoxin Concentrations: Nontoxic Patients

Authors (ref.)	Method	Dose (mg/day)	Mean Conc. (ng/ml)	Mean Conc. All Doses (ng/ml)
Beller et al.[7]	Radioimmunoassay			20
Bentley et al.[9]	ATPase inhibition	0.05	13	
		0.1	22	
		0.2	47	
Brooker and Jelliffe[18]	Enzymatic displacement			31.8
Lowenstein and Corrill[71]	[86]Rb uptake			25
Lukas and Peterson[75]	Double isotope dilution derivative			20
Morrison and Killip[87]	Radioimmunoassay	0.1	25	
		0.2	44	
Oliver et al.[95]	Radioimmunoassay			about 20
Rasmussen et al.[98]	[86]Rb uptake	0.05	12	
		0.1	18.2	
		0.2	24.3	
Ritzmann et al.[101]	[86]Rb uptake			19
Smith[114]	Radioimmunoassay			17

are poorly correlated with renal function.[7,99,114] The similarity in values obtained by the various methods suggests that metabolites of digitoxin either are not present in large amounts in serum or that they affect the various assay systems in a similar manner.

Patients taking digitalis-leaf preparations have, in general, been found to have serum digitoxin concentrations similar to those of patients given crystalline digitoxin, whether measured by Na^+, K^+ adenosine triphosphatase inhibition[9] or by radioimmunoassay.[7,114] This is not surprising, in view of the fact that digitoxin is a major constituent of digitalis leaf.[86]

Data have only recently become available regarding plasma ouabain concentrations in human subjects. Selden and Smith measured plasma ouabain levels in normal volunteers in experiments designed to produce a steady state.[104] Intravenous doses of 0.25 mg given daily resulted in a mean plasma ouabain concentration of 0.51 ng/ml 24 hours after the last dose during the plateau phase reached after 5 days. The range was 0.41 to 0.64 ng/ml among the individuals studied.

Studies in Clinically Digitalis-toxic Patients

The relationship between serum digitalis concentrations and digitalis effects in toxic and nontoxic patients has attracted the interest of a number of investigators recently. This is a particularly complex subject because of the many variables which influence cardiac responses to digitalis glycosides.[125] Factors of known importance include serum potassium, sodium, calcium, and magnesium levels, acid-base balance, hypoxemia, thyroid functional status, and autonomic nervous system influences. Additional drugs, particularly those with antiarrhythmic properties, may exert modifying effects. The nature and severity of underlying heart disease are also of great importance in determining response to digitalis.[7,117]

Table 4 summarizes digoxin level data from studies published to date. Despite inevitable variation in assay methods, patient population characteristics, criteria for toxicity, and timing of blood samples, reasonably consistent results are apparent in most of these series, which comprise a total of more

Table 4. Serum or Plasma Digoxin Concentrations: Nontoxic and Toxic Patients

Authors (ref.)	Method	Mean Conc. Nontoxic	Mean Conc. Toxic	Statistical Significance
Beller et al.[7]	Radioimmunoassay	1.0	2.3	Yes
Bertler and Redfors[11]	[86]Rb uptake	0.9	2.4	Yes
Brooker and Jelliffe[18]	Enzymatic displacement	1.4	3.1	Yes
Burnett and Conklin[21]	ATPase inhibition	1.2	5.7	Yes
Chamberlain et al.[28]	Radioimmunoassay	1.4	3.1	Yes
Evered and Chapman[38]	Radioimmunoassay	1.38	3.36	Yes
Fogelman et al.[92]	Radioimmunoassay	1.4	1.7	No
Grahame-Smith and Everest[49]	[86]Rb uptake	2.4	5.7	Yes
Hoeschen and Proveda[56]	Radioimmunoassay	0.8–1.3	2.8	Yes
Morrison, Killip and Stason[88]	Radioimmunoassay	0.76	3.35	Not stated
Oliver, Parker and Parker[94]	Radioimmunoassay	1.6	3.0	Yes
Smith, Butler and Haber[112]	Radioimmunoassay	1.3	3.3	Yes
Smith and Haber[109]	Radioimmunoassay	1.4	3.7	Yes

than 1,000 patients. The mean digoxin concentrations observed in patients with toxic manifestations are about twofold higher than those of nontoxic patients, with the difference achieving statistical significance in all series except that of Fogelman et al.[42] The latter series appears to differ in other important respects as well, including the absence of a significant difference in renal function between toxic and nontoxic groups.

In our own experience, one of the most important single factors predisposing to digoxin toxicity has been impaired renal function. Mean concentration of blood urea nitrogen and incidence of uremia were both significantly higher in toxic than in nontoxic hospitalized patients.[109] Toxic patients in this series also tended to be older, a finding which may well have exerted its influence at least in part through diminished glomerular filtration rate and hence decreased digoxin excretion.[37] A high incidence of renal functional impairment was also evident in digoxin-toxic patients studied prospectively.[7] Figure 6 compares serum digoxin and digitoxin levels in toxic and nontoxic patients from this series. The differing relative prevalence of renal insufficiency among patients taking digoxin and digitoxin or digitalis leaf correlates well with available data regarding renal excretion of these drugs (vide infra). It is of considerable importance to note that doses of digoxin were not significantly higher in toxic patients in either of these series,[7,109] further implicating impaired excretion in the genesis of digoxin intoxication. It is apparent that advanced cardiac disease in and of itself can limit glomerular filtration rate leading to digoxin retention. Hoeschen and Proveda[56] and Evered and Chapman[38] have also observed a high prevalence of impaired renal function among digoxin-toxic patients.

Figure 7 summarizes the results of serum digoxin concentration measurements in a group of 110 hospitalized patients.[109] The mean serum digoxin level in toxic patients was higher than that of patients without toxicity at each of the three dosage levels. As can be appreciated from the magnitude of the standard deviation values, however, significant overlap of serum concentrations occurred between the toxic and nontoxic groups even when these were defined by strict criteria. Further studies of the same

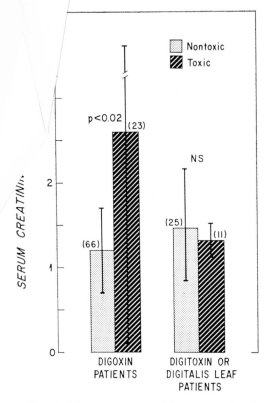

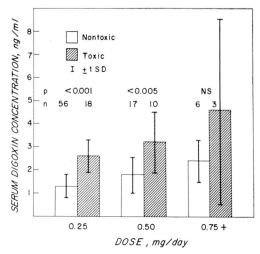

Fig. 6. Mean serum creatinine concentrations in nontoxic and toxic patients receiving digoxin (*left*) or digitoxin or digitalis leaf (*right*). A significant difference (p<0.02) in mean serum creatinine concentration was observed only in patients on digoxin. (From the data of Beller et al.[7])

Fig. 7. Mean serum digoxin concentrations in nontoxic and toxic hospitalized patients. Results are subdivided by daily maintenance dosages.[109] (Reprinted with permission from the Journal of Clinical Investigation.)

hospital population showed that patients with questionable digoxin excess (manifested by occasional ventricular premature beats, first-degree atrioventricular block, atrial fibrillation with occasional junctional escape beats, marked sinus bradycardia, or atrial fibrillation with relatively slow ventricular response) tended to have serum digoxin levels in the intermediate range with significant overlap with both toxic and nontoxic patients. Figure 8 compares serum digoxin concentrations in a group of 83 patients studied prospectively.[7] To exclude all possibility of bias, digoxin radioimmunoassay was performed on coded samples and compared with independent clinical diagnosis only after the termination of the study. A highly significant

difference in mean serum digoxin concentrations between toxic and nontoxic patients was found, but overlap is again apparent. Several other series have also shown significant overlap of levels in toxic and nontoxic patients.[18,28,38,94]

Brooker and Jelliffe have subjected their data to probit analysis, and have found that a serum digoxin concentration of 1.4 ng/ml, the mean for patients without rhythm disturbances by their method, was associated with a 10 per cent incidence of arrhythmias.[18] At 2.0 ng/ml the risk rose to 25 per cent, and reached 50 per cent at 2.9 ng/ml.

The available evidence, then, indicates that no arbitrary level can be selected which unequivocally distinguishes between toxic and nontoxic serum digoxin concentrations, and serum concentration data are of greatest usefulness when interpreted in the overall clinical context. Although uncommon, patients with digoxin levels below 1.0 ng/ml occasionally meet usual criteria for toxicity. At the other end of the spectrum, patients may occasionally require serum digoxin concentrations of 3.0 ng/ml or more to maintain

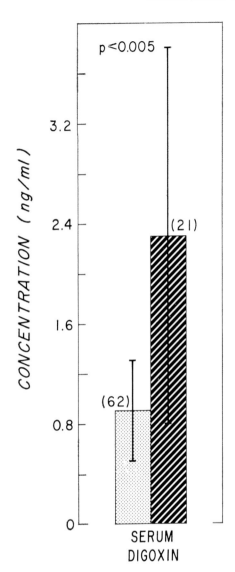

Fig. 8. Mean serum digoxin concentrations determined by radioimmunoassay in nontoxic (stippled bar) and toxic (cross-hatched bar) patients, with numbers in each group shown in parentheses. Vertical lines show one standard deviation above and below the mean. (From Beller et al.[7])

adequate control of supraventricular tachyarrhythmias (atrial flutter or atrial fibrillation) and tolerate these levels without toxic manifestations.

It must be realized, of course, that no absolute criteria for digitalis intoxication exist, since all of the disturbances of impulse forma-

tion and conduction caused by toxic doses of cardiac glycosides may also arise in the natural course of cardiac disease.[27,125] The presence of cardiac and/or pulmonary disease is commonly associated with a number of factors which tend to increase the slope of phase-4 spontaneous diastolic depolarization in cells of the His-Purkinje system,[108,128] to increase disparity of recovery times, enhancing probability of reentrant rhythm disturbances,[57,108] or to depress atrioventricular conduction.[108] Digitalis glycosides in sufficient doses are known to produce all of these electrophysiological effects,[57,61,129] increasing the likelihood of overt rhythm disturbance in a heart predisposed by organic disease with or without the additional risk factors previously mentioned. In our own experience, advanced cardiac disease has been significantly correlated with clinical evidence of toxicity. In the prospective study referred to previously,[7] 74 per cent of toxic patients were in functional class III or IV.

Similar considerations apply to the experience gained in a number of laboratories with serum digitoxin concentration measurements. Table 5 summarizes these results. As in the case of digoxin, significant differences in mean concentrations have generally been observed in patients with and without electrocardiographic manifestations of toxicity. Some degree of overlapping of values between toxic and nontoxic groups has been noted,[9,114] and, if anything, tends to be greater than in the case of digoxin. This may be due in part to the particular difficulty of establishing a definite diagnosis of digitoxin toxicity, since rhythm disturbances caused by this drug may be sufficiently prolonged to complicate application of the criterion of disappearance of the arrhythmia when the drug is withheld.

In the case of both digoxin and digitoxin, recent studies support the impression that pulmonary disease is associated with an increased risk of digitalis intoxication. Morrison and Killip[89] have reported that hypoxemia due to chronic lung disease resulted in overtly toxic rhythm disturbances at serum

Table 5. Serum or Plasma Digitoxin Concentrations: Nontoxic and Toxic Patients

Authors (ref.)	Method	Mean Conc. Nontoxic	Mean Conc. Toxic	Statistical Significance
Beller et al.[7]	Radioimmunoassay	20	34	Yes
Bentley et al.[9]	ATPase inhibition	23	59	Yes
Brooker and Jelliffe[18]	Enzymatic displacement	31.8	48.8	Not stated
Lukas and Peterson[75]	Double isotope dilution derivative	20	43–67 (range)	Not stated
Morrison and Killip[87]	Radioimmunoassay	25 (0.1 mg/day) 44 (0.2 mg/day)	53	Yes
Rasmussen et al.[98]	[86]Rb uptake	16.6	48.7	Not stated
Ritzmann et al.[101]	[86]Rb uptake	19	39–51 (range)	Not stated
Smith[114]	Radioimmunoassay	17	34	Yes

glycoside concentrations lower than those usually associated with toxicity in a population without marked hypoxemia. Beller et al.[7] similarly report a significantly increased prevalence of acute or chronic pulmonary disease among toxic compared with nontoxic patients.

Another process suspected of predisposing to digitalis toxicity is acute coronary-artery disease.[105] Measurements of serum digoxin and digitoxin levels in the setting of acute myocardial infarction have suggested that alterations in myocardial sensitivity may lower the toxic threshold to digitalis in the initial 24 hours.[90] Recent experimental studies in the dog have documented a marked inhomogeneity of early digoxin uptake by the acutely and chronically infarcted ventricle,[8] which may contribute to the alteration of normal response to the drug.

Further evidence supporting ischemic heart disease as a factor associated with an increased risk of digitalis intoxication comes from an evaluation of 367 digitalized patients in whom serum digoxin or digitoxin concentrations were obtained.[118] Among 279 patients without digitalis toxicity, the prevalence of coronary-artery disease as a primary diagnosis was 61 per cent. Of 88 toxic patients, the prevalence of coronary-artery disease was

somewhat higher at 75 per cent ($P = 0.05$). Patients at the extremes of the overlapping range of serum levels, however, yielded a more striking result. As summarized in Table 6, the prevalence of coronary disease was significantly higher among patients "sensitive" to cardiac glycosides (toxic at relatively low serum levels) compared with "resistant" patients (nontoxic at relatively high serum concentrations). Evered and Chapman[38] have also commented on a higher incidence of ischemic heart disease than of rheumatic heart disease among toxic patients in their series, while the reverse was true of patients without toxicity but with high plasma digoxin levels.

Chamberlain et al.[28] have presented further evidence of the interaction between intrinsic cardiac disease and response to digitalis. In a study of the relationship between ventricular response to atrial fibrillation and serum digoxin concentration, a relatively poor correlation was observed in 116 unselected patients. However, many of these patients had disease of the atrioventricular conduction system with slow ventricular rates on or off digoxin. When the evaluation was restricted to those with rapid rates off digoxin, a much better correlation was noted.

A useful means of evaluating the difficult

Table 6.

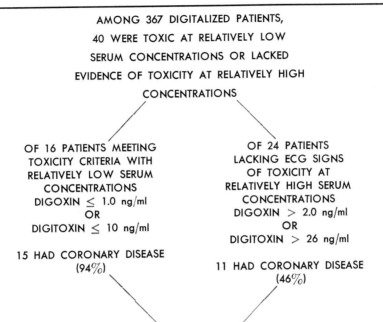

AMONG 367 DIGITALIZED PATIENTS,
40 WERE TOXIC AT RELATIVELY LOW
SERUM CONCENTRATIONS OR LACKED
EVIDENCE OF TOXICITY AT RELATIVELY HIGH
CONCENTRATIONS

OF 16 PATIENTS MEETING
TOXICITY CRITERIA WITH
RELATIVELY LOW SERUM
CONCENTRATIONS
DIGOXIN $\leq$ 1.0 ng/ml
OR
DIGITOXIN $\leq$ 10 ng/ml

15 HAD CORONARY DISEASE
(94%)

OF 24 PATIENTS
LACKING ECG SIGNS
OF TOXICITY AT
RELATIVELY HIGH SERUM
CONCENTRATIONS
DIGOXIN $>$ 2.0 ng/ml
OR
DIGITOXIN $>$ 26 ng/ml

11 HAD CORONARY DISEASE
(46%)

$p < 0.01$

clinical problem of individual myocardial sensitivity to digitalis is the acetyl strophanthidin tolerance test.[73,125] Barr et al. correlated tolerance to this rapidly acting cardioactive steroid aglycone with serum digoxin concentration in a series of hospitalized patients receiving maintenance doses of digoxin.[3] Acetyl strophanthidin tolerance was significantly correlated with serum digoxin concentration, as in the case of the animal experiments referred to above.[2] Despite this correlation, however, varying acetyl strophanthidin sensitivity was observed among individuals with comparable serum digoxin levels, suggesting a clinical role for this approach in selected cases.

Although not a direct measurement of cardiac glycoside concentration, the determination of salivary electrolyte composition has attracted attention recently as a means of identifying digitalis-toxic patients.[135] Salivary potassium and calcium concentrations were found to be higher in digitalis-toxic patients than in a group without toxicity, and

the product of potassium and calcium concentrations gave still better separation of the two groups.

THE ROLE OF DIGITALIS ASSAY TECHNIQUES IN STUDIES OF THE CLINICAL PHARMACOLOGY OF CARDIAC GLYCOSIDES

Despite some remaining uncertainty as to the ultimate role of serum digitalis measurements in the management of individual patients, there is no doubt that these techniques will continue to be highly useful in the investigation of various special problems in the clinical pharmacology and toxicology of cardiac glycosides. In this section, studies representative of recent advances in this field will be reviewed.

Cardiopulmonary Bypass

Digoxin handling by patients undergoing cardiopulmonary bypass has been assessed by the use of radioimmunoassay methods. Coltart et al.[30] demonstrated negligible losses of digoxin from the body during bypass. Hemodilution due to oxygenator prime caused an initial fall in mean serum digoxin concentration from 1.5 to 1.1 ng/ml after 2 hours of bypass, but this returned to an average of 1.7 ng/ml on the first postoperative day with reequilibration of the large tissue-bound digoxin stores. Because of the high degree of tissue binding of the drug, digoxin left in the oxygenator and discard sucker bottle at the end of bypass amounted to no more than 3 µg. It must be recognized, of course, that bypass does have metabolic consequences which may cause increased myocardial sensitivity to cardiac glycosides. In addition, any alteration in renal function must be taken into account in the selection of further maintenance doses. Morrison et al.[88,91] have reported a similar experience, and animal experimental studies using tritiated digoxin have documented directly the constancy of myocardial digoxin concentration during cardiopulmonary bypass in the dog.[79]

Gastrointestinal Digoxin Absorption

A persisting problem in the clinical pharmacology of digoxin results from uncertainty regarding completeness of absorption from the gastrointestinal tract. This is compounded by recent warnings from the U.S. Food and Drug Administration that a number of lots of digoxin have required recall because of excessive variation in digoxin content from tablet to tablet.[51] Studies employing the direct administration of tritiated digoxin have yielded useful data,[34,50] but this approach is not applicable to studies of the drug in the tablet form used clinically. White et al.[132] have studied the time course of absorption of digoxin tablets in normal subjects. Plasma digoxin levels peaked at about one hour in fasting subjects, falling to the final excretory plateau after about 5 to 6 hours. After a meal, the same subjects had slightly lower and later peaks but plateau levels were unchanged. A crossover study of 21 patients receiving daily maintenance doses showed no significant difference in steady-state plasma digoxin concentrations when the drug was taken fasting or in the postprandial state. The rapid appearance of digoxin in the blood documented in this study suggests that, at least for the preparation tested (Lanoxin), the oral route of administration is adequate for most patients without gastrointestinal disease who require digitalization.

In contradistinction to the pattern in normal subjects, patients with malabsorption syndromes have been shown to have poor and erratic gastrointestinal absorption of digoxin. Heizer et al.[53] found that patients with sprue, short bowel syndrome, radiation enteritis, and marked hypermotility had low serum digoxin concentrations by radioimmunoassay when given usual oral maintenance digoxin doses. Two patients with steatorrhea due to pancreatic insufficiency maintained serum digoxin levels comparable to those of normal control subjects, suggesting that qualitatively or quantitatively abnormal mucosa rather than steatorrhea per se caused the abnormality in absorption.

The problem of bioavailability of various different digoxin tablet preparations has also been studied by radioimmunoassay. Lindenbaum et al.[69] showed a marked variation in serum digoxin concentrations during the first 6 hours after oral administration of digoxin tablets from different manufacturers, and variation was also present between two lots from a single manufacturer. One preparation gave a peak serum digoxin level only one-seventh that of the highest peak observed, with a twofold difference persisting at the end of 6 hours. Although these data cannot be extrapolated to predict total absorption of the various preparations, the observed variability in time course of absorption has obvious clinical implications.

Studies in the Pediatric Age Group

Digoxin doses usually given to infants and children are relatively larger than adult doses on a mg/kg or mg/M² body surface area basis. Willerson et al. studied serum digoxin concentrations by radioimmunoassay in infants and children, and found that the levels encountered were significantly higher than those of an adult population.[133] These higher doses and blood levels were well tolerated, and toxicity was not encountered in this series. Modification of the radioimmunoassay technique to deal with 0.1-ml serum samples facilitated this study.[113] Similar results have been reported by Hayes et al.[52] Their infant group had a mean serum digoxin level of 2.7 ng/ml for nontoxic patients, compared with a mean of 4.5 for infants with clinical evidence of toxicity. Older children had values comparable to those of the adult population. Soyka has also found higher serum digoxin concentrations in infants and young children.[123]

Increasing recognition of possible indications for in utero digitalization such as fetal atrial tachycardia led Rogers et al. to study human fetal and neonatal serum digoxin concentrations together with maternal levels.[102] Pregnant women with rheumatic heart disease receiving maintenance digoxin were studied. Their mean serum digoxin concentration at delivery was 0.6 ng/ml, while both fetal cord blood and 12-hour neonatal levels averaged 0.5 ng/ml, documenting the transplacental passage of the drug and the potential feasibility of intrauterine digitalization.

Studies Following Suicidal and Accidental Digitalis Ingestion

A significant variation in the usual time course of serum digoxin decline was observed by radioimmunoassay in a series of patients who took very large doses of digoxin accidentally or with suicidal intent.[117] Serum half-times between 4 and 48 hours postingestion were considerably shorter than those observed with ordinary doses of digoxin.[33] Figure 9 shows the time course of serum digoxin concentration following the ingestion of 5 mg of digoxin by a 51-year-old man with coronary-artery disease. Values shown span a time

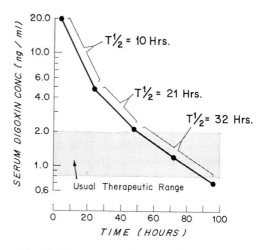

Fig. 9. Time course of serum digoxin concentration decline in a patient who ingested 5 mg of digoxin with suicidal intent. Abbreviated half-times in the initial 4 to 48 hrs after ingestion were seen in several other patients as well.[117] (Reprinted with permission from Circulation.)

course from 4 to 96 hours after the ingestion. The half-life reaches the expected value of 32 hours only after 48 hours, when the serum level has declined to near the usual therapeutic range. The reason for this phenomenon remains uncertain, but it may be that the relationship between tissue and serum levels is altered in favor of a higher serum:tissue ratio, resulting in the presentation of a relatively greater proportion of the total body digoxin store to the kidney per unit time for clearance.

Pébay-Peyroula et al. have also accumulated an interesting experience in the assay of serum digitalis glycoside concentrations following massive overdosage, usually due to self-poisoning.[97] Digitoxin and lanatoside C concentrations were measured by the red cell rubidium uptake inhibition method, using atomic absorption spectrophotometry for rubidium quantitation.[16] Extraordinary plasma levels of more than 1,000 ng/ml occurred initially in patients who had ingested 10 and 15 mg of digitoxin. Although plasma digitoxin levels sometimes fell rapidly, a patient without prior heart disease who had taken 15 mg of digitoxin still had a concentration of 700 ng/ml on the fourth day—and recovered! There were two fatalities among the 5 patients who had ingested 10 mg of digitoxin. A total of 4 deaths occurred among 22 patients in this series, and of these 3 had preexisting heart disease. Thus, the experience of these investigators is in accord with that of Smith and Willerson,[117] who found that all but the most massive ingestions were relatively well tolerated by patients without underlying heart disease, in marked contrast to patients with diseased hearts.

Miscellaneous Studies

Rasmussen and co-workers have carried out extensive clinical studies of serum digitoxin concentrations[98] using Gjerdrum's modification of the red cell ^{86}Rb uptake inhibition assay.[46] Digitoxin kinetics in patients with impaired renal function were studied by this group.[99] During both the absorption phase and maintenance therapy, serum digitoxin concentrations of patients with poor renal function were lower than those of the control group, but most of the differences noted were attributable to different concentrations of serum proteins in the two groups. The reported lack of correlation between renal function and digitoxin elimination is in agreement with the findings of other workers.[9,114]

The important area of interactions between digitoxin and other drugs has been reviewed recently by Solomon and Abrams.[120] Serum digitoxin concentration measurements by the red cell ^{86}Rb uptake inhibition method have been used to study the effects of drugs such as phenobarbital and phenylbutazone, which appear to accelerate hepatic digitoxin metabolism.[121,122] Effects of steroid-binding resins on the metabolism of both digoxin and digitoxin have been studied by the ^{86}Rb method,[4,5] by radioimmunoassay,[48] and by direct measurement of tritiated glycosides.[24,25,120] Caldwell et al.[25] have shown a significant decrease in the serum half-life of digitoxin in human subjects during treatment with cholestyra-mine, with more rapid return to base-line values of digitoxin-induced changes in left ventricular ejection time and Q-S$_2$ intervals. This change was presumed to be mediated by interruption of the enterohepatic circulation of digitoxin by cholestyramine.

Spurrell et al.[124] have studied the effect of digoxin on atrioventricular conduction in 19 patients with known conduction system disease. Despite histories of transient complete heart block in the course of myocardial infarction or chronic intermittent heart block, there was no incidence of return to second- or third-degree block precipitated by "therapeutic" levels and in some cases high serum digoxin levels for 7 days. Thus, following recovery of normal conduction, there was no evidence of increased sensitivity to digoxin in these patients.

A final example of the applicability of digitalis assays to studies of the clinical pharmacology of cardiac glycosides may be found in the work of Selden and Smith,[104] who used a radioimmunoassay technique[116] to study the pharmacokinetics of ouabain in dogs and man. After a single intravenous dose of ouabain, plasma levels of the drug fell rapidly, reaching a phase of slow exponential decline after 7 hours. The half-life of this excretory phase was 18 hours in dogs and 21 hours in normal human subjects. As shown in Figure 10, repeated intravenous administration of ouabain to human subjects for nine successive days produced a plateau of plasma concentration and urinary excretion after 4 to 5 days, confirming plasma and urinary half-lives in the 19- to 24-hour range. The renal ouabain clearance pattern was similar to that of creatinine, with a mean ratio of ouabain to creatinine clearance of 0.81. Plasma half-life data were in good agreement with prior estimates of duration of pharmacological effect as estimated by systolic time intervals[131] and slowing of the ventricular response to atrial fibrillation.[47] The duration of effect of ouabain thus bears a close relationship to the plasma half-life of the drug, as is the case for digoxin and digitoxin.

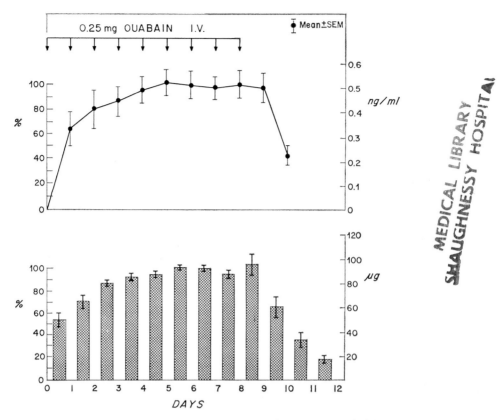

Fig. 10. *Top*: Mean plasma ouabain concentration just prior to daily intravenous administration of 0.25 mg to three normal human subjects.[104]   The vertical axis shows per cent attainment of the steady-state plateau. *Bottom*: Mean 24-hour urinary ouabain excretion during the same experiment. (Reprinted with permission from Circulation.)

CONCLUDING REMARKS

Recent technical advances have placed measurement of clinically relevant serum or plasma cardiac glycoside concentrations within reach of the well-equipped hospital clinical laboratory. A rapidly expanding literature concerning both methods and clinical application of these measurements indicates that mean digoxin and digitoxin levels are significantly higher in patients with clinical evidence of toxicity compared with nontoxic patients. It must be emphasized, however, that overlap exists in a gray area of intermediate concentrations wherein multiple factors influencing individual response demand that serum level data be interpreted in the overall clinical context. Type and

extent of underlying cardiac disease appear to be especially important determinants of the effect of any given serum or myocardial digitalis level.

In our own experience, serum digoxin and digitoxin concentration data have been particularly useful in the evaluation of patients unable to give an adequate history of type and/or dose of cardiac glycoside taken, and in complex clinical situations such as those following cardiac surgery in which cardiac and renal function may fluctuate considerably and digitalis dosage schedules tend to be more irregular than usual. The needed dose in the digoxin-resistant patient with malabsorption syndrome,[53] or in apparent patient resistance to digoxin with preparations of decreased bioavailability,[69] may be effectively assessed by the use of serum level measurements.

Further experience will dictate the ultimate role of serum digitalis measurements in the management of the individual problem patient. There seems no doubt, however, that the methods discussed in this review will continue to be highly useful in attacking many of the residual problems in the clinical pharmacology of cardiac glycosides.

REFERENCES

1. Akera, T., Larsen, F. S., and Brody, T. M.: Correlation of cardiac sodium- and potassium-activated ATPase activity with ouabain-induced inotropic stimulation. J. Pharmacol. Exp. Ther., *173*:145, 1970.
2. Barr, I., et al: Correlation of the electrophysiologic action of digoxin with serum digoxin concentration. J. Pharmacol. Exp. Ther., *180*:710, 1972.
3. Barr, I., et al: Correlation of serum digoxin level with acetyl strophanthidin (AS) tolerance. Ann. Intern. Med., *74*:817, 1971.
4. Bazzano, G., Gray, M., and Bazzano, G. S.: Treatment of digitalis intoxication with a new steroid-binding resin. Clin. Res., *18*:592, 1970.
5. Bazzano, G., and Bazzano, G. S.: Cholestipol and cholestyramine in the treatment of digitalis intoxication. Clin. Res., *19*:305, 1971.
6. Beermann, B., Helstrom, K., and Rosen, A.: Fate of orally administered ^{3}H-digitoxin in man with special reference to the absorption. Circulation, *43*:852, 1971.
7. Beller, G. A., et al: Digitalis intoxication: A prospective clinical study with serum level correlations. New Eng. J. Med., *284*:989, 1971.
8. Beller, G. A., et al.: Inhomogeneity of digoxin uptake in the infarcted canine left ventricle. Circulation, in press.
9. Bentley, J. D., et al.: Clinical application of serum digitoxin levels—a simplified plasma determination. Circulation, *41*:67, 1970.
10. Bertler, A., and Redfors, A.: An improved method of estimating digoxin in human plasma. Clin. Pharmacol. Ther., *11*:665, 1970.
11. Bertler, A., and Redfors, A.: Plasma levels of digoxin in relation to toxicity. Acta Pharmacol., *29*(Suppl. III):281, 1971.
12. Besch, H. R., Jr., et al.: Correlation between the inotropic action of ouabain and its effects on subcellular enzyme systems from canine myocardium. J. Pharmacol. Exp. Ther., *171*: 1, 1970.
13. Binnion, P. F., et al.: Plasma and myocardial digoxin concentrations in patients on oral therapy. Brit. Heart J., *31*:636, 1969.
14. Bloom, P. M., Nelp, W. B., and Tuell, S. H.: Relationship of excretion of tritiated digoxin to renal function. Amer. J. Med. Sci., *251*: 133, 1966.
15. Boston Collaborative Drug Surveillance Program: Relation between digoxin arrhythmias and ABO blood groups. Circulation, *45*:352, 1972.
16. Bourdon, R., and Mercier, M.: Dosage des heterosides cardiotoniques dans les liquides biologiques par spectrophotometric d'absorption atomique. Ann. Biol. Clin., *27*:651, 1969.
17. Bretschneider, H. J., et al.: Arterielle konzentration, arterio-venose differenz im coronarblut und organ verteilung von C^{14}-markiertein lanatoside C nack rascher intravenoser injection. Arch. Exp. Path. Pharmakol., *244*: 117, 1962.
18. Brooker, G., and Jelliffe, R. W.: Serum cardiac glycoside assay based upon displacement of ^{3}H-ouabain from Na-K ATPase. Circulation, *45*:20, 1972.
19. Brown, D. D., and Abraham, G. N.: Plasma digoxin levels in normal human volunteers. Circulation, *44*:11, 1971.
20. Burnett, G. H., and Conklin, R. L.: The enzymatic assay of plasma digitoxin levels. J. Lab. Clin. Med., *71*:1040, 1968.
21. Burnett, G. H., and Conklin, R. L.: The enzymatic assay of plasma digoxin. J. Lab. Clin. Med., *78*:779, 1971.
22. Butler, V. P., Jr., and Chen, J. P.: Digoxin-specific antibodies. Proc. Nat. Acad. Sci., *57*:71, 1967.
23. Butler, V. P., Jr.: Digoxin radioimmunoassay. Lancet, *1*:186, 1971.
24. Caldwell, J. H., and Greenberger, N. J.: Interruption of the enterohepatic circulation of digitoxin by cholestyramine. I. Protection against lethal digitoxin intoxication. J. Clin. Invest., *50*:2626, 1971.
25. Caldwell, J. H., Bush, C. A., and Greenberger, N. J.: Interruption of the enterohepatic circulation of digitoxin by cholestyramine. II. Effect on metabolic disposition of tritium-labeled digitoxin and cardiac systolic intervals in man. J. Clin. Invest., *50*:2638, 1971.
26. Caldwell, P. C., and Keynes, R. D.: The effect of ouabain on the efflux of sodium from a squid giant axon. J. Physiol., *148*:8P, 1959.
27. Chamberlain, D. A.: Plasma digoxin concentration as a guide to therapeutic requirements. In: *Biological Effects of Drugs in Relation to Plasma Concentrations* (Davies, D. S., and Prichard, B. N. C., Eds.). Proceedings of Symposium, British Pharmacological Society. New York, Macmillan, in press.
28. Chamberlain, D. A., et al.: Plasma digoxin concentrations in patients with atrial fibrillation. Brit. Med. J., *3*:429, 1970.

29. Coiner, D., et al: Serum cardiac glycoside assay method and possible clinical use. J. Nucl. Med., 9:377, 1968.
30. Coltart, D. J., et al.: The effect of cardiopulmonary bypass on plasma digoxin concentrations. Brit. Heart J., 33:334, 1971.
31. Doherty, J. E., and Perkins, W. H.: Tissue concentration and turnover of tritiated digoxin in dogs. Amer. J. Cardiol., 17:47, 1966.
32. Doherty, J. E., Perkins, W. H., and Flanigan, W. J.: The distribution and concentration of tritiated digoxin in human tissues. Ann. Intern. Med., 66:116, 1967.
33. Doherty, J. E.: The clinical pharmacology of digitalis glycosides: a review. Amer. J. Med. Sci., 255:382, 1968.
34. Doherty, J. E., et al.: Tritiated digoxin: XIV. Enterohepatic circulation, absorption, and excretion studies in human volunteers. Circulation, 42:867, 1970.
35. Doherty, J. E., Perkins, W. H., and Wilson, M. C.: Studies with tritiated digoxin in renal failure. Amer. J. Med., 37:536, 1964.
36. Dutta, S., et al.: The uptake and binding of six radio-labelled cardiac glycosides by guinea pig hearts and by isolated sarcoplasmic reticulum. J. Pharmacol. Exp. Ther., 164, 10, 1968.
37. Evered, D. C., Chapman, C., and Hayter, C. J.: Measurement of plasma digoxin concentrations by radioimmunoassay. Brit. Med. J., 3:427, 1970.
38. Evered, D. C., and Chapman, C.: Plasma digoxin concentrations and digoxin toxicity in hospital patients. Brit. Heart J., 33:540, 1971.
39. Ewy, G. A., et al.: Digoxin metabolism in the elderly. Circulation, 39:449, 1969.
40. Ewy, G. A., et al.: Digoxin metabolism in obesity. Circulation, 44:810, 1971.
41. FDA Drug Bulletin. U.S. Food and Drug Administration, Washington, October 1971.
42. Fogelman, A. M., et al.: Fallibility of plasma-digoxin in differentiating toxic from non-toxic patients. Lancet, 2:727, 1971.
43. Friedman, M., and Bine, R., Jr.: A study of the rate of disappearance of a digitalis glycoside (lanatoside C) from the blood of man. J. Clin. Invest., 28:32, 1949.
44. Friedman, M., St. George, S., and Bine, R., Jr.: The behavior and fate of digitoxin in the experimental animal and man. Medicine, 33:15, 1954.
45. Friedman, M., and Bine, R., Jr.: Employment of the embryonic duck heart for the detection of minute amounts of a digitalis glycoside (lanatoside C). Proc. Soc. Exp. Biol. Med., 64:162, 1947.
46. Gjerdrum, K.: Determination of digitalis in blood. Acta Med. Scand., 187:371, 1970.
47. Gold, H., et al.: Comparison of ouabain with strophanthidin-3-acetate by intravenous injection in man. J. Pharmacol. Exp. Ther., 94: 39, 1948.
48. Goldfinger, S. E., Heizer, W. D., and Smith,

T. W.: Malabsorption of digoxin in malabsorption syndromes. Gastroenterology, 58: 952, 1970.
49. Grahame-Smith, D. G., and Everest, M. S.: Measurement of digoxin in plasma and its use in diagnosis of digoxin intoxication. Brit. Med. J., 1:826, 1969.
50. Hall, W. H., and Doherty, J. E.: Tritiated digoxin XVI: Gastric absorption. Amer. J. Dig. Dis., 16:903, 1971.
51. Han, J.: The concepts of reentrant activity responsible for ectopic rhythms. Amer. J. Cardiol., 28:253, 1971.
52. Hayes, C. J., et al.: Serum digoxin studies in infants and children. Bull. N.Y. Acad. Sci., 47:1226, 1971.
53. Heizer, W. D., Smith, T. W., and Goldfinger, S. E.: Absorption of digoxin in patients with malabsorption syndromes. New Eng. J. Med., 285:257, 1971.
54. Henderson, R. R., et al.: Serum digoxin levels in a cardiac outpatient population: A prospective clinical study. Circulation, 44:11, 1971.
55. Herrera, F. C.: Action of ouabain on sodium transport in the toad urinary bladder. Amer. J. Physiol., 210:980, 1966.
56. Hoeschen, R. J., and Proveda, V.: Serum digoxin by radioimmunoassay. Canad. Med. Assoc. J., 105:170, 1971.
57. Hoffman, B. F., and Singer, D. H.: Effects of digitalis on electrical activity of cardiac fibers. Progr. Cardiov. Dis., 7:226, 1964.
58. Hoffman, J. F.: The red cell membrane and the transport of sodium and potassium. Amer. J. Med., 41:666, 1966.
59. Jelliffe, R. W.: A chemical determination of urinary digitoxin and digoxin in man. J. Lab. Clin. Med., 67:694, 1966.
60. Kliman, B., and Peterson, R. E.: Double isotope derivative assay of aldosterone in biological extracts. J. Biol. Chem., 235:1639, 1960.
61. Kosowsky, B. D., et al.: The effects of digitalis on atrioventricular conduction in man. Amer. Heart J., 75:736, 1968.
62. Kuschinsky, K., et al.: Accumulation and release of ^{3}H-digoxin by guinea-pig heart muscle. Brit. J. Pharmacol., 30:317, 1967.
63. Kuschinsky, K., Lullman, H., and van Zwieten, P. A.: The binding of ^{3}H-peruvoside by guinea pig isolated atria. Arzneimittelforschung, 18:1602, 1968.
64. Kuschinsky, K., Lullman, H., and van Zwieten, P. A.: The binding of ^{3}H-digitoxigenin by guinea-pig atrial tissue. Brit. J. Pharmacol., 34:613, 1968.
65. Langer, G. A.: The intrinsic control of myocardial contraction—ionic factors. New Eng. J. Med., 285:1065, 1971.
66. Larbig, D., and Kochsick, K.: Radioimmunochemische Bestimmung von digoxin in menschlichen serum. Klin. Wschr., 49: 1031, 1971.

67. Lee, K. S., and Klaus, W.: The subcellular basis for the mechanism of inotropic action of cardiac glycosides. Pharmacol. Rev., 23: 193, 1971.

68. Lely, A. H., and van Enter, C. H. J.: Noncardiac symptoms of digitalis intoxication. Amer. Heart J., 83:149, 1972.

69. Lindenbaum, J., et al.: Variation in biologic availability of digoxin from four preparations. New Eng. J. Med., 285:1344, 1971.

70. Lowenstein, J. M.: A method for measuring plasma levels of digitalis glycosides. Circulation, 31:228, 1965.

71. Lowenstein, J. M., and Corrill, E. M.: An improved method for measuring plasma and tissue concentrations of digitalis glycosides. J. Lab. Clin. Med., 67:1048, 1966.

72. Lown, B., Cannon, R. L., and Rossi, M. A.: Electrical stimulation and digitalis drugs: Repetitive response in diastole. Proc. Soc. Exp. Biol. Med., 126:698, 1967.

73. Lown, B., and Levine, S. A.: Current Concepts in Digitalis Therapy. Boston, Little, Brown, 1954.

74. Luchi, R. J., Park, C. D., and Waldhausen, J. A.: Relationship between myocardial ouabain content and inotropic activity. Amer. J. Physiol., 220:906, 1971.

75. Lukas, D. S., and Peterson, R. E.: Double isotope dilution derivative assay of digitoxin in plasma, urine and stool of patients maintained on the drug. J. Clin. Invest., 45:782, 1966.

76. Lukas, D. S.: Some aspects of the distribution and disposition of digitoxin in man. Ann. N.Y. Acad. Sci., 179:338, 1971.

77. Lukas, D. S., and DeMartino, A. G.: Binding of digitoxin and some related cardenolides to human plasma proteins. J. Clin. Invest., 48: 1041, 1969.

78. Lullmann, H., and Van Zwieten, P. A.: The kinetic behavior of cardiac glycosides in vivo, measured by isotope techniques. J. Pharm. Pharmacol., 21:1, 1969.

79. Molokhia, F. A., et al.: Constancy of myocardial digoxin concentration during experimental cardiopulmonary bypass. Ann. Thorac. Surg., 11:222, 1971.

80. Marcus, F. I.: Metabolic factors determining digitalis dosage. In: Basic and Clinical Pharmacology of Digitalis. Springfield, Charles C Thomas, 1972.

81. Marcus, F. I., et al.: The effect of acute hypokalemia on the myocardial concentration and body distribution of tritiated digoxin in the dog. J. Pharmacol. Exp. Ther., 178:271, 1971.

82. Marcus, F. I., et al.: Metabolism of tritiated digoxin in renal insufficiency in dogs and man. J. Pharmacol. Exp. Ther., 152:372, 1966.

83. Marcus, F. I., et al.: Administration of tritiated digoxin with and without a loading dose: A metabolic study. Circulation, 34:865, 1966.

84. Marks, B. H.: Factors that affect the accumulation of digitalis glycosides by the heart. In: Basic and Clinical Pharmacology of Digitalis (Marks, B. H., and Weissler, A., Eds.). Springfield, Charles C Thomas, 1972.

85. Marks, B. H., et al.: Distribution in plasma, uptake by the heart, and excretion of ^{3}H-ouabain in human subjects. J. Pharmacol. Exp. Ther., 145:351, 1964.

86. Moe, G. K., and Farah, A. E.: Digitalis and allied cardiac glycosides. In: The Pharmacological Basis of Therapeutics, 3rd ed. (Goodman, L. S., and Gilman, A., Eds.). New York, Macmillan, 1965.

87. Morrison, J., and Killip, T.: Radioimmunoassay of digitoxin. Clin. Res., 18:668, 1970.

88. Morrison, J., Killip, T., and Stason, W. B.: Serum digoxin levels in patients undergoing cardiopulmonary bypass. Circulation, 42: 110, 1970.

89. Morrison, J., and Killip, T.: Hypoxemia and digitalis toxicity in patients with chronic lung disease. Circulation, 44:II-41, 1971.

90. Morrison, J., and Killip, T.: Serial serum digitalis levels in patients with acute myocardial infarction. Clin. Res., 19:353, 1971.

91. Morrison, J., and Killip, T.: Serial serum digitalis levels in states of altered myocardial metabolism. Bull. N.Y. Acad. Med., 47:1230, 1971.

92. Odell, W. D., and Daughaday, W. H., Eds.: Principles of Competitive Protein-binding Assays. J. B. Lippincott, Philadelphia, 1971.

93. Okita, G. T.: Distribution, disposition, and excretion of digitalis glycosides. In: Digitalis (Fisch, C., and Surawicz, B., Eds.). New York, Grune and Stratton, 1969.

94. Oliver, G. C., Parker, B. M., and Parker, C. W.: Radioimmunoassay for digoxin. Technique and clinical application. Amer. J. Med., 51:186, 1971.

95. Oliver, G. C., Jr., et al.: The measurement of digitoxin in human serum by radioimmunoassay. J. Clin. Invest., 47:1035, 1968.

96. Oliver, G. C., et al.: Absorption and transport of digitoxin in the dog. Circ. Res., 29:419, 1971.

97. Pébay-Peyroula, F., Gaultier, M., and Nicaise, A. M.: Assay of digitalis glycosides: Its application in clinical toxicology. Clin. Tox., 4:419, 1971.

98. Rasmussen, K., Jervell, J., and Storstein, O.: Clinical use of a bio-assay of serum digitoxin activity. Europ. J. Clin. Pharmacol., 3:236, 1971.

99. Rasmussen, K., et al.: Digitoxin kinetics in patients with impaired renal function. Clin. Pharmacol. Ther., 13:6, 1972.

100. Repke, K.: Metabolism of cardiac glycosides. In: Proceedings First International Pharmacological Meeting, Vol. 3 (Wilbrandt, W., Ed.). Oxford, Pergamon Press, 1963.

101. Ritzmann, L. W., et al.: Serum glycoside levels in digitalis toxicity. Circulation, 40:111, 1969.

102. Rogers, M. C., et al.: Human fetal and neonatal digoxin studies. Circulation, *44*:52, 1971.

103. Schatzmann, H. J.: Hertzglykoside als Hemmstoffe fur den aktiven kallumund Natrium—transport durch die Erythrocytenmembran. Helv. Physiol. Pharmacol. Acta, *11*:346, 1953.

104. Selden, R., and Smith, T. W., with the technical assistance of Findley, W.: Ouabain pharmacokinetics in dog and man: Determination by radioimmunoassay. Circulation, *45*:1176, 1972.

105. Selzer, A.: The use of digitalis in acute myocardial infarction. Progr. Cardiov. Dis., *10*: 518, 1968.

106. Shapiro, S., et al.: The epidemiology of digoxin: A study in three Boston hospitals. J. Chronic Dis., *22*:361, 1969.

107. Shapiro, W., Narahara, K., and Taubert, K.: Relationship of plasma digitoxin and digoxin to cardiac response following intravenous digitalization in man. Circulation, *42*:1065, 1970.

108. Singer, D. C., and Ten Eick, R. E.: Pharmacology of cardiac arrhythmias. Progr. Cardiov. Dis., *11*:488, 1969.

109. Smith, T. W., and Haber, E.: Digoxin intoxication: The relationship of clinical presentation to serum digoxin concentration. J. Clin. Invest., *49*:2377, 1970.

110. Smith, T. W., et al.: Studies on the localization of the cardiac glycoside receptor. J. Clin. Invest., *51*:1777, 1972.

111. Smith, T. W., and Haber, E.: Current techniques for serum or plasma digitalis assay and their potential clinical application. Amer. J. Med. Sci., *259*:301, 1970.

112. Smith, T. W., Butler, V. P., Jr., and Haber, E.: Determination of therapeutic and toxic serum digoxin concentrations by radioimmunoassay. New Eng. J. Med., *281*:1212, 1969.

113. Smith, T. W.: The clinical use of serum cardiac glycoside concentration measurements. Amer. Heart J., *82*:833, 1971.

114. Smith, T. W.: Radioimmunoassay for serum digitoxin concentration: Methodology and clinical experience. J. Pharmacol. Exp. Ther., *175*:352, 1970.

115. Smith, T. W., Butler, V. P., Jr., and Haber, E.: Characterization of antibodies of high affinity and specificity for the digitalis glycoside digoxin. Biochemistry, *9*:331, 1970.

116. Smith, T. W.: Ouabain-specific antibodies: Immunochemical properties and reversal of Na^+, K^+-activated adenosine triphosphatase inhibition. J. Clin. Invest., *51*:1583, 1972.

117. Smith, T. W., and Willerson, J. T.: Suicidal and accidental digoxin ingestion: Report of five cases with serum digoxin level correlations. Circulation, *44*:29, 1971.

118. Smith, T. W.: Contributions of quantitative assay techniques to the understanding of the clinical pharmacology of digitalis. Circulation, *46*:188, 1972.

119. Solomon, H. M., and Reich, S. D.: A source of error in digoxin radioimmunoassay. Lancet, *2*:1038, 1970.

120. Solomon, H. M., and Abrams, W. B.: Interaction between digitoxin and other drugs in man. Amer. Heart J., *83*:277, 1972.

121. Solomon, H. M., Abrams, W. B., and Reich, S. D.: Interactions between digitoxin and other drugs in vitro and in vivo. Clin. Res., *18*:344, 1970.

122. Solomon, H., et al.: Induction of the metabolism of digitoxin in man by phenobarbital. Clin. Res., *19*:356, 1971.

123. Soyka, L. F.: Clinical pharmacology of digoxin. Ped. Clin. N. Amer., *19*:241, 1972.

124. Spurrell, R. A. J., Harris, A. M., and Howard, M. R.: Effect of digoxin on A–V conduction. Brit. Med. J., *3*:563, 1971.

125. Surawicz, B., and Mortelmans, S.: Factors affecting individual tolerance to digitalis. In: *Digitalis* (Fisch, C., and Surawicz, B., Eds.). New York, Grune and Stratton, 1969.

126. Turba, F., and Scholtissek, C.: Digitalis preparations labeled with radioactive carbon. Arch. Exp. Path. Pharmakol., *222*:206, 1954.

127. *The United States Pharmacopeia*, 17th revision, 1965, pp. 191–197.

128. Vassale, M.: Automaticity and automatic rhythms. Amer. J. Cardiol., *28*:245, 1971.

129. Vassale, M., Karis, J., and Hoffman, B. F.: Toxic effects of oaubain on Purkinje fibers and ventricular muscle fibers. Amer. J. Physiol., *203*:433, 1962.

130. Watson, E., and Kalman, S. M.: Assay of digoxin in plasma by gas chromatography. J. Chromatogr., *56*:209, 1971.

131. Weissler, A. M., et al.: Assay of digitalis glycosides in man. Amer. J. Cardiol., *17*:768, 1966.

132. White, R. J., et al.: Plasma concentrations of digoxin after oral administration in the fasting and postprandial state. Brit. Med. J., *1*:380, 1971.

133. Willerson, J. T., et al.: Serum digoxin levels in children. Amer. J. Cardiol., *26*:666, 1970.

134. Withering, W.: An account of the foxglove and some of its medical uses, with practical remarks on dropsy and other diseases. In: *Classics of Cardiology* (Willius, F. A., and Keys, T. E., Eds.). New York, Dover Publications, 1941.

135. Wotman, S., et al.: Salivary electrolytes in the detection of digitalis toxicity. New Eng. J. Med., *285*:871, 1971.

Chapter 4

ADVANCES IN CONGENITAL
HEART DISEASE

Celia M. Oakley, M.D.

The last few years have brought spectacular surgical advances particularly for the neonate with severe or complex cardiac deformities and in the correction of the transposition syndromes and truncus arteriosus. Diagnostic skills have grown concurrently, especially the use of noninvasive methods for screening purposes, for serial studies and often to provide complementary information not gained from catheterization and angiocardiography. Belatedly a better appreciation of the natural history of many congenital cardiac defects is being realized, so that the cardiologist can answer the question "Should it be done?" as well as "Can it be done?"

Nearly every congenital cardiac anomaly is now within the scope of modern surgical techniques either for correction or for significant palliation. The heart is the pump; in congenital heart disease the adequacy of its contractile function is not usually a problem. The minimum basic material required for radical correction of the central anatomical derangements can be said to be: (1) the presence of two ventricles, (2) adequate development of the main pulmonary arteries to the lungs, and (3) the absence of severe pulmonary vascular obstructive disease.

Many of the relatively simple congenital defects which permit life until childhood have been correctable for the last fifteen years.[27] Recent improvements in operating conditions have aided both surgical efficiency and subsequent patient survival. Extracorporeal circulation can be managed with relative safety in infancy.[26] Alternatively, without the need for circulatory bypass, the Kyoto method of deep hypothermia provides the surgeon with a dry flaccid heart while "core" rewarming avoids the development of postoperative metabolic acidosis.[9,10,117] These technological advances plus the gradual accretion of experience have transformed the outlook for the neonate and infant. However, the severity or complexity of the anomalies makes full preoperative diagnosis mandatory to decide whether palliative or radical correction is to be attempted, and in what form.

The greatly expanded surgical potential has brought an urgent need for more accurate prognosis, a more precise appreciation of the likely natural history and above all an un-biased appraisal of the current "local" surgical risks in terms of the individual patient and his future.

Some heart defect is present in nearly 1 per cent of live newborn children.[22,105] More than a quarter of them die in the first month of life and another quarter fail to survive the first year.[22,102] Because many deaths occur in the neonatal period and the operative mortality is high, the newborn infant has been regarded as poor surgical material. This is untrue. Deaths occur because the abnormalities are incompatible with independent life, let alone growth and activity, unless something is done to improve the perfusion of vital organs. The infant with congenital heart disease is frequently normally developed and nourished at birth and the possibility of successful surgery depends to a considerable extent on making a diagnosis and decision before deterioration multiplies the risk.

The increasing sophistication and completeness of laboratory diagnosis have paved the way for the development of noninvasive methods which now complement catheterization and in some instances render it unnecessary. Ultrasound techniques or isotopic scanning of the heart chambers can in some instances obviate the need for further hemodynamic study by defining lesions unlikely to be amenable to surgical treatment. For example, ultrasound recording can be used to pick out hypoplastic left heart syndromes.[91] Asplenia syndromes can be recognized by the detection of Howell-Jolly bodies in the peripheral blood and by radioisotope scanning over the centrally placed liver.[136]

In 1966 the introduction of balloon atrial septostomy by Rashkind[126] transformed the early prognosis for infants with transposition of the great arteries and intact ventricular septum. What was hitherto the most fatal yet most common form of transposition now yields a high proportion of survivors because these children are suitable for future radical correction by the Mustard intra-atrial vein-

switch procedure which carries a remarkably low risk in this group.

Reconstruction of a right ventricular outflow tract to the pulmonary artery in conditions where this is defective or absent has become possible by the Rastelli technique.[93,128] The three major anomalies which have now become responsive to treatment are: (1) truncus arteriosus, (2) transposition of the great arteries with severe pulmonary stenosis, and (3) atresia of the main pulmonary artery or valve (extreme tetralogy of Fallot).

Many controversial aspects of management remain and are evolving. These include the indications for staged palliative versus early definitive correction of Fallot's tetralogy, pulmonary-artery banding versus early primary closure in ventricular septal defect, the timing of radical correction of transposition after early successful septostomy, the best age for the repair of the supracardiac form of total anomalous pulmonary venous drainage. The answers to these problems largely depend on local experience and surgical results. Other vexing questions such as whether to close "small" atrial or ventricular septal defects, where to draw the line in pulmonary stenosis, or which children with aortic-valve stenosis can safely be deferred reflect our still imperfect knowledge of natural history.

PROGRESS IN SCREENING AND NONINVASIVE TECHNIQUES

Two new types of screening methods have advanced greatly in recent years and now each is an important noninvasive technique to assess congenital cardiovascular malformations. These are radioisotope scintillation scanning and reflected ultrasound scanning of the heart.

Radioisotope Scintillation Scanning (Nuclear Angiocardiography)

METHOD

Gamma-emitting radioisotopes have been used in the past to detect the distribution and amount of pulmonary blood flow in a non-invasive manner.[41,42] The techniques have also been used to determine indirectly the levels of pulmonary venous and arterial pressures. The use of oxygen-labeled carbon dioxide, which has a half-life of only two minutes, has proved a reliable means of detecting left-to-right shunts.[41]

More recently, intravenous 99m technetium has been used for radioangiography employing a scintillation camera with pinhole collimator and a computer-tape storage system to define chamber and great-artery position, approximate chamber volume and the distribution of pulmonary arterial blood flow in neonates and infants and children with congenital heart disease.[63,64,85,161]

99m technetium has a half-life of only six hours and is used in the form of sodium pertechnetate. The radiation hazard is low, with a dose for infants of 150 μc per pound.[64] A bolus of about 1 ml is injected intravenously and followed by a flush of saline. The detector of the scintillation camera is placed over the anterior chest wall and Polaroid camera exposures are made from the visual scintillation-camera display at a rate of approximately one image per second. This is relatively slow compared with conventional angiocardiography but the route of the circulation can be followed and the position of cavae, right atrium, the ventricular chambers and great arteries can be seen. It is possible to concentrate either on a single cardiac chamber or on a portion of either lung, and pulmonary vascular dilution curves can be analyzed to detect even the presence of a very small left-to-right shunt.

APPLICATION

The radionuclide angiocardiograms so obtained permit the recognition of many anomalies including transposition, corrected transposition and hypoplastic left heart.[63,64,161] Subdiaphragmatic total anomalous pulmonary venous drainage can be recognized by the accumulation of radionuclide in the liver after its clearance from the lungs and followed by recirculation to the heart. Not only is differentiation from respiratory distress syndrome or other lung conditions readily made but a positive diagnosis is obtained. In this example scanning can indicate surgery before further deterioration occurs and without the need for catheterization and angiography.

The ability to detect quite small left-to-right shunts[64] and the repeatability of the method seem to offer a means of following the natural history of ventricular septal defect (VSD) in large groups of children.

Previous methods of external precordial scintillation scanning have often led to inaccurate interpretations because of the frequent inclusion in the mapping field of more structures than desired, with consequent difficulties in accurate analysis. Radioisotope images can closely reflect the findings observed by contrast angiography, including the large right atrium in Ebstein's malformation, aneurysmal dilatation of the pulmonary arteries in cases of congenital absence of the pulmonary valve, persistence of a left superior vena cava or absence of an inferior vena cava. The technique facilitates the preliminary recognition of complicated cardiac malpositions in the asplenia syndromes with visceral heterotaxia.

The compromise in image resolution compared with x-ray angiocardiograms is well compensated for by the simplicity, speed and safety of the method. As a screening method and as a means of serial evaluation of the natural history of congenital cardiac disease, it offers important complementary information to conventional angiocardiography.

Ultrasound Cardiography in Congenital Heart Disease

Technological advances have brought tremendous improvement in the resolution and detail which it is possible to obtain in reflected ultrasound cardiograms. The position and size of the cardiac chambers, the presence of a ventricular septum and the disposition of the great arteries can now be studied.[124] In addition to the movement of the mitral valve, which provides information about the function of the left ventricle[91] (as well as direct evidence of disease affecting the mitral valve itself), the movements of the tricuspid and aortic valves can also be recorded. In infancy and childhood a 3.5 megaHertz source of ultrasound is used; reflected ultrasound is displayed on a storage oscilloscope and either photographed or continuously recorded with a moving film camera onto paper.

In a single ventricle, the presence of only one atrioventricular valve and the absence of a ventricular septum can be determined.[25] The relative sizes of the ventricles can also be estimated, and in some instances an abnormal direction of movement of the interventricular septum may give evidence of increased volume loading of the right ventricle as in atrial septal defect.[39]

In Ebstein's anomaly of the tricuspid valve, a gross and diagnostic delay in tricuspid-valve closure can be shown.[31] This movement of the tricuspid valve corresponds with the midsystolic sound well known as an auscultatory phenomenon in Ebstein's anomaly (Fig. 1A). The late closure is attributable to the taking up of slack in the redundant septal cusp and occurs whether or not the ECG shows right bundle branch block or a preexcitation pattern.

In aortic-valve stenosis the mobility and thickness of the abnormal valve cusps can be recognized and the severity of the stenosis can be assessed. In discrete subaortic stenosis posterior bulging of the septal ridge can be

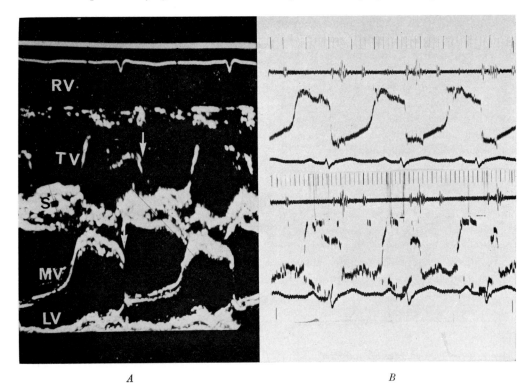

A   B

Fig. 1. Ultrasound records from a patient with Ebstein's anomaly. *A*: The ECG shows the anterior wall of the right ventricle (RV), the anterior cusp of the tricuspid valve (TV), the ventricular septum (S), the anterior cusp of the mitral valve (MV) and the posterior wall of the left ventricle (LV). Closure of the tricuspid valve (arrow) is delayed compared with closure of the mitral valve (arrow). *B*: Simultaneous phonocardiogram shows that mitral-valve closure (upper trace) coincides with the first heart sound and that tricuspid-valve closure (lower trace) coincides with the systolic click. (Reproduced with permission from The British Heart Journal.)

detected; absence of any abnormal systolic movement in the apposing anterior mitral cusp is noteworthy and contrasts with hypertrophic obstructive cardiomyopathy (HOCM).

In HOCM the anterior mitral cusp shows a characteristic reopening movement in mid-systole.[123,123a] At this time the anterior mitral cusp moves into the outflow pathway and approximates to the septal echoes which are abnormally prominent. In patients with HOCM who have no outflow-tract obstruction, this characteristic and diagnostic systolic opening movement is absent or slight, but the diagnosis can be made from ultrasound records by the abnormal septal echoes and abnormality in the diastolic phase of mitral-valve movement. Incompliance of the left ventricle where this is diffusely involved by abnormal myocardial hypertrophy in HOCM leads to delay in left ventricular filling and slowing of the diastolic closure slope, thus resembling mitral stenosis except that the valve cusp is not thickened. Conversely, in HOCM with outflow-tract obstruction both mitral regurgitation and focal hypertrophy permit a faster diastolic closure slope in the normal or low-normal range.

There is no doubt that with further refinements in recording methods ultrasound will find a place in the routine precatheterization screening of infants and children with congenital cardiac lesions.

In the normal heart the continuity between the anterior cusp of the mitral valve and the aortic root is readily appreciated, as the ultrasound transducer follows the anterior mitral cusp superiorly until the aortic root is reached. In transposition the aortic root echoes are displaced anterior to the mitral cusp, a finding which is diagnostic of transposition.

The recognition of transposition and of hypoplasia of the left heart, for example, instantly defines one group requiring urgent therapeutic catheterization with balloon septostomy and distinguishes it from a second group which need not be investigated further once the diagnosis is made. In this way, ultrasound will facilitate the more efficient use of the catheterization laboratory and will protect parents and medical staff from the burden of therapeutically fruitless investigations in sick neonates.

THE TRANSPOSITION SYNDROMES

Many recent anatomical studies have greatly clarified this hitherto difficult subject.[37,38,46,150,151,152,155] As radically corrective or at least palliative operations can now be offered to nearly all patients with transposition, a full structural and physiological diagnosis is required of the cardiologist in all cases: the anatomical type, the presence and size of septal defects, ventricular outflow obstruction or single ventricle and the state of the pulmonary vascular resistance.

DEFINITION

Transposition means that the great arteries are "placed across" the ventricular septum and thus arise from the wrong ventricles, the aorta from the right ventricle and the pulmonary artery from the left ventricle.

INCIDENCE

Transposition of the great arteries is one of the most common causes of congestive heart failure in cyanotic infants.[102,105] It is the leading cause of death due to congenital heart disease in the first two months of life, and accounts for 15 to 20 per cent of the congenital cardiac abnormalities examined at autopsy in infants less than one month of age. There is a distinct male dominance of between 2:1 and 4:1. Complete transposition is relatively uncommon in firstborns, the birth weights are normal or high, and there is an increased incidence of maternal diabetes.[102]

NECESSARY SEMANTICS

Transposition refers to reversal of the anteroposterior relationship of the great arteries without right-left reversal so that in transposition the *aorta* is anterior.

Inversion refers to right-left reversal without

anteroposterior reversal, as in a mirror image. The word is used in reference to the *ventricles*.

Visceroatrial situs describes the position of the viscera, venae cavae and atria. Situs solitus is the normal situation, with the liver, inferior vena cava and right atrium on the right; situs inversus is the opposite, with the liver, inferior vena cava and right atrium on the left.

Levocardia means that the heart is mainly in the left hemithorax. *Dextrocardia* means that the heart is mainly in the right hemithorax—nothing else. Hence levocardia solitus (the normal situation), levocardia inversus (isolated levocardia), dextrocardia inversus, and dextrocardia solitus (isolated dextrocardia) are all self-explanatory terms.

The transposition syndromes can usefully be divided into:

1. Transposition with two ventricles
    complete simple transposition (*d-transposition*)
    physiologically corrected transposition (*l-transposition* or inverted transposition)
    transposition of the aorta only (*double-outlet right ventricle*).
2. Transposition with single ventricle.
3. Transposition with asplenia or polysplenia (so-called visceral heterotaxia).

Complete Transposition With Two Ventricles

The maximum possible different arrangements of two atria, two ventricles and two transposed great arteries are only eight. This was pointed out with clarity over 30 years ago (Fig. 2).

Since each arrangement can occur in either situs solitus or situs inversus (S and I in Fig. 2) this leaves only four possibilities: 1, 5, 3 and 7. Fortunately, 3 and 7 are so rare that they can virtually be discarded (except by collectors). This leaves only 1 and 5 plus their counterparts in dextrocardia inversus.

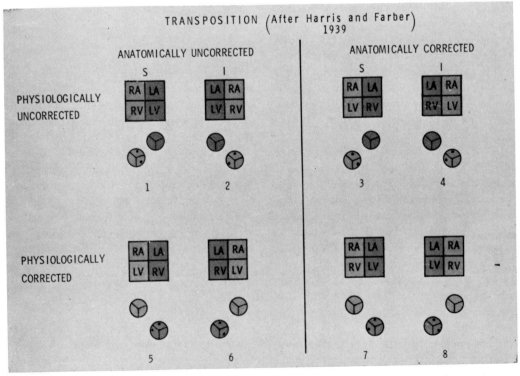

Fig. 2. The possible dispositions of the cardiac chambers and great arteries in transposition (see text). S = solitus, I = inversus. (After Harris, J. S., and Farber, S.: Arch. Path., *28*:427, 1939.)

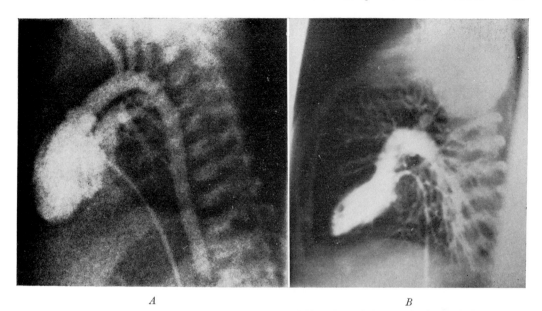

A   B

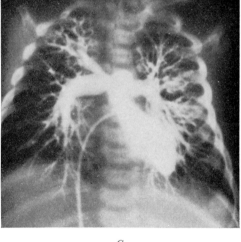

C

Fig. 3. Complete simple transposition. *A*: Right ventricular injection; lateral projection shows sub-aortic conus, high aortic valve and filling of the posterior pulmonary artery via a patent ductus. The ventricular septum is intact. *B*: Left ventricular injection; lateral projection. *C*: Left ventricular injection; frontal view. The lungs are grossly over-filled.

COMPLETE OR D-TRANSPOSITION (1 in Fig. 2)

This is the common form of complete transposition in situs solitus.[46,121] The transposed aorta is anterior and "normally" placed to the right of the pulmonary artery (because it arises from the right ventricle and passes straight up without crossing the pulmonary artery as it does in the normal heart). In essence the heart is normal but the great arteries are misconnected. Thus the systemic venous blood is directed through the right ventricle into the aorta and the pulmonary venous blood through the left ventricle into the pulmonary artery (Fig. 3).

CORRECTED OR L-TRANSPOSITION

In *physiologically* corrected transposition (5 in Fig. 2) there is inversion of the ventricles so that the aorta (still anterior and arising from the morphological right ventricle) receives the pulmonary venous blood via the

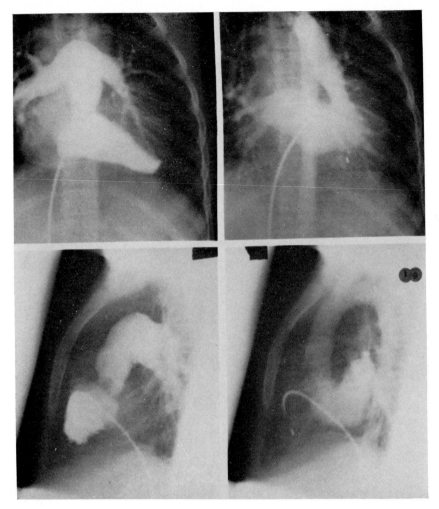

Fig. 4. Corrected transposition to show the ventricular inversion. Frontal views above, left lateral below, after contrast injection into "right" ventricle (on the left). The "right" ventricle is elliptical, smooth walled and lies inferoanteriorly. The pulmonary valve is low and the pulmonary artery arises centrally. On the right the left atrium and "left" ventricle are opacified in later frames. The "left" ventricle lies posterosuperiorly and has an infundibulum from which the aortic valve arises. The ascending aorta forms the upper part of the left-hand border of the heart shadow. The ventricular septum is intact.

left atrium, as in the normal heart. Because of the ventricular inversion the left ventricle and mitral valve lie on the right and transfer venous blood from right atrium to pulmonary artery and the right ventricle and tricuspid valve are to the left. The aorta therefore ascends on the left side (Fig. 4).[139]

In *anatomically* corrected forms of transposition (3 and 7 in Fig. 2) the aorta lies anteriorly but arises from the morphological

left ventricle. In 3, the associated ventricular inversion means that the morphological *left* ventricle carries venous blood from the right atrium to the aorta.

In 5 the circulation is normal (the transposition is also physiologically corrected) but the aorta is still said to be transposed because it is anterior, having been carried upward and forward on top of a subaortic conus. In this exceedingly rare situation, the conus (infundibulum) has developed with the left instead of the right ventricle.

In summary, for both the solitus and inversus situations there are two anatomically and physiologically uncorrected forms (types 1 and 2), two anatomically corrected forms (types 3 and 4), two physiologically corrected forms (types 5 and 6), and two anatomically and physiologically corrected forms (types 7 and 8).

In practice, only types 1 and 5 need be considered in the solitus situation and only types 6 and 2 in the inversus situation (in order of probability).

THE STRUCTURAL DIAGNOSIS

The full structural diagnosis to determine the exact chamber relationship requires recognition of: (1) visceroatrial situs (find the liver), (2) the ventricular "loop" (find the right ventricle), and (3) the conotruncal relationship (find the origin of the aorta).

The visceroatrial situs is readily deter-

mined, since the inferior vena cava is always on the same side as the liver and leads to the sinus venosus which is incorporated into the right atrium.

The ventricular "loop" means the relationship of the two ventricles. In situs solitus, a d-loop means normally placed ventricles with the right ventricle on the right of the left ventricle, as in complete transposition (d-transposition) (Fig. 3). An l-loop means ventricular inversion with the right ventricle on the left of the left ventricle as in corrected or l-transposition (Fig. 4).

The conotruncal relationship is defined by noting the whereabouts of the conus (infundibulum) and aorta. In the normal heart the conus is subpulmonary. In transposition the conus is, with rare exceptions, subaortic. It is recognized angiographically because it subtends the higher semilunar valve and is part of the *right* ventricle. The crista supraventricularis is part of the conus muscle; the most common site for a ventricular septal de-

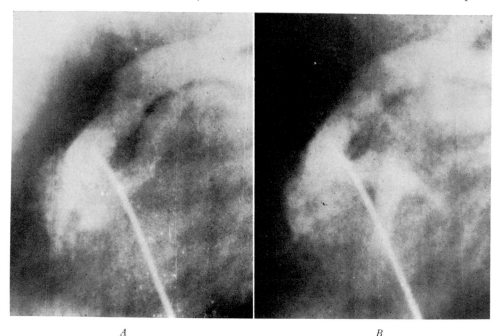

A   B

Fig. 5. Complete transposition with VSD. Right ventricular cineangiogram lateral views. *A*: Systole. The right ventricle fills the aorta anteriorly and the pulmonary artery posteriorly through a VSD. The separation of the high aortic valve from the VSD by the crista supraventricularis is well seen. *B*: Diastole. The upper and lower margins of the VSD are seen.

4

fect both in transposition and in hearts with normal origin of the great arteries is below this. In transposition, therefore, a ventricular septal defect is usually closely related to the pulmonary valve but separated from the aorta by the infundibulum of the right ventricle (Fig. 5).

This methodology applies equally to dextrocardia. In the usually complex situations of isolated dextro- and levocardia, the approach is still the same: the determination of the position of the atria, the relationship of the ventricles to the atria, whether there is a single ventricle, and the origins of the great arteries in relation to the conus and ventricles.

PHYSIOLOGY

In complete transposition the pulmonary and systemic circulations are completely separate and run parallel instead of in series as in the normal heart (Fig. 6). For survival, some systemic venous blood must be diverted from its route back to the aorta and cross over through a septal defect or patent ductus into the pulmonary circuit ("effective pulmonary flow"). Similarly, some blood that has passed through the lungs must be deflected across to the systemic circuit ("effective systemic flow"). The quantity of blood passing each way must be equal over short periods of time; otherwise one of the circuits would soon contain all the blood. Obviously the greater the volume of this equal and bidirectional shunting, the better the patient will be. Equally obviously, the volume of blood in the pulmonary or systemic circuits has nothing to do with the amount of blood that is shunted. The lungs can be greatly overfilled when the effective blood flow is very small (Fig. 3b). Thus, gross pulmonary plethora can exist in a baby who is deeply cyanotic with complete simple transposition. Less obviously, the pulmonary circuit can rarely be oligemic in such a baby.

In simple transposition the resistance to blood flow through the lungs and through the systemic vascular bed determines the pressure in the left and right ventricles. In the absence of pulmonary stenosis or a large ventricular communication, the left ventricular pressure is usually low and the right ventricular pressure is at systemic level.

Complete Transposition Without Ventricular Septal Defect (Simple Transposition)

While the ductus arteriosus is patent, a right-to-left shunt occurs across it (Fig. 3a). Increased pulmonary venous return to the left atrium then insures a left-to-right shunt at atrial level across either an atrial septal defect or a stretched foramen ovale. When the duct closes, or when it is small, the shunt across an isolated atrial septal defect is bidirectional; the left-to-right component occurs in systole when the atrioventricular valves are closed and the right-to-left component occurs in diastole. The right atrium receives blood in systole because the right atrium is believed to be more distensible than the left atrium, and the right atrium returns blood to the left side in diastole because the blood tends to flow toward the more distensible low-pressure left ventricle. These phasic flows have been beautifully shown by cineangiography.

In complete transposition the left ventricular systolic pressure is determined by the pulmonary vascular resistance or by the presence and severity of pulmonary stenosis. A low pulmonary vascular resistance favors a high pulmonary blood flow with volume overload of the left heart. In the presence of significant pulmonary stenosis or a high pulmonary vascular resistance, the pulmonary blood flow decreases but the left ventricular systolic pressure is high.

In the presence of a big ventricular septal defect or patent ductus arteriosus, the left ventricular pressure equals but does not exceed the right ventricular pressure. Increased blood flow through the lungs causes a rise in left atrial pressure and in the left ventricular diastolic pressure with a left-to-right shunt across the ventricular septal defect during diastole. During systole, the low

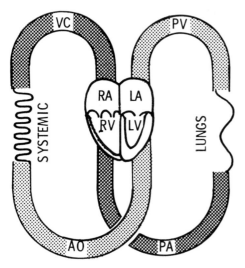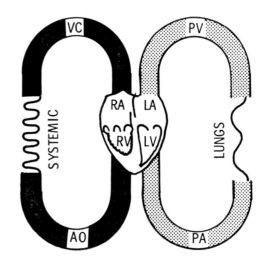

Fig. 6. The circulation in transposition (on the right) compared with the normal on the left. "Effective" pulmonary and systemic blood flows depend on equal and opposite right-to-left and left-to-right shunts.

pulmonary vascular resistance permits a right-to-left shunt from the right ventricle into the systemic circuit. The driving pressure is similar in the two circuits, but the relative flows vary independently of each other according to the status of the resistance vessels in each circuit.

In transposition the systemic arterial blood is composed mainly of recirculated systemic venous blood plus some shunted pulmonary venous blood (effective systemic flow). Similarly, pulmonary arterial blood is composed mainly of recirculated pulmonary venous blood plus some shunted systemic venous blood (effective pulmonary blood flow). A decrease in effective pulmonary blood flow will cause a fall in systemic mixed venous saturation. This in turn will cause a fall in systemic arterial saturation, systemic vasodilatation and an increase in recirculated systemic blood flow.

Advances in the Diagnosis of Complete Transposition

Confirmation of the clinical diagnosis can be made by ultrasound or isotope scintillation scanning. Full diagnosis depends essentially on good-quality selective ventricular

angiography (Fig. 3) with injections into the right and left ventricles. This will reveal the relationship of the ventricles to each other and of the great arteries to them. Venous catheterization from the leg can verify the presence of a normal inferior vena cava and the atrial location, and balloon septostomy can be carried out if transposition is confirmed. Passage of the catheter across the atrial septum to the left ventricle is almost always possible in the neonate, although not necessarily in the older patient with transposition. Unless there is significant left ventricular outflow-tract obstruction, the pulmonary artery can nearly always be reached.

The catheter is looped in the left atrium with the tip in a right pulmonary vein. Then by pushing the loop down through the mitral valve into the left ventricle, the tip of the catheter is brought out of the pulmonary vein into the left ventricle where it points upward and posteriorly toward the pulmonary artery into which it can then be advanced.[24]

The presence and size of ventricular septal defect and the presence and severity of pulmonary stenosis or pulmonary vascular obstruction can thereby be assessed. The blood flows and resistances in the two circuits can also be calculated.

Management of Transposition

EARLY MANAGEMENT OF COMPLETE TRANSPOSITION WITHOUT VENTRICULAR SEPTAL DEFECT

In the neonate the absence of atrial septal defect in transposition is nearly always associated with higher left atrial pressure than right atrial pressure, absence of any increase in saturation in the right atrium, and fully saturated blood in the left atrium.

It is agreed that atrial septostomy is indicated in the neonate with transposition whether or not a ventricular septal defect is present. In simple transposition, creation of a big atrial septal defect by the Rashkind technique[126] is usually ideal because it allows adequate bidirectional shunting without allowing transmission of pressure from the high-pressure systemic circuit in the right ventricle to the low-pressure pulmonary circuit and left ventricle. In most cases the systemic arterial oxygen saturation can be brought to around 70 per cent by this means, thus alleviating hypoxemia and metabolic acidosis and providing fairly adequate palliation until the child is older.

Occasionally balloon septostomy does not result in improvement because, despite the creation of a generous atrial septal defect, mixing at atrial level fails to occur. The reason for this nonmixing is not understood, but it may be related to low pulmonary blood flow and volume so that insufficient blood is returned to the left atrium to activate a bidirectional shunt; further, nonmixing may be related to synchrony of left and right atrial contraction so that the expected potential pressure gradients between the two atria during the cardiac cycle fail to develop. Whatever the reason, failure of atrial septostomy to relieve hypoxemia is an indication for early radical correction. It is obviously useless to proceed to surgical creation of an atrial septal defect. The modern modifications of the closed operation for this purpose developed by Blalock and Hanlon in 1950 now are used only in older babies in whom atrial communication has been proved to be inadequate or absent and in whom the atrial septum is too tough to be ruptured by the balloon catheter.[121]

EARLY MANAGEMENT OF COMPLETE TRANSPOSITION WITH BIG VENTRICULAR SEPTAL DEFECT

Although the physiology in complete transposition with a large ventricular septal defect is quite different, some improvement usually follows atrial septostomy. Banding of the pulmonary artery is advisable subsequently. In these children the left ventricular and pulmonary-artery pressures are at systemic level and there is a high blood flow through the lungs to the left atrium. As in uncomplicated ventricular septal defect in infancy, heart failure is apt to develop as the pulmonary vascular resistance falls and pulmonary blood flow increases, with overfilling of the left atrium. Venting the left atrium by septostomy reduces the risk of pulmonary edema. The consequent left-to-right shunt at this level, together with relief of pulmonary congestion, usually improves the arterial oxygen saturation.

Children with transposition and large ventricular septal defects can develop pulmonary vascular obstruction remarkably early in life.[95] Although the mechanisms are not understood, they almost certainly have to do with the combination of high pulmonary-artery pressure, high pulmonary blood flow and high pulmonary venous pressure. It is possible, but unproven, that the high pulmonary-artery saturation or high hematocrit may also have something to do with this reaction. Most probably it is a combination of many of these associations.[121] Whatever the explanation, the pulmonary blood vessels must be protected in such children either by pulmonary-artery banding[162] or by radical correction before the development of irremediable pulmonary vascular obstruction. If atrial septostomy is not carried out first, pulmonary-artery banding alone, by reducing pulmonary blood flow and the return of blood to the left heart chambers, grossly curtails bidirectional shunt-ing. The resulting increase in cyanosis is often lethal; if it is not, the banding is prob-ably inadequate to protect the lung vessels.

Radical Correction in Simple Transposition without Pulmonary Stenosis

The results of surgical treatment of com-plete transposition have improved immeasur-ably since the adoption of the venous correc-tion procedure described by Mustard and his associates from Toronto in 1964.[1,34,36,71,90,106,107] This operation is technically easier to perform than the venous switch developed earlier by Senning.[134] In it the systemic and pulmonary venous return are transposed by the placement of an intra-atrial baffle after the atrial septum is removed. The baffle is placed within the resulting common atrium so that blood from the pulmonary veins en-tering posteriorly has access only to the tri-cuspid valve and right ventricle. Systemic venous blood returning through the superior and inferior venae cavae is retained pos-teriorly and conveyed behind venous con-duits to the mitral valve and left ventricle (Fig. 7).

Early problems with atrial dysrhythmias and conduction defects have led to some modifications in the technique. The sinus pacemaker must be carefully protected during the right atriotomy and superior vena caval cannulation. Secondly, the coronary sinus blood is permitted to enter the right ven-tricle with the pulmonary venous blood by placing the baffle to the left of it, thereby avoiding the atrioventricular node and main bundle.

Initially pericardium was used for the baffle; however, as pericardium thickens, contracts and even calcifies, nowadays Dacron is usually preferred. The atrial wall to which the baffle is sutured is thought to provide sufficient growing material to prevent future problems from inadequate atrial size.

It has been suggested that tricuspid re-gurgitation may also create problems. This fear seems groundless, however, as tricuspid regurgitation does not develop in other con-ditions in which right ventricular hyper-tension exists from birth (for example in the the Eisenmenger syndrome or untreated tetralogy of Fallot).

Results are now very good in patients with intact ventricular septa,[36,83] but in small in-fants and in patients with large ventricular septal defect or severe pulmonary stenosis the operative mortality rate is still high and the results are less favorable.

Using the Kyoto technique of profound hypothermia in the first year of life, Barratt-Boyes has had dramatic successs in the neonate and now advocates elective repair of complete transposition without septal de-fect.[9,10] When symptoms demand, he has operated on children with large ventricular septal defect in the neonatal period. Using conventional extracorporeal circulation with moderate hypothermia, the Mayo Clinic group have found a big difference in the mor-tality rate for the repair of transposition be-tween children above and below the age of two years.[36] They repaired 20 simple trans-positions without ventricular septal defect with the loss of only one patient in the older group. In the same age group, the mortality rate was 45 per cent in 40 patients with

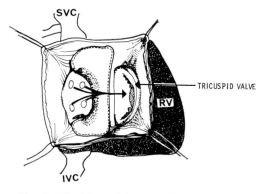

Fig. 7. The Mustard intra-atrial vein switch. The baffle is in place and the arrow shows how blood from the pulmonary veins posteriorly is directed over the baffle to the tricuspid valve. Blood from the SVC and IVC is channeled behind the baffle toward the mitral valve. The coronary-sinus ostium is retained in the arterial atrium.

transposition and large ventricular septal defect and/or severe pulmonary stenosis. Below the age of two years, three out of five patients with intact ventricular septum and no pulmonary stenosis survived, but all four patients with large ventricular septal defect or severe pulmonary stenosis died.

The timing of repair of simple transposition depends on a number of considerations. If a baby has been improved by atrial septostomy and the left ventricular pressure is low, then it is safe to postpone further correction until he has reached an age and weight where the surgical mortality is acceptable. Two circumstances demand early complete repair: the failure of adequate mixing despite a good septostomy, and a precipitous rise in pulmonary-artery pressure. Even with an intact ventricular septum, severe pulmonary vascular changes can occasionally occur as early as the first or second year of life. Since pulmonary vascular damage cannot be recognized until it has to some extent already happened, this risk has led to the adoption of elective repair in the first year at some centers. Serial cardiac catheterization is necessary to detect any rise in left ventricular pressure. If it is found, distinction must be made by pulmonary-artery catheterization between left ventricular outflow-tract obstruction at subvalvular level and pulmonary hypertension. A rise in left ventricular systolic pressure to half the systemic pressure or above, in the absence of pulmonary stenosis, implies an urgent need for early operation.

CORRECTION OF TRANSPOSITION WITH INTACT VENTRICULAR SEPTUM AND PULMONARY STENOSIS

This may be at valvular, subvalvular or combined valvular and subvalvular levels.[138] Significant pulmonary stenosis limits pulmonary blood flow and thus limits the benefits to be gained from atrial septostomy. When the stenosis is at valvular level, early repair by the Mustard technique can be carried out with pulmonary valvotomy through the pulmonary artery.[34] Stenosis at subvalvular level is a completely different problem. The type of stenosis closely resembles that in discrete subaortic stenosis: the mitral valve is intimately involved. Sometimes subvalvular narrowing is seen to appear and progress in patients with simple transposition who had no obstruction. This has been attributed to a bulging of the septum from the high-pressure right ventricle toward the low-pressure left ventricle (Fig. 8). By the time the left ventricular pressure has begun to rise as a result of the outflow-tract obstruction, septal hypertrophy and a fibromuscular bridge on the septum have rendered the obstruction permanent. If the peak systolic left ventricular-pulmonary gradient is less than 50 mm Hg, it can usually be safely ignored. If it is greater than 50 mm Hg, it is important but often impossible to alleviate surgically because of its diffuse muscular nature, the involvement of the mitral valve, the difficulties of access and danger of coronary damage. In such patients, as in those with an open ventricular septum and severe pulmonary stenosis, a Rastelli type of procedure may have to be the mode of final repair.[128] Until the child is big enough to accept an adult-sized prosthesis, a Blalock-Taussig aortopulmonary shunt is the preferred method of treatment. In all cases the placement of a shunt should be preceded by a Rashkind procedure.

RADICAL CORRECTION OF TRANSPOSITION WITH LARGE VENTRICULAR SEPTAL DEFECT

Before radical correction the status of the pulmonary vascular bed must be assessed with precision.[95] Since flows and resistances can vary independently in the two circuits, the Mayo Clinic workers believe that calculations of flow and resistance ratios can be misleading. They suggest that pulmonary arteriovenous difference is the best guide, but the margins for error can be small. Patients with a difference below 2.0 volumes per cent do not have severe pulmonary vascu-

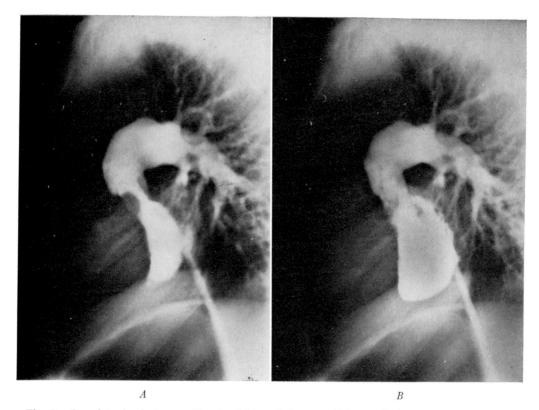

A   *B*

Fig. 8. Complete simple transposition in child aged 2 years. Left ventricular injection; lateral views. *A*: Systole. Septum bulging toward the low-pressure left ventricle and narrowing below the pulmonary valve outlined posteriorly by the anterior cusp of the mitral valve. *B*: Diastole. The narrowing of the left ventricular outflow tract is no longer visible.

lar disease and are certainly operable. A difference of 2.6 volumes per cent or more is indicative of severe pulmonary vascular disease precluding operation, and one between 2.0 and 2.5 volumes is "borderline." Patients in the operable range (when not anemic) have a pulmonary-artery oxygen saturation of 87 per cent or above. Correlation of degree of pulmonary vascular disease with pathology in fatal surgical cases showed that the 7 patients in the "operable" category by the above criteria showed Heath and Edwards changes[70] of grade 3 or less while the 4 patients with a pulmonary arteriovenous difference between 2.4 and 2.8 volumes per cent showed grade-4 changes, that is, "plexiform" dilatations indicating irreversible arteriolar disease.[79]

CORRECTION OF TRANSPOSITION OF THE GREAT ARTERIES WITH VENTRICULAR SEPTAL DEFECT AND PULMONARY STENOSIS

For children with transposition, a big ventricular septal defect (VSD) and pulmonary stenosis, neither heart failure nor profound cyanosis need develop because good mixing can occur at ventricular level. When pulmonary stenosis is more severe and hypoxemia is the problem, the arterial saturation can be improved by a Blalock-Taussig operation. The presence of pulmonary stenosis protects the lungs from the development of the pulmonary vascular obstructive changes which occur early in patients with transposition and VSD alone. When pulmonary stenosis is at valve level, closure of the ventricular communication and pulmonary valvotomy can be carried out at the same time as the Mustard procedure.

With mild or moderate pulmonary stenosis a Mustard procedure can be carried out as a first stage, leaving the VSD and pulmonary stenosis. The unfavorable bloodstreaming of uncorrected transposition is thereby corrected and improvement of arterial oxygen saturation is to be expected, leaving no pressing indications for completing surgical correction until the child is older and bigger. This method of management presupposes that the pulmonary stenosis will prove operable or sufficiently mild to leave uncorrected.

Although benefits can be gained from a systemic-pulmonary shunt in children with severe left ventricular outflow obstruction, marked cyanosis usually persists and later aortic homograft reconstruction of the right ventricular outflow tract with intracardiac correction of the aortic transposition will be needed, using the procedure of Rastelli[128] (Fig. 9, and see section on truncus arteriosus).

Repair of the ventricular septal defect with the creation of an intracardiac tunnel can be difficult. If the VSD is significantly smaller than the aortic orifice or even absent altogether, a sufficiently big VSD must be created by excising enough of the muscular interventricular septum to avoid left ventricular outflow-tract obstruction after the conduit is formed. In truncus arteriosus the VSD lies immediately below the trunk valve with no intervening tissue, whereas in transposition the VSD is usually separated from the aortic valve by the conus. When such a defect is also partially overhung by the tricuspid-valve septal cusp with the papillary muscle of the conus attached to its superior border,[77] the operation may be difficult.

Obviously the Rastelli technique is necessary only in patients with uncorrectable pulmonary outflow-tract obstruction. Such patients have thick-walled pressure-loaded left ventricles well adapted to sustaining the weight of the systemic circuit after correction. The Rastelli technique is inapplicable to patients with simple transposition in whom the left ventricle is a thin-walled low-pressure high-flow chamber, and thus poorly adapted to bearing a sudden systemic pressure load.

TRUNCUS ARTERIOSUS

Truncus arteriosus was not surgically correctable until successful application in 1967 of the reconstructive procedure developed by Rastelli at the Mayo Clinic.

In truncus arteriosus a single great artery or truncus leaves the heart through a single semilunar valve into which both ventricles empty through a high ventricular septal defect placed immediately beneath the truncus. The truncus receives blood from both ventricles and supplies blood to the coronary arteries and to both the pulmonary and systemic circulations. The embryology and anatomy of truncus arteriosus have recently

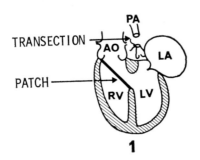
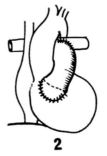
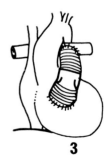

Fig. 9. The Rastelli operation. 1: A patch across the VSD connects the aortic root with the LV. The main pulmonary artery has been ligated and transected. 2 and 3: The completed operation from the front, showing an aortic homograft with anterior mitral cusp (2) and a Dacron graft with aortic homograft mounted in middle portion (3).

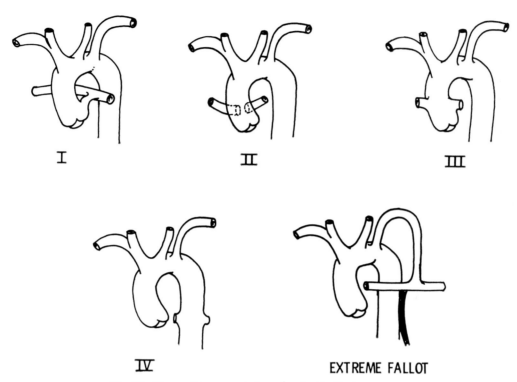

I   II   III

IV   EXTREME FALLOT

Fig. 10. Types of truncus arteriosus (see text). In the extreme
Fallot with pulmonary atresia a Blalock shunt is shown.

been described and clarified by De la Cruz[37]
and Van Praagh.[154]

The classification of Collett and Edwards
in 1949[29] has recently gained in virtue because the anatomical variations upon which
it was based now have important surgical
implications (Figs. 10 and 11):

Type 1: The truncus gives off a short main pulmonary artery which divides into right
and left pulmonary-artery branches.
Type 2: The right and left pulmonary arteries
arise independently from the *posterior*
wall of the truncus.
Type 3: The right and left pulmonary arteries
arise independently from the *lateral*
walls of the truncus.
Type 4: The pulmonary arteries are absent and
the ascending "truncus" gives rise only
to the coronary arteries. The arterial
supply to the lungs is from bronchial
arteries which arise from the descending aorta.

The total absence of pulmonary arteries in
type-4 truncus has led some to question the

propriety of the designation. Since no typical
truncus arteriosus resembling any of the
clinical types occurs at any stage in the development of the normal fetus and Van
Praagh has suggested that the so-called
truncus usually represents mainly an aortic
remnant,[154] this argument does not seem important. The main disadvantage is that
type-4 truncus is clinically different and
usually resembles pulmonary atresia with
VSD or an extreme Fallot's tetralogy in having a diminished pulmonary blood flow.

It would have been helpful to use the
term "pseudotruncus" to describe type 4,
but unfortunately this term has already been
applied (far less appropriately) to the most
severe form of Fallot's tetralogy with pulmonary atresia. At this extreme end of the
Fallot spectrum a main pulmonary artery
arises from the right ventricle but is im-
perforate either at or below the valve; the
main pulmonary artery may be represented

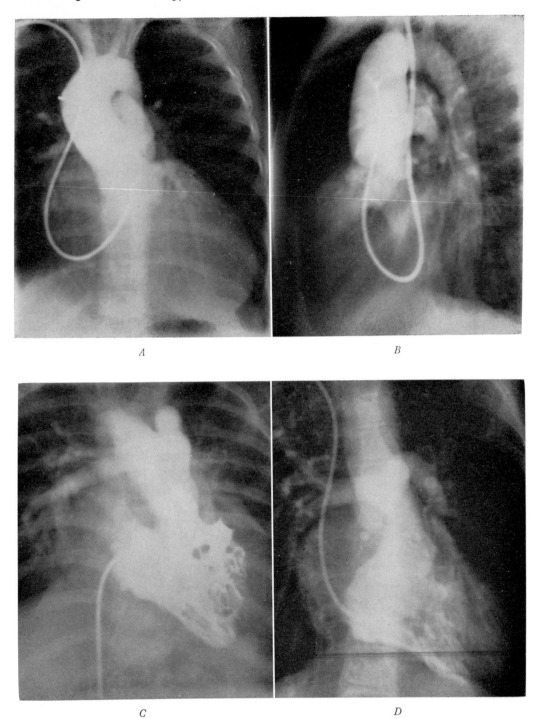

Fig. 11. Types of truncus arteriosus. *A*: Contrast injection into truncus type I (frontal view). *B*: Left lateral view of same patient. Posterior main pulmonary artery and complex quadricuspid truncal valve with some opacification of both ventricles due to reflux. *C*: RV injection frontal view, type I with rightward-turning arch. *D*: RV injection frontal view, type II.

merely by a fibrous thread. The main right and left pulmonary arteries are always present in this form of extreme tetralogy and they are supplied with blood either by systemic collaterals or by a Blalock-Taussig surgical anastomosis, rarely by a natural ductus (Fig. 10).

In type-4 truncus the main right and left pulmonary arteries are absent, as is the main stem pulmonary artery; enlarged bronchial arteries or other branches of the aorta convey blood direct to the intrapulmonary arteries of the lung. Type-4 truncus is therefore far less amenable to any sort of surgical aid, either palliative or radical, than is the extreme tetralogy with pulmonary atresia which can usually be corrected (Fig. 10).

Other variations of truncus occur:

Hemitruncus

The pulmonary artery to one lung derives from the right ventricle in the normal way and the pulmonary artery to the other lung comes from the ascending aorta.

Mixed Types

The pulmonary artery to one lung may be absent altogether, this lung being supplied by collateral vessels (half type 3 and half type 4).

Associated Anomalies

Truncus arteriosus may be associated with atresia, hypoplasia, coarctation or with total interruption of the aortic arch, in which case the descending aorta is filled through a large ductus arteriosus which forms an effective bypass between the ascending trunk and the descending aorta. Occasionally the ductus is small, causing a "coarctation," and occasionally tracheal compression is caused by the vascular ring thus formed. A right truncal arch is present in 20 to 25 per cent of reported cases.

Van Praagh pointed out that truncus arteriosus is not a form of transposition because (1) fibrous continuity between the truncal valve and the mitral valve is present in every case, and (2) single ventricle virtually never occurs in association with it. In most truncus valves there are only three cusps, as in the normal aortic valve. Occasionally the valve may be quadricuspid, bicuspid, or have six cusps, in which case cusp deformity and incompetence of the truncal valve are common (Fig. 11b). Rarely, the truncal valve may be stenosed.

Physiology

The physiological consequences of the condition depend upon the presence and size of the pulmonary artery and upon the resistance to flow through the lungs. Truncus arteriosus shares with transposition and total anomalous pulmonary venous drainage the diagnostically useful combination of cyanosis with increased pulmonary blood flow. Exact similarity between the saturations of the blood in the pulmonary arteries and the aorta is to be expected but is not invariably found. Especially in type-1 truncus the pulmonary arteries tend to receive a larger share of the blood from the right ventricle, and the saturation of aortic blood may exceed that of pulmonary-artery blood.

The pulmonary arteries are usually large. The pulmonary vascular resistance falls in infancy although it is high in the neonatal period. Excessive pulmonary blood flow results in pulmonary edema and congestive failure, but the systemic arterial saturation is relatively high. Banding of the pulmonary arteries may have to be considered. This carries a high mortality,[85,145] however, presumably because of the increased hypoxemia which inevitably results from banding the pulmonary arteries sufficiently tightly to influence pulmonary-artery pressure and also because of the contribution of truncal-valve incompetence[57] to heart failure. Excessive pulmonary blood flow at systemic pressure and perhaps the heart failure itself often lead to an early rise in pulmonary vascular resistance so that pulmonary blood flow falls, heart failure disappears but cyanosis increases and may even be recognized for the first time. Survival beyond infancy is thereby insured, and improvement can be quite abrupt. This may result in a favorable situation with the child clinically pink and virtually asymptomatic; when the pulmonary resistance rises higher, however, diminished pulmonary blood flow will be associated with deepening cyanosis.

A close correlation has been found between incompetence of the truncal valve and the development of heart failure in infancy.[57] This failure is not influenced by pulmonary-artery banding, and the early mortality is high. In the absence of severe truncal-valve incompetence, many babies with truncus arteriosus survive infancy. Mild reflux through the truncal valve is compatible with survival and need not interfere with subsequent radical surgery.

Natural stenosis at the origin of the pulmonary-artery branches from the truncus can in rare circumstances so regulate the pulmonary blood flow that heart failure is avoided. The narrowing can result in a lower pressure in the distal pulmonary arteries and pulmonary vascular disease will be less likely to develop.

In type-4 truncus blood flow to the lungs is usually small; in some instances, however, bronchial arteries may be large and supply the lungs with so much blood that cyanosis may be slight and heart failure may occur as in a typical truncus.[100] In other cases, although the bronchial arteries are large and profuse, there may be stenoses at the junction between the bronchial arteries and the lung vessels, giving rise to loud continuous murmurs over the lungs.[100,119]

Investigation of Patients With Truncus Arteriosus

In the laboratory investigation of a patient with a suspected truncus arteriosus, it is now much more important than it used to be to establish the exact anatomy of the truncus and to measure accurately the pulmonary blood flow and the pressure in each of the pulmonary arteries. Retrograde arterial catheterization, using a preshaped catheter, usually permits entry into each of the pulmonary arteries if the catheter fails to enter from the venous route and right ventricle. The unwarranted assumption of similar oxygen saturations in the pulmonary artery and aorta, when the pulmonary-artery saturation is in fact considerably lower, can result in the calculation of a falsely low pulmonary vascular resistance. This could lead to the submission for surgery of patients with inoperable severe pulmonary vascular obstruction. Retrograde "aortography" also aids recognition and quantitation of incompetence of the truncal valve. Mild regurgitation does not preclude surgery.

Some patients with type-4 truncus may be suitable for the Rastelli operation provided there is for each lung a bronchial or other systemic artery of sufficient size to serve as a distal end for the pulmonary-artery anastomosis. In such cases it is doubly important to cannulate each of the major relevant systemic arteries to the lungs and, if the pressure is identical to that in the aorta, to try to establish whether or not there is a stenosis at the point of junction with the pulmonary-artery radical. The lung in such patients may be served in part by arteries providing blood at high pressure and in part by a low-pressure perfusion through an obstructed systemic collateral vessel. It seems most unlikely that many patients with this type of anomaly will really prove amenable to complex surgical correction but, since no other operation is usually practicable, such patients should be investigated in detail.

The prognosis in truncus is dependent upon the anatomical type, the pulmonary-artery blood flow, the competence of the truncal valve and the availability of modern corrective surgery to that patient. Truncus is most lethal in the infant with truncal-valve incompetence or large pulmonary-artery branches and very high pulmonary blood flow. Improvement may follow treatment of heart failure, or may occur spontaneously from the unpredictable phenomenon of narrowing of the resistance vessels of the lungs. Surgical banding of large pulmonary arteries in the infant who may not otherwise survive possibly still is justified, but the surgical mortality is high.[59,162] The patient who survives infancy with a high pulmonary blood flow can expect reasonably normal activities during childhood, but these relatively asymptomatic patients benefit most from radical corrective surgery. The relatively low mortality of the corrective operation in childhood should stimulate vigorous efforts to keep infants and young children alive until they reach a size when the operation can be carried out.

Treatment of Truncus Arteriosus

Radical correction by the Rastelli operation or a modification of it is now possible and can be offered to patients provided that: (1) they have reached a reasonable size, and (2) they are free from severe pulmonary vascular obstructive disease. The operation has three parts[92,93] (Fig. 9):

1. The main pulmonary artery or right and left pulmonary-artery branches are separated from the truncus at their origins and the truncus, now the aorta, is repaired.
2. Through a circular ventriculotomy in a coronary-free portion of the anterior wall of the right ventricle, the ventricular septal defect is closed in such a way that the left ventricle communicates only with the aorta. In truncus this is often easier than in transposition because of the position of the VSD immediately under the truncus valve.
3. A long homograft of ascending aorta containing a mounted aortic homograft is inserted between the defect in the anterior wall of the right ventricle and the main pulmonary artery or arteries to form a new right ventricular outflow tract, pulmonary valve and main pulmonary artery.

Because of the difficulty in obtaining these long homografts and for other reasons, some surgeons now prefer to use a prosthetic conduit made of knitted Dacron with a valve-bearing area of woven Dacron containing the aortic homograft.

The new pulmonary valve can be placed either low down at the level of the right ventriculotomy or high up toward the junction of the graft with the patient's pulmonary artery. One of the difficulties of the operation can be closure of the sternum over the new right ventricular outflow tract. This protrudes anteriorly and distortion of the new valve can sometimes be best avoided by placing the pulmonary valve higher up the conduit toward the pulmonary arteries.

The operation has been attended by magnificent early results at the Mayo Clinic, where it was developed. McGoon and his colleagues recently reported that they had carried out 91 of these operations, 45 of them for the correction of truncus arteriosus and the others for transposition with pulmonary stenosis or pulmonary atresia. The operative mortality was only 10 per cent for patients aged between 5 and 12 years, but was 50 per cent for patients younger than 5 or older than 12.[92] It was suggested that operation be planned during the optimal age period whenever possible. Many children with truncus arteriosus will need surgery earlier, however, because they are developing pulmonary vascular obstructive disease which by the age of 5 years could preclude repair altogether. Because of the large size of the truncus arteriosus, children as young as 2 years have been submitted to the Rastelli procedure, with the successful placement of a graft sufficiently big to last for several years. Such children of course will need to have a new conduit fitted at least once during their growing period.

The problem of securing survival of the infant with a truncus arteriosus so that he can benefit later from corrective surgery remains. An 80 per cent mortality from pulmonary-artery banding is probably a worse alternative than leaving the infant to work out his own salvation under medical measures.

Long-term Results

Long-term results of the Rastelli procedure are still awaited, but the Mayo Clinic group have had only one late death and this was apparently unrelated to the heart disease. Calcification of the aortic homograft has been almost invariable, but this is not serious provided the calcification is restricted to the aorta and does not extend onto the cusps of the aortic homograft valve to cause pulmonary stenosis.

TOTAL ANOMALOUS PULMONARY VENOUS DRAINAGE

Total anomalous pulmonary venous drainage (TAPVD) accounts for between 1 and 4 per cent of cardiac malformations in the newborn.[43,131] About three quarters of children with TAPVD have died by the age of one year and only a very few survive to adult life without surgical correction.[19] Although this lethal condition is eminently curable, the high mortality has only recently improved.[30,60] Application of the Japanese technique of deep hypothermia with total circulatory arrest has been associated with a dramatic change in the surgical results,[40] but another essential prerequisite for surgical success is early diagnosis.[55] The early problems of recognition which led to late referral and late treatment are clear in published series, where the diagnosis was proved at autopsy rather than by hemodynamic studies and surgery.

In TAPVD the pulmonary veins are con-nected to the systemic venous system instead of to the left atrium. The malformation may occur alone (most frequently) or in association with other complex anomalies. Out of 75 children with TAPVD seen at the Hospital for Sick Children, Great Ormond Street, London, 58 had no other cardiac defects, yet only 25 per cent of these survived infancy;[14] of the 15 per cent discovered in the neonatal period, none survived. The experience at the Children's Hospital in Boston was similar, 60 per cent of 75 children having no other major defects but many exhibiting cyanosis within the first month and most developing heart failure within the first three months of life.[55] These facts dictate the need for an aggressive diagnostic and surgical approach. Most patients are of normal birth weight but few gain thereafter. Only 5 of the 39 Boston patients who survived to three months of age were above the tenth percentile for weight.

In TAPVD the pulmonary veins usually come together to form a common channel before making their abnormal anatomical attachment. Neill divided TAPVD into three groups: intracardiac, supracardiac and infracardiac (Fig. 12).[110]

In the intracardiac type the pulmonary

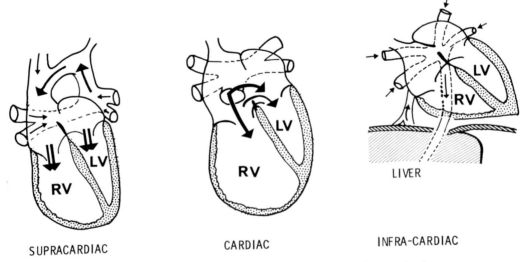

SUPRACARDIAC   CARDIAC   INFRA-CARDIAC

Fig. 12. Total anomalous pulmonary venous drainage (see text). In the "cardiac" type shown drainage is into the coronary sinus.

veins are connected directly to the right atrium or enter the coronary sinus. In the common supracardiac type the pulmonary veins are connected to a left vertical vein (often incorrectly referred to as a left superior vena cava) which drains into the left innominate vein (Fig. 13). In the infracardiac type all pulmonary veins travel below the diaphragm to join the portal vein or one of its radicals. This type is lethal in the neonate because severe obstruction to pulmonary venous return is invariably present. This obstruction is largely caused by the sheer length of the common pulmonary vein, but the vein may also be kinked as it passes through the diaphragm to join a branch of the portal vein. In some children TAPVD may be mixed: the pulmonary veins from the left lung may join to drain into the left vertical vein and the pulmonary veins from the right lung may drain into the superior vena cava or right atrium.

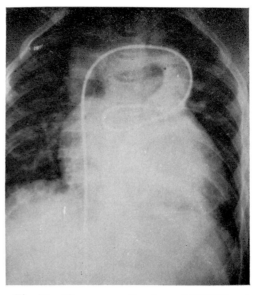

Fig. 13. The supracardiac form of TAPVD. A venous catheter from the leg has been passed up the SVC into the left innominate, down the vertical vein and into the confluence of the pulmonary veins. Contrast was injected into the origin of the vertical vein.

Physiology

In TAPVD all the venous return comes to the right side of the heart, and the left-sided chambers are filled only by means of a right-to-left shunt through an intra-atrial communication. This is often only a patent foramen ovale and, if it is small, flow to the left atrium could theoretically be obstructed, left ventricular output seriously curtailed. The importance of obstruction to blood flow at the foramen ovale has been the subject of considerable discussion in relation to the improvement likely to be achieved by a balloon septostomy.

Since the pulmonary venous blood joins with systemic venous blood at or before the right atrium, the oxygen saturation tends to be similar in all four chambers of the heart and in the two great arteries. Cyanosis may be clinically undetectable if the pulmonary blood flow is high in uncomplicated TAPVD, but is invariable in children who are in trouble with pulmonary hypertension and heart failure. It is surprising that complete mixing of the venous streams sometimes does

not occur, and streaming can be particularly marked in TAPVD to the coronary sinus. In this type the highly oxygenated coronary sinus blood may pass preferentially through the nearby tricuspid valve while the poorly oxygenated caval bood flows preferentially through the atrial communication to the left side of the heart (Fig. 12). The deep cyanosis of such patients despite a high pulmonary blood flow mimics transposition and can give rise to diagnostic difficulty. The distinction can, however, be made rapidly with angiography.

Pulmonary venous obstruction (PVO) is very common in most infants with TAPVD[55] and is invariable in the infracardiac type. In any type the common pulmonary vein may be stenotic at the site of its abnormal systemic connection, and in the common supracardiac type the vertical vein can be pinched as it ascends between the left main bronchus and the pulmonary artery.

Pulmonary arterial hypertension in TAPVD is common and it is often severe at an early age.[88] It has several apparently causal associations (but as in other forms of congenital heart disease its mechanism is not fully understood). These are: (1) elevated pulmonary venous pressure, (2) increased pulmonary blood flow, (3) hypoxemia and metabolic acidosis secondary to heart failure and a low systemic blood flow.

Severe early intimal proliferation and medial hypertrophy have been demonstrated in the pulmonary arterioles of some of these children.[88] A severe degree of pulmonary arterial hypertension has been shown to affect adversely both the natural course of the anomaly and the operative mortality.

Inadequate size or "stenosis" of the foramen ovale could result in left ventricular starvation with a low systemic cardiac output. Whether from this cause or not, underdevelopment of the left side of the heart has been invoked as a cause of high operative mortality including postoperative pulmonary edema. However, Cooley and his associates in Houston recorded a relatively normal systemic cardiac output prior to correction and reasoned that the left heart should therefore be able to maintain a normal cardiac output after repair.[30] Their view was upheld recently by Gomes and his colleagues from the Mayo Clinic, who found that postoperative acute pulmonary edema was uncommon after one-stage correction.[61]

Diagnosis

The clinical features of TAPVD in the infant have been emphasized recently.[55]

PULMONARY VENOUS OBSTRUCTION

Infants have signs of pulmonary hypertension with a relatively small heart, no murmurs, a low cardiac output and eventually severe right ventricular failure. Contrary to frequent statements, normal respiratory variation of the second heart sound is usual, being noted in 52 of 75 patients in Boston, but the pulmonary component tends to be loud.[55] In those patients with severe pulmonary venous obstruction (PVO), particularly when it is subdiaphragmatic, the heart is of normal size but diffuse pulmonary venous congestion gives the lungs a ground-glass appearance radiographically. The apparent lack of signs of cardiac abnormality sometimes delays referral and leads to a mistaken diagnosis of respiratory distress syndrome (despite clinical context). The radiographic picture of the severe pulmonary edemous obstruction with a normal-sized heart is seen not only when anomalous drainage is subdiaphragmatic but is compatible with obstructed drainage at any level; the site must be determined. Precordial scintillation scanning may prove to be useful in these particularly sick infants but is not yet widely available.[161]

Cardiac catheterization is therefore still usually important, even when the diagnosis is known or strongly suspected, in order to demonstrate the site of connection of the pulmonary vein. This is usually easily done, as a high oxygen saturation in hepatic venous blood, blood from the left innominate vein, or coronary sinus blood is rapidly established and is virtually diagnostic of the site of entry of the pulmonary veins. Selective injection of contrast medium into the pulmonary artery usually shows the anatomical mode of anomalous connection in the venous phase, but injection directly into the chamber which receives the common pulmonary vein is preferable when this can be done. The investigator is tempted to inject excessive amounts of contrast material because of the great dilution which is to be expected, but the dangers of large doses of contrast have recently been emphasized.[148]

Recognition of obstruction at the atrial septum is easy if the right atrial pressure exceeds that in the left atrium, but the absence of such a pressure gradient does not exclude the possibility because of the greater size and distensibility of the right atrium compared with the left. In cases of doubt, the diagnostic procedure should be followed directly with a therapeutic one by the passage of a Rashkind balloon septostomy catheter through the

foramen to enlarge the hole.[135] This maneuver can be difficult and potentially
hazardous because of the relatively small size
of the left atrium compared with the right,
and particularly difficult if the right atrial
pressure is high: the septum will then bulge
toward the left atrium. In babies with subdiaphragmatic drainage, the maneuver is
unlikely to be helpful because the main problem is severe obstruction to the common
pulmonary vein.

ABSENCE OF PULMONARY VENOUS OBSTRUCTION

Here the clinical picture is quite different.
Pulmonary blood flow is excessive, cyanosis is
not obvious and, although congestive heart
failure can appear early, it may be delayed
or not appear at all. Those few children in
whom symptoms may be absent even into
childhood are included in this group. In
marked contrast to those with PVO, they
show a pulmonary ejection systolic murmur,
a tricuspid diastolic flow murmur and a
gallop rhythm which may sound quadruple
because of wide splitting of the second heart
sound. Sometimes a continuous murmur is
heard over the anomalous venous trunk, but
its presence does not necessarily indicate
stenosis at the venous connection site. Most
of these patients have supracardiac TAPVD
but the distension of the supracardiac veins
which gives the well-known "snowman"
contour to the cardiac silhouette is usually
absent in the newborn, does not develop until 3 to 6 months of age or later and is then
easily missed because of its relative lack of
density compared with the heart shadow.
Where such a contour is thought to be present
in infants with this anomaly, it is usually the
result of thymic enlargement rather than of
distended systemic veins.

Treatment

Emergency surgical correction should be
arranged whenever the infradiaphragmatic
type of TAPVD is recognized or when the
PVO is severe. Patients without PVO can
usually be managed medically, especially
when there is a significant gradient between
the right ventricle and pulmonary artery.

In infants less than a year old who have
intractable congestive heart failure, surgical
treatment is needed if they are to survive.
Atrial septostomy has been associated with
alleviation of the heart failure in some cases,
the improvement being attributed to an increase in left atrial and ventricular filling
with a decrease in flow to the lungs and in
pulmonary arterial pressure.[135] It therefore
seems appropriate to consider balloon septostomy in all symptomatic infants with this
diagnosis at the time of initial cardiac
catheterization. If the patient has a good
response with resolution of the congestive
heart failure, a total corrective procedure can
be delayed until the age of 3 to 5 years when
it can be accomplished at a lower risk.
Prompt operative correction is indicated if a
good response is not obtained by balloon
septostomy.

Staged surgical procedures, designed to
leave a vent for the left atrium to prevent
postoperative pulmonary edema, have not
appreciably reduced the infant mortality
rate[107] and the need for a second operative
procedure obviously makes for additional
risks. Gomes and his colleagues attributed
their relative success to care in avoiding obstruction to the pulmonary veins during
operation by immediate opening of the common venous trunk after institution of bypass.
These workers favor a one-stage procedure
using cardiopulmonary bypass with moderate
hypothermia.[61] The operative mortality is
closely correlated to age, being high in
children younger than one year. Other
adverse factors are a high pulmonary-
artery pressure and a systemic arterial oxygen
saturation below 80 per cent. Using deep
hypothermia with surface cooling and total
circulatory arrest, Dillard and his colleagues
were the first to report successful results in
young, critically ill infants. Four such children weighing between 3.7 and 6.5 kg survived the operation.[40]

Survivors of complete correction of TAPVD

have excellent relief of symptoms, they can usually be regarded as cured and their outlook for the future is good.

VENTRICULAR SEPTAL DEFECT (VSD)

New knowledge and persisting problems in ventricular septal defect can be considered under the following headings:

1. Incidence and Recognition
   In infancy
   Incomplete diagnosis
   Associated anomalies.
2. Natural History
   Prognosis of VSD in infancy
   Spontaneous closure
   Prognosis of VSD beyond infancy
   Infective endocarditis
   Complications of big defects
     Aortic regurgitation
     Pulmonary vascular obstruction.
3. Natural History Modified by Treatment
   Management of the infant
   Indications for VSD closure beyond infancy
   Surgical sequelae.

Incidence of Ventricular Septal Defect and Recognition in Infancy

Isolated ventricular septal defect (VSD) is the most common congenital cardiac anomaly at birth;[22] it accounts for 30 per cent of all cardiac abnormalities at this time, about 2 per 1,000 live births.[72,73]

The incidence of VSD in premature babies may be four or five times higher than the incidence in full-term babies, but there seems to be no difference in the frequency or age of development of symptoms between premature and full-term babies with VSD.[72]

Recognition of VSD in the newborn may be long delayed or absent. The reasons have been previously explained: lack of obvious cyanosis, early absence of a murmur, the prevalence of "nonspecific" signs such as failure to gain weight and recurrent respiratory infections, and failure to appreciate the significance of tachypnea, inspiratory recession and excessive sweating.

Recent work has shown that the failure to gain weight is caused both by poor feeding and by the high metabolic cost of breathing.

Tachypnea, sternal elevation with intercostal recession and repeated infections result from overfilled, edematous and incompliant lungs. Increased sweating is necessary for adequate dissipation of heat by an organism with a high metabolic rate but low cutaneous blood flow. The increased sympathetic drive which maintains systemic blood pressure through vasoconstriction is responsible also for the excessive sweating.[109]

INCOMPLETE DIAGNOSIS

VSD may be associated with other defects or may exist as part of a more complex anomaly: atrial septal defect, pulmonary stenosis, patent ductus arteriosus or discrete subaortic stenosis. Neither the signs nor the hemodynamic consequences of the other anomaly are likely to be obscured when the VSD is a small one, but surgical disaster can follow failure to recognize a complicated VSD. Whenever a big VSD is diagnosed, it is necessary to exclude: (1) associated conditions, (2) unusual or multiple VSDs, and (3) more complex anomalies.

1. Associated conditions:
   Patent ductus arteriosus
   Preductal coarctation or actual interruption of the aortic arch
   Abnormalities of the mitral valve or left ventricle.
2. Unusual or multiple defects:
   Multiple muscular defects: "Swiss cheese septum"
   Total absence of the muscular septum: "incomplete common ventricle"
   Supracristal or bulboventricular defect.
3. VSD as part of a complex anomaly:
   Double-outlet right ventricle
   Single ventricle
   Ventricular inversion: "corrected transposition"
   Truncus arteriosus.

Aortography in the lateral or slight left anterior oblique projection should always be included in the investigation of any big VSD in order to recognize or exclude patent ductus arteriosus, coarctation, transposition, truncus arteriosus and abnormalities of the aortic root.

Patent Ductus Arteriosus

There may be an early diastolic murmur (EDM). With pulmonary vascular obstruction, the pulmonary circuit is filled at ventricular level and very little further shunting occurs at aortopulmonary level. In the diagnosis of an EDM accompanying VSD, aortic or pulmonary incompetence and pulmonary-artery branch stenosis must be considered. The last causes a systolic murmur which spills over into early diastole but its wide transmission over the lungs should cause suspicion.

Preductal Coarctation

Preductal coarctation and total interruption of the aortic arch give rise to similar physiological faults. Although in infancy preductal coarctation is common and readily suspected (by the early development of severe heart failure associated with variable femoral pulses which come and go), when the condition appears beyond infancy the femoral pulses are usually neither small nor delayed and both the coarctation and the patent ductus may be clinically silent.[143] In infancy the variability of the femoral pulses is attributable to lability of the pulmonary vascular resistance. When the left atrium becomes overfilled the pulmonary resistance rises; the right ventricle sends more blood to the feet, and so the femoral pulses appear. Then the pulmonary edema lessens so the pulmonary resistance falls, the proportion of right ventricular blood going to the lungs increases and the femoral pulses become impalpable again.

Beyond infancy the presence of a preductal coarctation complex may be suspected when catheterization reveals a left-to-right shunt at ventricular level but femoral-artery desaturation. The presence of the right-to-left shunt at aortopulmonary level may be missed if the systemic arterial sample is taken from the upper limb only.

Right ventriculography will show opacification of the descending aorta without opacification of the ascending aorta, but only aortography reveals the anatomy of the coarctation.

Before the VSD can be closed, the coarctation must be corrected and the ductus ligated. Absence of a collateral circulation around the coarctation site necessitates left atriofemoral bypass to maintain the integrity of the spinal cord if the duct is clamped first; this is not necessary if the duct can be retained until the coarctation has been dealt with.

Abnormalities of the Mitral Valve or Left Ventricle in VSD

Left ventricular (LV) outflow-tract obstruction caused by discrete subaortic stenosis or, less often, by aortic-valve stenosis or simple coarctation can be responsible for a persistent left-to-right shunt despite a very high pulmonary vascular resistance.

Mitral-valve abnormality (either congenital mitral regurgitation or obstruction at or above the mitral valve) may also be missed clinically. An apical pansystolic murmur or excessive left ventricular loading disproportionate to the size of the left-to-right shunt in a patient with a high pulmonary resistance may give the clue to a mitral leak. A disproportionate apical mid-diastolic bruit may similarly give away mitral obstruction.[75]

The site and size of a VSD are best determined by retrograde LV angiography in a slight left anterior oblique projection 20 to 30° from lateral, which puts the septum in profile. Especially if cineangiography is used the margins of the defect or the presence of more than one defect can be defined. Absence or fenestration of the muscular septum is suspected when the VSD seems to extend down to the inferior border of the right ventricle (the toe of the LV extends further down and may give a false impression that a septum exists) (Fig. 14).

A VSD in the endocardial cushion region is best suspected from the electrocardiogram (ECG) but cannot be distinguished angiographically from the more usual type of infracristal defect. Isolated VSD of this type is associated with neither mitral regurgitation

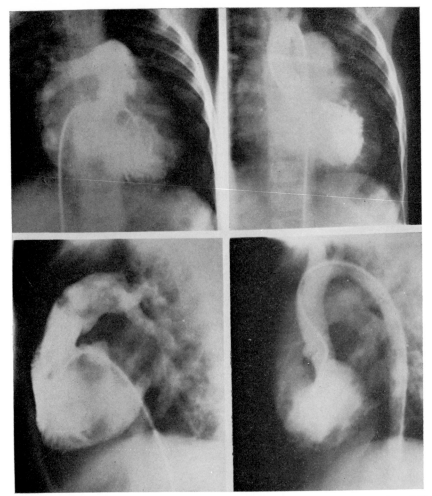

Fig. 14. Total infracristal VSD (incomplete common ventricle). RV injection on the left; LV injection on the right. Frontal views above and lateral below. *Below left*: Outline of the aortic cusp is seen. *Below right*: Broad band of contrast leaving the LV is limited above by the crista but below only at the apex of the ventricle. This huge defect was successfully patched (girl aged 5 years).

nor deformity of the LV outflow tract. The ECG shows left anterior hemiblock but usually no right bundle branch block.

A defect in the membranous septum between the LV and right atrium or associated with tricuspid regurgitation is suspected from evidence of a shunt also at atrial level; LV angiography in the frontal view proves this if right atrial opacification is seen.

A supracristal VSD is best recognized in a frontal or slight right anterior oblique projection when the defect is seen to enter the infundibulum of the right ventricle just below

the pulmonary valve. The resulting dilatation of the infundibulum may be visible on plain films. In the usual left anterior oblique view LV angiogram the margins of the defect are not seen in contrast to infracristal VSD. This poor definition, together with instant opacification of the pulmonary artery without prior filling of the body of the right ventricle, indicates a supracristal VSD. Aortography frequently shows aortic regurgitation into both ventricles with deformity of a prolapsed right coronary cusp (Fig. 15).

A "bulboventricular" defect is teardrop

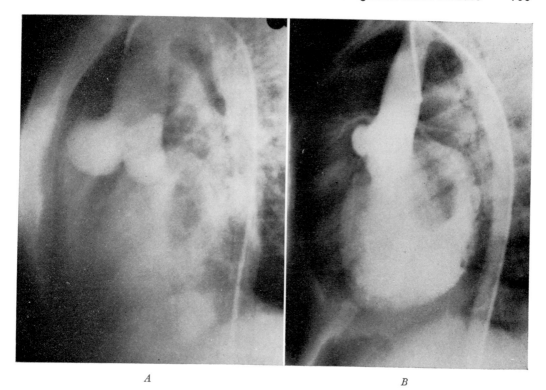

A   B

Fig. 15. VSD with aortic regurgitation and prolapsed right coronary cusp. Aortograms left lateral view. A: Supracristal VSD. B: Infracristal VSD. The deformity and angulation of the prolapsed cusp is easily recognized. The gross aortic regurgitation shown in B was corrected by closure of the VSD alone. (Reproduced with permission from Thorax.)

shaped, involving both the posteroinferior and anterosuperior portions of the septum. The crista is "split" by the defect and hypoplastic. The narrow end of the defect extends to the pulmonary-valve ring.

Double-outlet Right Ventricle (DORV)

This defect of the infracristal type without right ventricular outflow-tract obstruction need not differ physiologically from an uncomplicated big VSD. Although the aortic root arises anteriorly from the right ventricle, the valve approximates to the VSD during ventricular contraction; thus the LV empties mainly into the aorta during systole, with the spillover into the RV providing shunted blood in systole and diastole. RV blood is channelled solely into the pulmonary artery

and cyanosis is absent. Usually the VSD is big; if it is not as big as the aortic valve, however, LV outflow-tract obstruction results.[86] DORV can be suspected if the systolic murmur of VSD is transmitted into the neck and the ECG may show left-axis deviation of the mean frontal QRS. The diagnosis is made from an LV angiogram in the right anterior oblique view, which best shows the lack of continuity between the anterior mitral cusp and aortic root and the forward displacement of the aorta. Intracardiac repair with a patch to connect the aorta only with the LV through the VSD is not difficult, provided the surgeon recognizes the condition. Sometimes the VSD may first need to be enlarged in order to relieve or to avoid LV outflow stenosis[86] or to relieve pulmonary stenosis.[61]

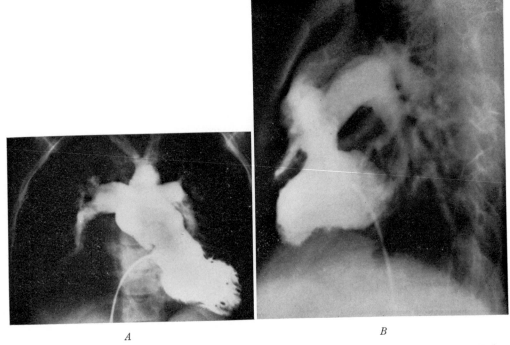

A   *B*

Fig. 16. Single ventricle, common type, with absent RV. The aorta arises anteriorly from the infundibulum which is connected to the LV by a "bulboventricular foramen." The pulmonary artery arises from the LV which receives both atrioventricular valves. Pulmonary blood flow is excessive. *A*: Frontal view, *B*: lateral view.

Single Ventricle

Here transposition of the aorta is almost invariable, but a high pulmonary blood flow can result in lack of detectable clinical cyanosis. In the most common variety the aorta arises from the infundibulum but the remainder of the right ventricle is absent. The big LV receives blood from both atrioventricular valves or a common atrioventricular valve. Blood enters the aorta via the infundibulum through an anteriorly placed "bulboventricular foramen" which is sometimes stenotic (Fig. 16). Preliminary diagnosis can be made by echocardiography. Only palliative treatment is possible and pulmonary-artery banding inevitably leads to an increase in cyanosis. Patients with moderate pulmonary stenosis or moderate increase in pulmonary vascular resistance can live for many years.

Corrected Transposition (Fig. 4)

This is usually but not invariably associated with a VSD.[139] The arterial ventricle may be hypoplastic with an incompetent atrioventricular valve. Clinical diagnosis of the presence of ventricular inversion is usually possible from the ECG, which shows Q waves in V_1 with absence of Q in V_5 and V_6, sometimes complete heart block but with narrow complexes, and a near-normal ventricular rate. The chest radiograph nearly always shows a bulge on the left heart border which is usually high, caused by the levoposed ascending aorta. Occasionally the bulge is at left ventricular level, caused by a misplaced or enlarged left atrial appendage and likely to be misdiagnosed as due to ventricular enlargement. Pulmonary stenosis may coexist at valvular or subvalvular level. As in d-transposition, the latter is hard to correct.

Ventricular angiography with injection into the venous ventricle reveals an elliptical smooth-walled anteroinferior ventricle which is readily recognizable as a morphological left ventricle. The arterial ventricle is posterosuperior and coarsely trabeculated, resembling a right ventricle; the aorta arises from its infundibulum to the left of the pulmonary artery and anterior to or beside the pulmonary artery in the lateral view. This ventricle may be hypoplastic or absent except for its infundibulum. In the lateral view the great arteries are seen to "cross over," the aorta passing forward and the pulmonary artery diving backward. This view also best shows the odd plane of the interventricular septum.

Surgical repair of VSD in corrected transposition has carried a high mortality because of: (1) failure to recognize single ventricle, hypoplasia of the arterial ventricle or incompetence of its atrioventricular valve, (2) difficulties of access because of the abnormal coronary distribution, and (3) the induction of heart block. With recognition of these problems, there seems to be no reason why VSDs in carefully selected cases should not be successfully corrected in the future.

Natural History

PROGNOSIS OF VSD IN INFANCY

Only a small proportion of babies with VSD develop symptoms. Hoffman and Rudolph found 10 of 62 (15 per cent) were seriously affected[72] and Ash in a clinical series found that 21 per cent of 165 infants showed evidence of trouble.[5]

The mortality of VSD during infancy may average 0.2 per 1,000 live births, or 10 per cent.[73,102] Earlier series have often quoted a higher figure, but this is probably because many children in whom the VSD had closed spontaneously had never been diagnosed. Since the typical murmur of VSD usually does not appear before the end of the first week, many babies with this defect may be discharged from an obstetric unit without the

suspicion of congenital heart disease having been aroused. Hoffman and Rudolph found that the typical systolic murmur had been heard during the first week in only 23 of 31 infants with VSD among a consecutive series of babies all of whom had been followed carefully from birth.[72] They also found that 10 of these VSDs closed spontaneously before one year of age; if they had not been detected prior to closure, the estimated mortality rate of VSD in their series would have been 4 out of 21 (19 per cent) instead of 4 out of 31 (13 per cent).[73]

Not only is the harsh pansystolic murmur of VSD rarely audible within the first week, but heart failure is uncommon before the second week. Often the first symptoms appear even later, at the end of the first month. Onset is explained by the gradual increase in pulmonary vascular capacity which ensues after a delayed fall in fetal resistance to flow through the lungs. Low output failure and pulmonary edema may supervene consequent upon too great a diversion of left ventricular blood through a big VSD into the lungs.

The babies who get into difficulty have higher pulmonary blood flows, larger pulmonary systemic blood-flow ratios and higher pulmonary-artery pressures than asymptomatic babies, and the height of the left atrial pressure showed a positive correlation both with pulmonary blood flow and with the presence of symptoms.[72]

Most symptomatic infants with big VSDs improve under medical management, although some will die, usually before the end of the first year. Survival can be aided in a number of ways. Some improve with real or relative decrease in the size of the defect or even complete closure. Ash found that half of 18 infants who survived congestive failure had normal or only slightly raised pulmonary-artery pressure when subsequently submitted to cardiac catheterization.[5]

Clinical improvement may also occur despite a persistently big defect. The development of muscular outflow-tract obstruction at infundibular level can cut down pulmonary-artery pressure and flow into the lungs.[54] Rarely, this becomes severe enough to cause reversal of the shunt with development of cyanosis—the so-called acquired tetralogy of Fallot. More commonly, pulmonary blood flow is cut down by the development of pulmonary vascular obstructive changes.[2,78,159]

Spontaneous Closure

Spontaneous closure of the ventricular septal defect was first suggested in 1918 by Parkes Weber in a paper entitled "Can the clinical manifestations of congenital heart disease disappear with the general growth and development of the patient?,"[120] and also specifically in the same year by French in Guy's Hospital Gazette in a paper entitled "The possibility of a loud congenital heart murmur disappearing when a child grows up."[50] The first patient to be fully documented by cardiac catheterization was reported by Azevedo in Acta Cardiologia, Brussels,[6] and in 1960 Evans, Rowe and Keith first presented evidence that spontaneous closure may indeed be a frequent occurrence.[49]

Spontaneous closure of VSD is now known to be common in infancy,[3,13,17,21,72, 81,101,102,157] and between 25 and 50 per cent of VSDs present at birth close completely or almost completely.[72,89] Many but not all of these closures occur during infancy. No difference has been found in the incidence of spontaneous closure between premature and full-term infants with VSD; children who were born prematurely continue to have a higher incidence. Spontaneous closure may be achieved by fibrous proliferation or by adherence of a right ventricular muscle bundle such as the moderate band. Less commonly, the septal cusp of the tricuspid valve may overlie the defect and adhere to it.[45,141]

All cases of isolated VSD registered between 1950 and 1965 were reviewed at the Hospital for Sick Children in Toronto—a total of 1,513 cases, of whom 633 had had cardiac catheterization (95 per cent of the clinical diagnoses being subsequently confirmed in those who were catheterized).[89] The incidence of spontaneous closure was found to be about 25 per cent. Nearly 90 per cent of the 190 VSDs which subsequently closed had done so by the age of 8 years, and the majority closed before 3 years of age. The oldest patient was between 16 and 21 years at the time of spontaneous closure.

Small defects close most frequently, but big defects may also close. In Hoffman and Rudolph's infant series defects closed or became smaller in 32 of 62 (52 per cent), and this included 8 closures among 35 babies with big defects.[72] Keith's group in Toronto found that 13 (7 per cent) of patients whose defects ultimately closed had been in congestive heart failure at some time during infancy.

Epidemiological and autopsy studies suggest that there is a significant incidence of anatomical closure of VSD even later in life. Ventricular septal defect constitutes only 7 per cent of congenital cardiac defects in adults, compared with 20 per cent in children (and 30 per cent at birth). This difference cannot be explained by childhood mortality. In Minnesota 1,603 adult bodies between 39 and 90 years were examined postmortem for evidence of spontaneous VSD closure. No history suggesting VSD had been elicited in any of the patients, but definite evidence of a previous VSD which had closed spontaneously was found in 7 (an incidence of one in 225 necropsies).[141] Closure had been achieved by a plug of dense fibrous tissue in 5 of the cases and by adherence of the septal cusp of the tricuspid valve in 2. In these latter cases, the possibility that the closure represented the mode of healing of infective endocarditis was suggested.

Spontaneous closure of the VSD has also been reported to occur after banding of the pulmonary artery[44,160] and when the VSD was physiologically advantageous in tricuspid atresia and double-outlet right ventricle.[125]

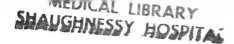

PROGNOSIS OF VSD BEYOND INFANCY:
A CONTINUING FALL IN THE NUMBERS

The majority of deaths in children with VSD were found by Hoffman to be due to prematurity, gastroenteritis or other malformations, rather than to the VSD per se.[73] He and others have concluded that death due to VSD is not common in childhood.[81,104,159] Hoffman found 35 instances of VSD in autopsy data from 141,057 persons over 20 years, a prevalence rate of 0.31 per 1,000, so death from VSD is equally uncommon in adults. The difference between the death rate in infancy (0.22 per 1,000) plus the death rate in adults (0.31 per 1,000) and the overall incidence of VSD at birth (2 per 1,000) could represent the disappearance of VSD at a rate of about 1.5 per 1,000 from largely unrecognized spontaneous closures. The usual estimated prevalence in young schoolchildren is only 1 per 1,000,[69,105] and a further difference in the prevalence of VSD between younger and older schoolchildren[103] is also consistent with the view that spontaneous closure may occur frequently throughout childhood.

Hoffman cites other evidence of a high spontaneous closure rate of VSD in children of school age.[73] Since about 40 per cent of all children born with congenital heart disease die before the time of school entry and the mortality rate for VSD in this period lies between 10 and 20 per cent, the proportion of VSDs in the surviving children with congenital heart disease should be higher than it is at birth. At birth there are 300 children with VSD among every 1,000 infants with congenital heart disease; 400 of these 1,000 will be dead by five years, but only 30 to 60 of the children with VSD will have died. Consequently, among the 600 survivors with congenital heart disease there should be 240 to 270 VSDs, and by five years of age 40 to 45 per cent of all children with congenital heart disease should have VSDs—nearly 3 per 1,000 instead of the 1 per 1,000 actually found.

The physiological consequences of isolated ventricular septal defect depend upon the size of the defect and the pulmonary vascular resistance. A small defect causes little or no functional disturbance and the pressures in the right heart are normal.[132] With a larger interventricular communication, the left-to-right shunt increases, but with little or no change in pulmonary-artery pressure. In such patients the physiological derangement is essentially due to volume overload of the left ventricle.

For small VSDs, the risks are few[130] and there is no evidence that a low pulmonary-artery pressure associated with a small VSD tends to rise in later life.[4] Atrial fibrillation is less common than in adult patients with atrial septal defect, except in patients with a shunt into the right atrium. Because of this and a possible risk of progressive tricuspid regurgitation, this type of defect should usually be closed.

Bloomfield postulated that a defective septum, whether open or spontaneously closed, may adversely affect left ventricular function;[13] this has not been verified. No evidence of left ventricular dysfunction has been found in children investigated after successful closure of VSD, nor has otherwise unexplained left ventricular failure been seen in older patients with small VSDs. There is therefore no reason to anticipate the late advent of heart failure in the older patient with a small VSD, nor that the acquired diseases of aging will be any less well tolerated.

A large defect results in obligatory equilibration of systolic pressure in the two ventricles which behave physiologically as a common chamber. Blood is ejected into the systemic and pulmonary circuits at the same pressure. The amount of flow depends upon the relative vascular resistances in the two circuits. A low pulmonary vascular resistance results in a high pulmonary blood flow and even in deprivation of systemic blood flow.

In children with big VSDs, the high neonatal pulmonary vascular resistance may regress normally after a slight delay compared with the normal, it may regress incompletely, or it may increase again after an initial complete or partial regression.[112]

Even when a VSD is initially big there is a strong tendency for the pulmonary blood flow and pulmonary-artery pressure to decline during the first few years of life, and this tendency may continue well beyond this period.[4] These changes probably result from a relative decrease in size of the defect due to differential growth, and they are accompanied by a fall in pulmonary vascular resistance.

The life expectancy of the adult with a big VSD is limited. Pulmonary vascular obstruction is usually progressive. In those with a persisting high pulmonary flow, heart failure may be seen between the ages of 25 and 40 years; such patients are rarely seen, however. On very rare occasions a high pulmonary vascular resistance may literally persist from the neonatal period, so that a bidirectional or right-to-left shunt (the Eisenmenger complex) is established in infancy. Much more often, a slow rise in pulmonary vascular resistance starts in childhood and determines the onset of cyanosis later in childhood or in adolescence or early adult life.

INFECTIVE ENDOCARDITIS

The risk of infective endocarditis (SBE) has often been cited as a reason for surgical closure of small VSDs, but the risk is now agreed to be small and not obviated by surgical closure.[137] SBE can complicate surgical closure or, rarely, even follow successful closure. A history of previous SBE is not regarded as an indication for surgery. The risk of hemodynamic deterioration is slight when SBE complicates a small VSD. Tricuspid regurgitation may follow infection of a small VSD situated close to the tricuspid valve, but aortic regurgitation is uncommon unless the valve was already incompetent. The aortic valvular leak antedates but predisposes to the infection, and the risk of aortic regurgitation is also not sufficient to recommend closure of the small uncomplicated VSD. The chance of infection with a big VSD is less than with a small VSD, presumably because

pressure gradients are absent. When aortic regurgitation already complicates VSD, the chances of infection are not only very high but the risk of deterioration is great.

COMPLICATIONS OF BIG DEFECTS

Two complications of VSD deserve special mention. These are aortic regurgitation and the development of pulmonary vascular obstructive changes.

VSD with Aortic Regurgitation

The association of ventricular septal defect with aortic regurgitation is well known.[80,108,113,133,149] Views still differ as to the pathogenesis and the best mode of management, but all agree that aortic regurgitation is one of the more common and serious complications of VSD. The VSD is usually large, and an unduly high number of defects lie anterosuperiorly to the crista supraventricularis rather than in the common position posteroinferior to the crista. Among 27 patients operated upon at the Royal Postgraduate Medical School from 1958 to 1967 with this combination of defects, 15 of the defects exceeded 1 cm per M^2 body surface area (or were bigger than the aortic root). The incidence of 7 patients with supracristal defects was 26 per cent and four times as high as the expected incidence. (The number of cases of VSD with aortic regurgitation occurring in this series of 229 surgically treated VSDs was rather high but many had been specially referred.)

In 19 of the 27 surgically treated patients, the regurgitation was associated with a prolapsed aortic right coronary cusp in all except one patient, in whom the noncoronary cusp had prolapsed. The prolapsed cusp was usually large, deep, patulous and thinned out, and there was often some abnormality also in the adjacent portion of the noncoronary cusp with thickening in the other cusps attributable to the effect of severe and sometimes longstanding aortic regurgitation.

The patients in whom no cusp prolapse was found were those with smaller defects.

In some of these the aortic regurgitation was less severe and its cause was not elucidated if the aorta was not opened. One patient had had infective endocarditis, while a bicuspid aortic valve was suspected in two others. In one patient there was no true aortic regurgitation but a ruptured aneurysmal right coronary sinus was leaking into the right ventricle. These findings were similar to those of Keck,[80] Scott et al.[133] and Plauth et al.[121] A gradient across the right ventricular outflow tract is common and seems in many patients to be accounted for by the prolapse of the aortic cusp through the defect into the right ventricular outflow tract.[108]

Pulmonary hypertension is uncommon in VSD with aortic regurgitation both because of partial plugging of a big defect by the prolapsed right coronary cusp and also because of the gradient across the right ventricular outflow tract associated with cusp prolapse. A large left-to-right shunt is common, particularly when it is augmented by the incompetent aortic valve shunting blood directly to the right ventricle via the VSD.

The incidence of infective endocarditis is high compared to its relatively low incidence in isolated VSD. The infection is a complication of the aortic regurgitation rather than the cause. Presumably the aortic regurgitation renders the patient more vulnerable to the development of infection.

The progressive nature of aortic regurgitation in patients with VSD has been stressed.

Management of VSD with Aortic Regurgitation

An early diastolic murmur should always be sought in any patient with a ventricular septal defect. The detection of aortic regurgitation is an indication for hemodynamic and angiographic study. Retrograde aortography is essential. In cusp prolapse this reveals the right coronary cusp and sinus of the aortic valve to be enlarged and deformed, forming an easily recognized berry-like projection from the anterior wall of the aorta. Aortic regurgitation may fill both ventricles when the VSD is supracristal, mainly the left

ventricle when the defect is infracristal. Aortic regurgitation coexisting but not directly associated with VSD can be differentiated by the relatively normal appearance of the aortic root and separation of the VSD from it. The coexistence of other lesions, particularly discrete subaortic stenosis, can also be recognized at this time.

If, on the basis of the investigations, the aortic regurgitation is thought *not* to be associated with a prolapsed cusp, both the VSD and the aortic regurgitation should be treated on their respective merits. If the VSD is large enough to warrant closure, it should be closed; otherwise the patient should be carefully followed and surgery deferred until aortic-valve replacement is necessary.

The association of aortic regurgitation with ventricular septal defect and cusp prolapse is an indication for early closure of the VSD, as the repair usually slows the progression of the aortic regurgitation and may delay the day when aortic-valve replacement will become necessary. In a few patients closure of the VSD will be associated with regression or even disappearance of aortic regurgitation. Opening of the aorta, plication of valve commissures or other conservative measures are not usually followed by better correction of the aortic regurgitation. Since such maneuvers undoubtedly add to morbidity and to the difficulties and hazards of future aortic-valve surgery, the operation should be confined to closure of the VSD unless aortic-valve replacement is already required.

There is still some conflict of opinion about the best management of this combination of lesions. Ellis et al. and Somerville et al. had a large proportion of small defects in their series[47,147] and Somerville came to the conclusion that repair or replacement of the aortic valve in addition to closure of the VSD was necessary to gain improvement. Valve prolapse was recognized in only a minority of her patients, although the majority were thought to have supracristal defects and prominence of the right coronary sinus was a frequent finding on aortography. Contrary to Somerville's recommendation that surgery should be deferred wherever possible until the time of skeletal maturity, our experience has indicated the low risks and benefits to be gained from dealing only with the VSD, in the hope that aortic-valve surgery may not be necessary or can be delayed until the patient has reached adulthood.[67]

Pulmonary Vascular Obstruction:
The Assessment of Operability

The factors which determine the development of pulmonary vascular obstruction (PVO) in VSD and its behavior after successful closure of the defect are still imperfectly understood. The development of a high pulmonary vascular resistance has been correlated with a high left atrial pressure as well as with a high pulmonary blood flow.[82] It is possible that a relatively small capacity or incompliant left atrium could contribute both to early heart failure in some infants and to the development of pulmonary vascular obstruction in others.

In general, all patients with severe pulmonary vascular obstruction have a large VSD, at least the size of the aortic-valve orifice. The pulmonary hypertension is obligatory and at systemic level, although at a stage when the left-to-right shunt is large, flow gradients may be recorded both across the VSD and across the right ventricular outflow tract to the pulmonary artery. When the pulmonary blood flow diminishes consequent upon the gradual development of obliterative changes in the resistance vessels, these flow gradients disappear and the systolic pressure becomes similar in left ventricle, right ventricle, pulmonary artery and aorta.

Assessment of operability depends ultimately on the hemodynamic data, although the physical signs provide valuable guidelines to the feasibility of VSD closure in a particular patient.[74]

Very few patients with severe pulmonary hypertension who remain in the operable range show arterial desaturation at rest because the vis a tergo caused by an excess of venous return to the left ventricle over venous return to the right ventricle keeps right ventricular blood out of the left ventricle and aorta. Mild desaturation on effort, however, may not preclude surgery. Patients in the operable range usually show some physical evidence of a left-to-right shunt. Left ventricular enlargement, a mitral diastolic and a right ventricular outflow-tract flow murmur should be sought but the absence of any or all of these does not invariably mean inoperability. On the other hand, the presence of a mitral diastolic flow murmur, a systolic murmur at the left sternal edge or a prominent left ventricle does not mean that the VSD can safely be closed either. Perhaps the most reliable physical sign is the persistence of a well-split second heart sound. This sign (in the absence of right bundle branch block) indicates prematurity of aortic-valve closure due to a shortened preejection and ejection period because of shunting through the VSD, together with delay in pulmonary-valve closure associated with increased flow from the right ventricle.

The ECG usually shows persisting evidence of left ventricular volume overload and the chest x-ray significant cardiac enlargement and pulmonary plethora, but these signs too can be misleading.

If the pulmonary blood flow is at least twice the systemic blood flow, the patient is likely to benefit from closure of the VSD and the operative mortality should be under 10 per cent. With a pulmonary blood flow of over 1.5 times the systemic flow, operation should usually still be carried out but mortality is likely to be higher and the ultimate benefit less predictable. When pulmonary: systemic vascular resistance ratio (rP:rS) is used, a figure exceeding 0.7:1.0 suggests inoperability.[23] It is preferable to measure oxygen consumption and to consider that a pulmonary vascular resistance of more than 10 units/M^2 indicates that a defect should not be closed. Possibly a simple calculation of pulmonary blood flow or even the saturation of blood in the pulmonary artery would be as useful. A pulmonary blood flow of more than 4 L/min/M² or a blood saturation over 80 per cent indicates that the defect may be closed. A test inhalation of 100 per cent oxygen often brings about an increase in left-to-right shunting in those borderline patients who are likely to benefit from VSD closure. This procedure is recommended in all cases.

In arriving at a decision whether or not to advise operation, age must be considered. The younger the patient, the more likely it is that the pulmonary vascular obstruction may be reversible. Thus the child younger than 2 or 3 years whose flows are almost balanced may not have immutable pulmonary arteriolar changes and closure should probably be advised. The same flows in a patient of 15 or 20 would preclude operation. It has not been the practice in our own center to use lung biopsy to aid the decision, although the gradation of changes described by Heath and Edwards[70] almost certainly bears more relation to postoperative progress than the measured hemodynamics. In the instances quoted the young child might show only mild reversible grade-2 changes in the pulmonary arterioles, whereas the young adult would be likely to show grade-4 changes (irreversible, and result of operation likely to be fatal).[79]

Pulmonary vasoconstriction can easily be provoked in children with VSD (and also in children with normal hearts) and this can be a source of error at the time of cardiovascular assessment if attention is not paid to the adequacy of ventilation during the study. Alveolar hypoventilation from overgenerous sedation or during general anesthesia can lead to hypercapnia and respiratory acidosis, which can result in elevation of pulmonary-artery pressure in children with small VSDs. The validity of the physiological data depends upon the normality of the patient's ventilation and gas exchange during the time of collection of the data. Whenever possible, a pulmonary venous blood sample should be obtained in order to check Po_2, Pco_2 and pH, or failing these a left atrial, left ventricular or aortic blood oxygen sample may be equally informative. This should be analyzed and the result reported while the catheter is proceeding. Inhalation of 100 per cent oxygen usually increases the left-to-right shunt[97] and assessment of oxygen responsiveness can be useful in the assessment of operability in borderline patients with pulmonary vascular disease.

The fall in pulmonary-artery pressure which follows closure of a big VSD is usually predictable and explicable solely by removal of the shunt. Loss of pulmonary vasoconstriction does not need to be invoked. Subsequently the pulmonary-artery pressure tends to remain about the same as it was at the completion of surgery but to rise further during exercise.[66]

There are now a few reports of progressive pulmonary hypertension leading eventually to death after successful VSD closure,[23] and postoperative cardiac catheterization should always be carried out in these patients. If the pulmonary-artery pressure remains significantly elevated at rest and particularly if the pressure rises further during exercise, sports should probably be prohibited as it is likely that high pulmonary-artery pressure favors progression of the vascular changes.

The prognosis of moderate pulmonary hypertension persistent after VSD closure is still not known.

Pregnancy and the Contraceptive Pill

It is well known that pregnancy carries a high maternal risk in patients with severe pulmonary vascular disease and cyanosis (Eisenmenger syndrome). The maternal mortality has been 100 per cent in such patients in our experience. The babies grow poorly, and there is a high fetal mortality as well.

Both pregnancy and contraceptive hormones have been associated with rapid progression of pulmonary vascular obstruction and are contraindicated in any patient with pulmonary hypertension.[115] Big VSDs which are operable should of course be closed before puberty, but if found in young women should be closed before pregnancy.

With the Eisenmenger syndrome, it is our practice to recommend surgical sterilization of women of childbearing age.

For girls who have significant pulmonary hypertension persisting after VSD closure, the decision about the wisdom of future pregnancy must be individual. Provided it is moderate rather than at systemic level and has not advanced since the time of operation, pregnancy cannot legitimately be denied to them. Contraceptive hormones should probably be avoided in all. Much more information is needed.

VSD WITH PULMONARY HYPERTENSION BELOW SYSTEMIC LEVEL

Any patient with significant pulmonary hypertension in association with a left-to-right shunt through a VSD should probably have the defect closed. In general, patients in this in-between category of VSD are relatively uncommon beyond infancy and young childhood. (Much more often, the pulmonary-artery pressure is roughly normal or at systemic level.) It can be argued and may be true that this intermediate group is composed of patients whose VSDs had previously been larger. Others have very high flows across a VSD which lies under the tricuspid-valve septal cusp; thus partial occlusion of the defect in systole may account for the pressure differential while its larger size in diastole explains the high flow across it.

In all these patients a check must be made that the pulmonary hypertension is real rather than caused by hypoventilation. Pulmonary hypertension of significant level can be considered as a systolic pressure at or above twice the normal maximum, i.e. 50 mm Hg or over, and clearly there must be a significant left-to-right shunt through the defect if the pulmonary hypertension is to be influenced by operation. A pulmonary-to-systemic flow ratio in excess of 2:1 at rest is suggested as a guide.

Management in Infancy

In infancy the development of heart failure is associated with a high pulmonary-artery pressure as well as left atrial hypertension from left atrial overfilling. Although at least half of the infants will improve with conservative treatment and later attain a lower pulmonary blood pressure, the ones who fail to improve require surgical help.

Pulmonary-artery banding has been practiced in such infants since it was first suggested by Damman and Muller in 1952. When this operation is successful the baby comes out of heart failure, growth is resumed and the pulmonary-artery pressure, the left atrial pressure and the pulmonary blood flow all fall (Fig. 17). Unfortunately, not all survivors show such improvement.[99] The best recorded surgical mortality for banding in isolated VSD lies between 5 and 12 per cent,[76] with a later mortality of 10 to 20 per cent for VSD closure and debanding including some unsatisfactory results because of unmodifiable pulmonary-artery stenoses. These are the best published figures and they add up to a total surgical mortality of at least 20 per cent for the staged procedure—an unfavorable comparison with the best published figures for primary VSD closure.[84] Others quote less favorable results from banding.[28] The preliminary mortality of banding is low only in centers with wide experience and excellent facilities for the postoperative care of infants, including assisted respiration. Banding therefore requires a highly specialized surgical team.

The pulmonary-artery banding operation is no longer considered an optimal surgical procedure for isolated VSD. For those infants who remain ill, primary VSD closure should now be available.[9,35,117,140] Kirklin's first figures for VSD closure in infancy were described a decade ago, and increasing numbers of reports now indicate primary intracardiac repair of VSD in infancy with a risk of under 10 per cent.[35,84,117,140]

In Great Britain well under 100 babies per year should require surgical help for VSD

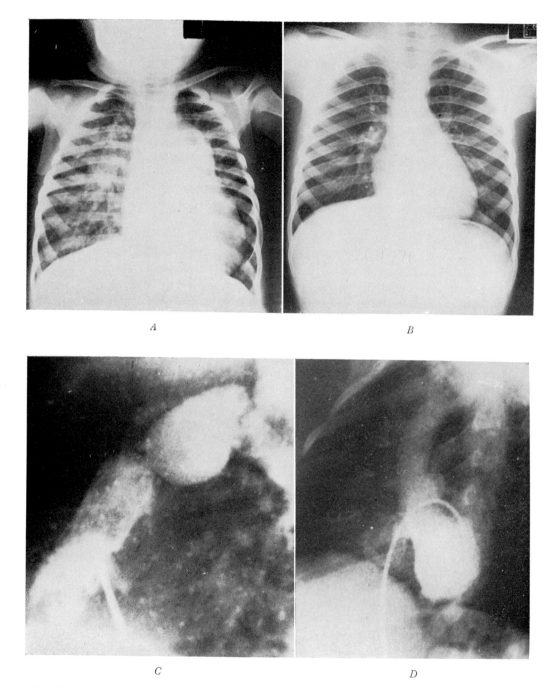

A   *B*

C   *D*

Fig. 17. Pulmonary-artery banding in isolated VSD. *A*: 8-month-old infant. *B*: Same child 4½ years later. Note almost normal chest x-ray with striking regression of main pulmonary-artery dilatation and lung vascularity. *C*: Same child, from RV cineangiogram, injection below the band. "Ghosting" of the aorta is seen. *D*: LV injection via foramen ovale shows the outline of a straightforward infracristal VSD. This has now been successfully closed and the pulmonary-artery band removed.

during infancy. When considered in conjunction with the other congenital cardiac anomalies requiring surgery in infancy, half a dozen centers would have a chance to acquire skill by doing perhaps 1 to 2 infant VSD closures per month.

The mechanism of improvement must be ascertained in any infant who comes out of heart failure and begins to flourish, because a very few will exhibit some progressive and excessive rise in pulmonary vascular resistance. These children should be submitted to VSD closure as soon as increasing pulmonary vascular resistance is recognized. Pulmonary-artery banding has been tried in this group, but it is impossible to tie the band tightly enough that the resistance to flow offered by the band exceeds that offered by the pulmonary arterioles. The result of banding in this group is therefore either surgical death or no change in hemodynamics. For most babies who improve after a difficult period in infancy, VSD closure can be planned after the age of two years when the operative mortality should lie between 1 and 5 per cent.

SUMMARY OF INDICATIONS FOR VSD CLOSURE

Closure of ventricular septal defects is indicated for:

1. The infant with a big VSD who fails to improve on a medical regimen.
2. Any VSD with pulmonary hypertension provided there is a significant left-to-right shunt.
3. VSD with right ventricular pressure at systemic level and outflow-tract obstruction.
4. VSD with aortic regurgitation (and cusp prolapse).
5. VSD with a left ventricular right atrial shunt or tricuspid regurgitation.

The natural history of VSD with a normal pulmonary-artery pressure is now known to be benign. There is no need to close such a defect, regardless of the size of the left-to-right shunt. Spontaneous late closure may still occur during the school years or even

later, but this possibility is not the reason for advocating a conservative approach.

Conversely, the presence of pulmonary hypertension resulting from obligatory equalization of pressures on each side of a big defect carries a bad prognosis, whether associated with high pulmonary blood flow or with pulmonary vascular obstruction and low pulmonary blood flow.

Heart failure in infancy does not necessarily lead to death or inoperability. If it looks as if either may result, however, primary closure of the defect in infancy is now preferred to banding, provided it can be done with a relatively low mortality rate.

The presence of pulmonary hypertension is the key to prognosis; surgical closure is likely to modify this favorably provided the pulmonary vascular obstruction is not greatly advanced.

ATRIAL SEPTAL DEFECT OF SECUNDUM TYPE

Natural History

The natural history of atrial septal defect (ASD) is incompletely known because of the relatively high incidence of discovery in individuals who are already well on in adult life. Many of these patients are over 40 or even in their 60s when the defect is discovered, either on account of a routine chest roentgenogram or because of the onset of symptoms. It is often stated, but is probably not true, that most older patients with atrial septal defect have disabling and progressive symptoms. The fact that many are asymptomatic at the time of accidental discovery strongly suggests that many others are never diagnosed at all. The situation then is the obverse of that in ventricular septal defect, in which a loud murmur is the hallmark (most children nowadays are discovered but have a relatively high incidence of spontaneous closure). In ASD the defect is relatively silent and not productive of symptoms in the young. Spontaneous closure, although documented, is probably very rare.

Atrial septal defect rarely appears during infancy. If an infant with symptoms is found to have a large left-to-right shunt at atrial level an additional left-sided lesion should be strongly suspected. This may be a coarctation, aortic stenosis, ventricular septal defect, patent ductus arteriosus or left ventricular myocardial disease. Endocardial fibroelastosis, often with mitral regurgitation, may lead to incompetence of the foramen ovale. Similarly, but rarely, an adult with rheumatic mitral-valve disease may acquire a left-to-right shunt from the same mechanism. Uncommonly an infant may be found to have only a secundum atrial septal defect and the early onset of left-to-right shunting may have to be attributed to unusually rapid regression of physiological right ventricular hypertrophy.

It is widely accepted that the left-to-right shunt in ASD results from the greater distensibility of the right ventricle compared with the left ventricle and usually has nothing to do with the size of the defect. The pulmonary hypertension which develops in a minority cannot be attributed to the direct transmission of sytemic pressures to the right side of the heart and hence to the pulmonary vessels. Pulmonary vascular disease in ASD is rare in childhood and, when seen, it frequently differs from pulmonary hypertension associated with ASD in older patients. The young person with pulmonary hypertension and a secundum ASD sometimes has a small heart, no significant left-to-right shunt, very little dilatation of the pulmonary-artery branches but very severe pulmonary vascular disease. Angiographically and histologically the findings resemble those observed in idiopathic or primary pulmonary hypertension. Such patients seem to have pulmonary hypertension from early in life, and it now seems likely that they possesss two dissociated abnormalities: one an ASD and the other "small-vessel" pulmonary hypertension. There is on the other hand a small but distinct group of older patients, nearly always female, with severe pulmonary hypertension at

or near to systemic level associated with the persistence of a large left-to-right shunt at atrial level.[164] These may be seen at any age but most commonly in middle life. The pulmonary-to-systemic flow ratio may exceed 3:1. Although the operative risk is fairly high, the result can be extremely rewarding (Fig. 18).

The development of complications in patients with ASD is unknown, but the development of atrial fibrillation nearly always brings deterioration and eventual congestive heart failure—as a rule not associated with significant pulmonary hypertension. Considerable cardiomegaly, atrial fibrillation and heart failure may be seen in patients with a persisting left-to-right shunt of some magnitude (Fig. 18), but also in patients who have little or no increase in pulmonary blood flow despite normal pulmonary-artery pressures. An hypothesis to explain the curious situation (in which the presence of a large ASD is easily confirmed but shunting is slight) can be put forward. With the onset of atrial fibrillation and dilated right heart chambers, tricuspid regurgitation develops and eventually becomes severe. The volume of blood which leaks back into the right atrium from the right ventricle in systole is exchanged for a volume of blood which was previously accepted from the left side as shunted blood. The volume capacity of the right ventricle is thereby satisfied, diastolic pressures in the two atria and ventricles equilibrate as before, but there is no longer a significant total left-to-right shunt. In such patients it is fruitless to close the ASD without repairing the tricuspid valve. The patient's symptoms are directly caused by tricuspid regurgitation, and restoration of tricuspid-valve competence might be expected to restore the previous large left-to-right shunt. Obviously this thesis has not been tested, but the combined operation of ASD closure with tricuspid-valve repair seems necessary. Conservative repair of the tricuspid valve rather than replacement is likely to be followed with more success in these patients than in patients with rheumatic

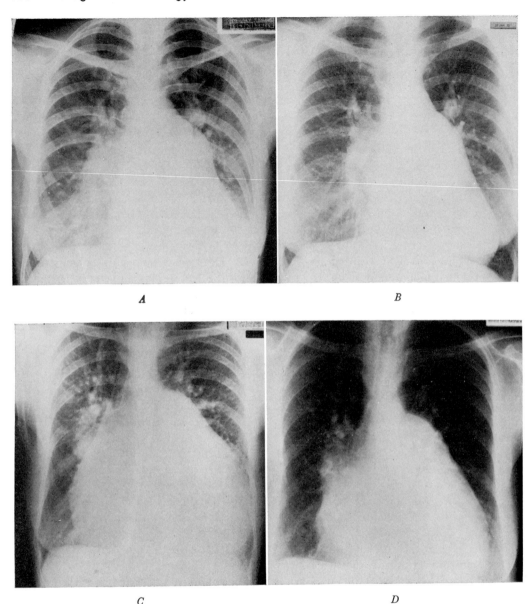

Fig. 18. Secundum ASD in the "elderly." *A*: Patient E.S. before repair. *B*: Four months after surgical repair. *C*: Patient G. S. before repair. *D*: Seven months after surgical repair.

heart disease, because the patient with ASD usually has a good right ventricle; his signs and symptoms stem directly from the valve reflux rather than from myocardial failure. Indeed, the evidence for the development of either left or right ventricular dysfunction in ASD is very slim. With the development of tricuspid regurgitation both the left and the right atria share the load. Similarly both ventricles share the same end-diastolic pressure, just as they do in uncomplicated ASD in the child. The effect of atrioventricular valve incompetence, therefore, whether it primarily affects the left or the right ventricle, is to increase atrial filling and to raise the height of the end-diastolic pressure in both ventricles.

The effect of mitral regurgitation will be to increase the left-to-right shunt. The effect of tricuspid regurgitation, however, is to diminish the left-to-right shunt. Cyanosis may develop. Since cyanosis does not stem from pulmonary vascular disease, it should not preclude surgery.

Mitral Regurgitation with ASD

Mitral regurgitation is diagnosed more often than it is actually present. The diagnosis of mitral-valve disease of rheumatic origin in patients with ASD led to undue prominence being given to the syndrome described by Lutembacher.[111] Murmurs at the apex often emanate from the tricuspid valve in ASD but they are heard at the apex because of the large size of the right heart chambers.

When mitral regurgitation is correctly recognized, reliable clinical distinction can be made from ostium primum defect by the electrocardiogram, which fails to show the left anterior hemiblock—an invariable finding in ostium primum. The mechanism of mitral regurgitation in secundum ASD is usually a congenital or acquired elongation of the chords of the anterior medial cusp with ballooning or floppiness of that cusp. As in defects of the atrioventricular canal, closure of the ASD should not be carried out unless the mitral regurgitation is also corrected or has been proved to be mild.

Lutembacher's Syndrome

ASD may be complicated by mitral stenosis but the combination exists less frequently than diagnosed. Rheumatic mitral stenosis is becoming rarer and congenital anomalies of the mitral valve are uncommon in secundum ASD. Acquired mitral regurgitation of nonrheumatic origin is probably more frequent than mitral stenosis.

Overdiagnosis of mitral-valve disease in ASD results from the dilatation of the right heart chambers; this renders pulmonary and tricuspid murmurs audible at the "mitral" area and even sometimes in the axilla.

Classically a raised left atrial pressure with ASD may be suspected from a raised cervical venous pressure. This sign may be absent, however, because the large size of the combined atrial chambers minimizes any increase in atrial pressure and the mitral-valve gradient may be small or absent. Conversely, when rarely the ASD is small, so that the left atrial pressure is not vented, a continuous murmur may be audible.

When mitral stenosis is suspected in ASD, mitral echocardiography is the most reliable clinical means of detection. For the reasons given above, it may prove superior even to pressure measurement.

Central Cyanosis in ASD

In anatomically isolated ASD, arterial desaturation may be associated with loss of left-to-right shunt from pulmonary hypertension or tricuspid regurgitation. It may also occur due to mixing within the left atrium despite a high pulmonary blood flow, which occurs when much of the inferior vena caval bloodstream is directed into the left atrium by a well preserved fetal eustachian valve. Patients can occasionally show clinical cyanosis and clubbing giving rise to diagnostic difficulties. More often, desaturation occurs only on exercise.

The development of a small right-to-left shunt at atrial level during exercise is common in atrial septal defect, and a right-to-left shunt has been used as a diagnostic tool during the performance of a Valsalva maneuver in suspected ASD.

Systemic Embolization in ASD

The presence of a potential or actual right-to-left shunt in ASD explains the low but real incidence of paradoxical embolism in this condition.

Indications for Surgical Closure

ASD closure is rarely indicated in infancy. Often it is useful to correct the cause of the left-to-right shunt, e.g. coarctation. The ASD is retained as a temporarily beneficial vent to the left atrium.

When ASD is recognized in childhood, it is usual to recommend surgical closure because the operative mortality rate is extremely low, below 1 per cent. The operation is curative, and the possibility of future trouble is avoided.

Most asymptomatic patients with ASD show remarkable stability over many years. Infective endocarditis is virtually unknown, and serial cardiac catheterizations tend to show no change. Although the incidence of congestive heart failure shows a significant increase after the age of 30 years, truly symptom-free patients over this age can safely be followed medically. The discovery of this lesion has usually been accidental; the congenital defect has had a fair test, and symptoms may never appear.

The preferred management is to refine the diagnosis by cardiac catheterization and then to review the patient annually. The development of symptoms or signs of change will not preclude the good surgical result and low surgical risk possible at an earlier stage. In ASD surgical closure can be carried out successfully in advanced age even when recognition and treatment were prompted by development of severe disability or complications (Fig. 18). Although earlier reports suggested that symptomatic benefit from ASD closure was limited in the older patient in whom medical management was preferable,[96] our experience has led us to a contrary view. Indeed, several recent reports indicate that the operative mortality rate can be low and the symptomatic benefit great in patients over 40 years of age.[33,56]

Markman has shown that patients with ASD rarely die before the fifth decade but believes that the incidence of symptoms increases substantially thereafter.[96] Certainly the onset of real symptoms often heralds progressive limitation, and the symptomatic patient with ASD should be considered for surgery almost regardless of age.

Incorrect Diagnosis

A diagnosis of uncomplicated atrial septal defect can usually be made with confidence on clinical grounds; rarely is it faulted by subsequent catheterization. The anatomy can, however, be complicated. Complicating anatomy can be divided into occult (those that cannot be diagnosed clinically and are usually missed also at catheterization) and overt (usually suspected clinically and readily confirmed at catheterization).

Occult Complications

Hemianomalous pulmonary venous drainage without atrial septal defect[52] may be occult if the abnormal drainage is directed into the right atrium. A clinical clue may be the presence of near-normal mobility of the two components of the second heart sound with respiration.

Cor triatriatum may be unobstructed because of free communication with the right atrium. This means that pulmonary venous blood enters the right atrium and a mixture of pulmonary and systemic venous blood then is returned to the lower chamber, the left atrium proper, via a patent foramen ovale. Arterial desaturation is obligatory in this situation but it may be slight and clinically inapparent. If the left ventricle receives a high proportion of pulmonary venous blood, as it may if the pulmonary blood flow is high, the degree of desaturation may be minimal. The presence of this condition is usually missed at the time of cardiac catheterization but, as with isolated cor triatriatum, it is best shown by angiocardiography in the frontal view. This anomaly can readily be corrected but it is potentially confusing for unprepared surgeons.

Overt Anatomical Complications

ASD of the sinus venosus type, with anomalous drainage of some of the right upper-lobe veins into the superior vena cava, can frequently be suspected from the chest x-ray;

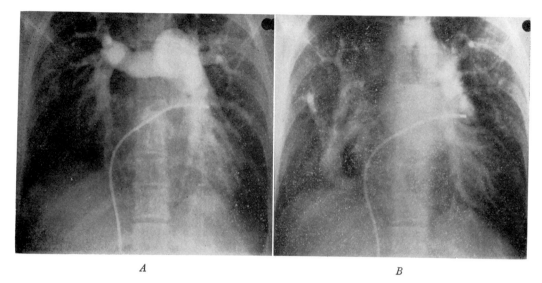

A   B

Fig. 19. "Scimitar" (see text). Right ventricular angiogram. *A*: Pulmonary arteriogram phase. *B*: Pulmonary venous phase. The left atrium is opacified but no contrast has reached right atrium (no ASD was present). The right pulmonary veins join to form a dilated common trunk which enters the IVC-RA junction.

a bulge may be seen at the junction of the superior vena cava and right atrium where the anomalous veins enter. Abnormal horizontal vascular shadows can sometimes be recognized in the right upper zone. Hemianomalous pulmonary venous drainage anywhere except into the right atrium proper can usually be suspected from the plain chest x-ray. Drainage into the left vertical vein of all venous blood from the left lung gives rise to a mediastinal bulge, most marked on the left (as in total anomalous drainage of the supracardiac type) but, as the superior vena cava is unlikely to be as dilated, the right half of the "snowman's head" may be inconspicuous.

When the pulmonary venous blood from the right lung drains into the right atrial-inferior vena caval junction, it usually gives rise to a "scimitar" shadow (Fig. 19) which is readily recognizable. Sometimes the anomaly is rendered invisible because of displacement of the cardiac mass into the right hemithorax. When dextrocardia solitus is seen in a patient with signs of ASD, the scimitar syndrome should be suspected.

In addition, in some but not in all cases, there may be hypoplasia of the right pulmonary artery, abnormalities in the bronchial anatomy of the right lung and a systemic arterial supply to part of the right lung.[65]

DISTINCTION FROM MITRAL-VALVE DISEASE

When atrial septal defect is associated with gross cardiomegaly in older patients, a clinical diagnosis of mitral-valve disease is sometimes made. The size of the heart may lead to a decision to assume medical treatment without proceeding to cardiac catheterization. The clinical diagnostic features which deny mitral-valve disease in such patients include:

1. Often rather mild disability in proportion to the heart size.
2. Total absence of left ventricular enlargement.
3. Absence of a mitral pansystolic murmur.
4. Absence of left atrial enlargement.
5. Presence of partial or complete right bundle branch block on ECG.
6. Increased caliber of the pulmonary arteries in the middle and peripheral lung fields in chest x-ray.
7. Pulmonary venous hypertension absent from chest x-ray.

ATRIAL SEPTAL DEFECT
OF PRIMUM TYPE
(ATRIOVENTRICULAR DEFECTS)

The anatomy of the mitral valve in endocardial cushion defect has been greatly clarified by the work of Baron[7,8] and the late Rastelli.[127] To Baron is largely owed the precision with which the anatomy of the ostium primum defect can now be recognized angiographically. Rastelli contributed particularly to the understanding of the complete form of persistent atrioventricular canal and provided the guidelines whereby operable forms of this serious defect may be distinguished and dealt with surgically.

Isolated defects of the ventricular part of the membranous atrioventricular septum (so-called cushion type of VSD) are rare, and the common defects are complex and involve multiple structures. These defects range from atrial septal defect of the primum type to a complete atrioventricular canal of Rastelli's type 3, in which the four cardiac chambers communicate with each other through a single large atrioventricular orifice across which a conjoined tricuspid and mitral septal cusp is slung.

In endocardial cushion defect, the atrioventricular septum (membranous septum) is absent. Because of this the cleft anterior leaflet of the mitral valve is displaced downward and forward. The resulting deformity of the left ventricular outflow tract can be recognized on angiocardiograms and the appearance is pathognomonic.

In normal individuals the right-hand border of the outflow tract of the left ventricle is formed by the membranous septum and is straight and smooth. In endocardial cushion defect the right border of the left ventricle is formed by the displaced anterior mitral leaflet. During systole this bulges toward the left atrium, imparting a serrated contour to the right margin. The cleft between the two halves of the leaflet can often clearly be seen (Fig. 20), with a mitral regurgitant jet. In diastole the leaflets disappear from sight as nonopaque blood from the left atrium enters the ventricle. The resulting narrowing of the outflow tract to the left ventricle seen in diastole is often referred to as a "gooseneck" deformity. It is less specific than the systolic appearance, because its presence depends on mobility of the abnormal

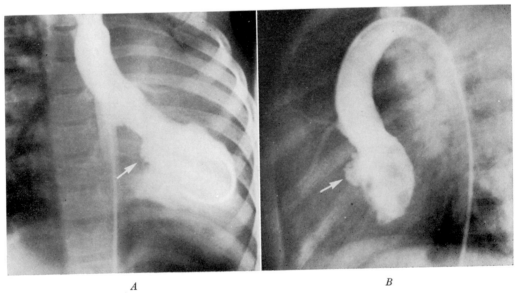

A   B

Fig. 20. Ostium primum ASD (see text). Retrograde LV angiogram. *A*: Frontal view. The cleft is arrowed. *B*: Lateral view. Contrast in the cleft mitral anterior cusp causes a frilly bulge on the anterior LV wall (arrow).

anterior leaflet; when movement is limited because of abnormal insertion or shortening of chordae, the "gooseneck" is not seen.

The presence of a "good" gooseneck therefore has important surgical implications. Correction of mitral regurgitation is essential to the successful outcome of operation. Mobility of the anterior leaflet means that there are sufficient leaflet tissue and normal chordae for a good functional correction. When the outflow tract remains broad in diastole because of poor movement of the leaflet, the prognosis for surgical correction of mitral regurgitation is less good. This finding should sway the physician toward deferring surgery if the patient is a young child in whom the placement of an artificial mitral valve would be particularly undesirable.

In the complete form of persistent atrioventricular (A–V) canal, an interatrial and interventricular communication and a complex common atrioventricular valve are found. Rastelli[127] divided these into three types dependent on differences in configuration, relationship and attachments of the anterior leaflet of the common valve: (1) The anterior leaflet is divided and attached to the ventricular septum, (2) the anterior leaflet is divided but not attached to the septum, and (3) the anterior leaflet is completely common and neither divided nor attached to the septum. In the first two types, the prospects for surgical correction are good and the appearance of the left ventricular outflow tract on angiography resembles that in the ostium primum type of defect except that there is an interventricular shunt. In the third type, with the anterior leaflet suspended across the A–V canal, the appearance of the outflow tract of the left ventricle is different. Instead of the scalloped right border with a single deep indentation at the site where the two halves of the anterior mitral leaflet coapt, a smooth simple right angle is seen in diastole. The horizontal component is formed by the undivided common leaflet slung across the A–V canal, the vertical component by contrast medium trapped under the posterior mitral leaflet. In systole the right border assumes an irregular contour, without the characteristic appearance described in the less complete types of canal. The detection of an interventricular component of an atrioventricular shunt is extremely difficult by angiographic means. Its presence can be inferred if the right and left ventricular pressures are equal, but the directional passage of the contrast—whether from left ventricle to right atrium (partial canal) or from left ventricle to right ventricle (complete canal)—is particularly difficult to define.

Prognosis and Indications for Operation in ASD of the Primum Type

The natural history of primum ASD without functional incompetence of the abnormal mitral valve is probably virtually identical to that in uncomplicated secundum ASD. It is arguable and unknown whether in later life the development of atrial fibrillation will bring with it the development of mitral-valve regurgitation. Certainly this possibility exists and can be used in favor of operation in asymptomatic patients with the uncomplicated defect. An argument against surgery is the slightly greater risk of closing the defect, either from the creation of mitral regurgitation where none existed or the creation of heart block. In fact, neither of these complications should arise in the 1970s. Much of the gloom surrounding the surgery of atrioventricular defects arises from the early unfortunate experience with them.

Regurgitation through the mitral valve may pass largely into the left atrium or directly into the right atrium. If the regurgitation is more than slight, the success of the operation depends on the surgeon's ability to reduce or eliminate it.[118] Failure to do so results in a postoperative increase in left atrial pressure, since the whole of the regurgitant volume has to be accommodated in the left atrial chamber rather than dissipated into both atria.

It is now possible to predict angiographically patients in whom the mitral valve is likely to prove amenable to repair.[146] In a proportion of patients in whom cusp and chordal tissue is deficient and abnormal, or in whom there has been previous infective endocarditis, mitral-valve replacement will be essential. Operation should obviously be deferred if possible until a small child is bigger or until increasing symptoms or developing heart failure force action.

Pulmonary hypertension is more common in A–V canal defects than in secundum ASD, for several obvious reasons: (1) the possibility of pulmonary venous hypertension if there is significant mitral regurgitation, (2) the presence of a ventricular defect in complete canal, and (3) the greater frequency of atrioventricular canal (particularly complete canal) in patients with Down's syndrome, who seem to display an unusual proclivity to the development of early pulmonary vascular obstruction.

ASD of the primum type can almost invariably be recognized from the ECG, which rarely fails to show the characteristic features of partial or complete right bundle branch block with left anterior hemiblock. There may also be a long P–R interval, related not to early trifascicular block but to right atrial dilatation. A similar ECG is seen in patients with common or single atrium; these patients have an ostium primum type of anatomy, associated with total absence of the interatrial septum. Angiographic findings are similar to those in uncomplicated ostium primum defect.

DISORDERS OF THE LEFT VENTRICULAR OUTFLOW TRACT

Aortic-valve Stenosis

Incidence and Natural History

Congenital aortic-valve stenosis is three or four times as common in boys as in girls. In at least half the cases, the stenosis is attributable in part to the fact that the valve is functionally bicuspid and cannot open fully;

the cusps are tethered across the diameter of the valve ring.

Bicuspid aortic valve is the most common congenital malformation of the heart, but the low incidence of early recognition means that it is not included in figures for congenital heart lesions present at birth. Its actual prevalence may be as high as 4 per 1,000 live births, and 4 out of 5 of those affected are male. Campbell calculated that 15 to 35 per cent of patients with lone aortic stenosis appearing in adult life have bicuspid valves.[20] As many as 25 per cent of these bicuspid valves are calcified by the age of 40 and 50 per cent are calcified in patients over the age of 50. With congenital aortic stenosis, virtually all valves are found to be calcified in patients over the age of 40.

Since congenitally abnormal aortic valves are liable to become calcified, and since calcification is associated with immobility and therefore with stenosis, it follows that even a minor deformity of the aortic valve can lead to serious aortic stenosis in the fifth or sixth decade. If a valve is relatively immobile and stenotic, it must also be regurgitant; therefore the incidence of aortic regurgitation in patients with congenitally abnormal valves increases from youth to older age. Nearly all calcified aortic valves are found to leak when investigated by aortography. The progressive deterioration from abnormal wear and tear due to design faults in underprivileged valves fully accounts for the large numbers of patients with lone aortic stenosis in middle and later life.

The overwhelming male predominance of older patients with calcific aortic stenosis is the same as the sex incidence of aortic-valve stenosis in childhood. It contrasts with the female preponderance of patients with mitral stenosis or multiple valve disease of rheumatic origin.

In rheumatic aortic stenosis associated with mitral-valve disease, the aortic valve has three symmetrical cusps which are thickened and contracted with stenosis due more to commissural fusion and fibrosis than to calcification, which is often slight or absent. The difference is easily distinguished angiographically as well as surgically from aortic stenosis of congenital origin, which in the adult is largely attributable to cusp immobilization rather than to commissural fusion.

AORTIC-VALVE STENOSIS AS A CAUSE OF HEART FAILURE IN THE NEONATE

In the neonate severe aortic-valve stenosis is rare but singularly lethal. It occurs early, within the first week. Unlike the older child, the infant tends to congestive heart failure with an extreme low-output state. Difficulty in palpating the peripheral pulses is one of the cardinal diagnostic features. Cyanosis is absent but tachypnea is striking. Hepatomegaly is usually found, and the heart is often grossly enlarged radiologically. The ECG shows florid evidence of left ventricular hypertrophy with extensive S-T depression and T-wave inversion. Hastreiter suggests that many of these infantile aortic-valve stenoses are really partial forms of the hypoplastic left heart syndrome.[68] Certainly the nature of the valve deformity may make surgical relief difficult or even impossible. The valve ring is often hypoplastic, the valve cusps are greatly thickened, and the commissures are difficult to identify or even absent, giving a unicommissural valve. The frequently associated left ventricular failure in these babies necessitates a full left heart study to prove the severity of the obstruction. Some degree of associated endocardial fibroelastosis is common, or there may be mitral regurgitation due to papillary muscle subendocardial ischemic necrosis. Relief is needed urgently. Most centers now prefer the use of cardiopulmonary bypass to venous inflow occlusion. Intervention is fully justified in the occasional infant with a relatively well-formed aortic valve, in whom a reasonable result can be obtained, although reoperation will probably be required relatively early in childhood.[18]

AORTIC-VALVE STENOSIS IN CHILDHOOD

In childhood, complete absence of symptoms is usual and the diagnosis is usually made from the chance finding of a murmur. Heart failure is rare in aortic stenosis, any symptoms are late and therefore of great importance when they develop. Sudden death may be the first and only sign, although

Table I. Increase in the Severity of Aortic-Valve Stenosis During Childhood

Patient		Age	Symptoms	ECG	Pressures mm Hg		Valve
					LV	GR	
PQ	1964	5	0	N	160 / 0 to 7	48	—
	1971	12	dyspnea + angina	S–T ↓	240 / 0 to 10	130	1 cm bicuspid
GS	1965	7	0	N	110 / 0 to 10	30	—
	1970	12	0	S–T ↓	220 / 0 to 12	110	9 mm bicuspid

N = Normal.
GR = Systolic pressure gradient across the aortic valve.

death usually occurs in patients who have exhibited good clinical evidence of severe stenosis.[58]

The condition is not static, even in childhood. Progressive increase in the severity of obstruction may occur during the growing period and before degenerative changes in the valve bring further deterioration in its function. Data from two patients in whom aortic stenosis progressed during childhood are shown in Table I. After completion of growth, valve function is likely to remain relatively stable until degenerative changes have become sufficiently marked to affect mobility. The development of symptoms and the risk of death obviously depend both on the severity of the obstruction and the functional response of the myocardium.

These facts explain the periods of life when the risks are greatest. In the neonatal period the left ventricular myocardium is unprepared by hypertrophy and the valve lesion is likely to be exceptionally severe. In childhood trouble may come because of a rapidly progressive increase in severity of obstruction. In later life symptoms may be heralded by deterioration in the valve or in the left ventricle, the latter due either to time alone with senescence changes in the myocardium[122] or to the development of coronary-artery disease.

INDICATIONS FOR SURGICAL TREATMENT

In the infant, as in the older patient with definite symptoms and proven severity, the need for operation is usually obvious; with a child, however, the decision is difficult. Open aortic valvotomy carries only a small risk in skilled hands, but at best it is only a palliative procedure; the nature of the valve deformity makes correction as such impossible. The surgeon is further hampered by the great danger of producing incompetence in the valve. It is indeed preferable to leave moderate stenosis than to create moderate incompetence. This often means that the surgeon must content himself with a millimeter or two split along the two main commissures, which fulfills the aim of the

operation—to render the child safe to grow up free from the dangers of sudden death and irremediable left ventricular myocardial damage.

Guidelines to the assessment of severity of aortic stenosis in children can be listed:

1. Any true symptom, particularly dizziness or syncope during or immediately after effort, is indicative of severe lesion. Angina is comparatively rare but equally sinister.
2. A long murmur, particularly a murmur which peaks late in systole, has been shown to be one of the best clinical indicators of a high gradient across the aortic valve. This is sometimes but not always accompanied by delay in aortic-valve closure, giving a reversed split of the second heart sound. Measurement of systolic time intervals can provide an even more sensitive guide, a combination of a prolonged ejection time with a shortened preejection period being specific for severe left ventricular outflow-tract obstruction. (Diseases of the left ventricle are marked by prolongation of the preejection period but shortening of the total ejection time.)
3. The chest radiograph usually does not help. It may be normal or show only poststenotic dilatation of the ascending aorta in patients with severe symptoms and clinical and catheterization evidence of severity. Aortography may be useful in revealing the type of valve deformity and in predicting the likelihood of a reasonable surgical result.[142]
4. The ECG is more useful in childhood than in the older age groups. Children with mild or moderate aortic stenosis tend to have normal electrocardiograms, apart from some increase in QRS voltage. If S-T segment and T-wave changes are found in the left ventricular leads of a child with aortic stenosis, it must be assumed that surgical relief is needed urgently[129] (Fig. 21). With a normal resting stroke volume, surgical relief is usually indicated if the peak gradient exceeds 75 mm Hg. Obviously, if symptoms or ECG changes are associated with a gradient of less than this, operation should still be advised. If a child is asymptomatic with a normal ECG both at rest and during exercise despite a gradient of 75 to 100 mm Hg, the situation is arguable; operation should probably be advised because childhood aortic valvotomy in this sort of patient may postpone the day when aortic-valve replacement is needed in adulthood.

The best to be achieved by open aortic valvotomy in childhood is a hemodynamically more efficient but still malformed valve which will continue to deteriorate in function. The purpose of the operation is to en-

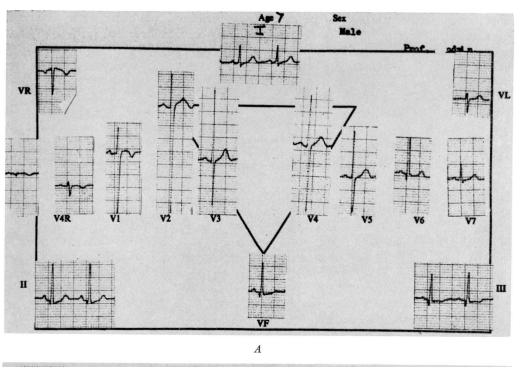

A

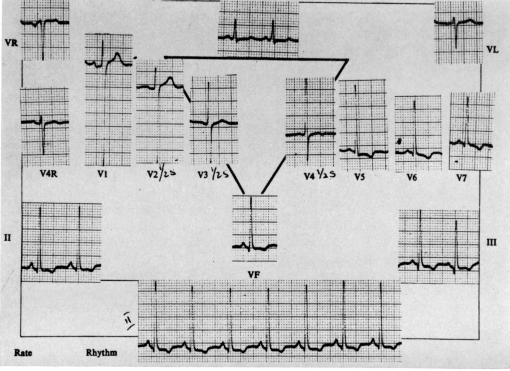

B

Fig. 21. Deterioration in ECG in congenital valvular AS (see text).

able these children eventually to take their places among adults with congenitally severe but now calcified aortic stenoses. When viewed this way, open aortic valvotomy can produce extremely gratifying results. In the best centers, the risks are under 5 per cent.[16] Unfortunately the severity of the design fault which led to a need for valvotomy in childhood permits only modest improvement from surgery and is followed by the relatively rapid development of degenerative changes,[20] so that some patients come back for aortic-valve replacement in the second decade of life. Even so, the benefits of open valvotomy are obvious, since children can survive until the aortic root is large enough to accept an adult-sized prosthesis.

Other Forms of Left Ventricular Outflow-tract Obstruction

Left ventricular obstruction at supravalvular and subvalvular level is far less common than aortic-valve stenosis, and the implications and natural history are different. The clinical signs which distinguish supravalvular aortic stenosis and hypertrophic obstructive cardiomyopathy have been emphasized and are now well known.[114,156]

Valve Stenosis

Upward ballooning of the mobile conjoined cusps in systole gives rise to an ejection click, with return of the valve to the closed position marked by an easily audible closure sound.

By contrast *in discrete subaortic stenosis* the pressure baffle provided by the subvalvular obstruction leads to impaired movement of the overlying normal valve. Moreover, jet effects and poststenotic dilatation involving the valve site may further interfere with valve function. The delayed, soft or absent aortic-valve closure sound, the frequent presence of an early diastolic murmur and the absence of an ejection click are thereby explained.

Supravalvular Aortic Stenosis

Associated congenital anomalies are common. The condition is frequently associated with peripheral pulmonary-artery stenoses and may occur in three settings:

1. In children with mental retardation and a characteristic facies.[11] An association with the severe form of infantile hypercalcemia has been proved in a few patients[12,53] and reproduced experimentally.[51]
2. In patients with the rubella syndrome. Rarely, supravalvular aortic stenosis may be associated with stenoses in other major vessels, both pulmonary-artery branches and systemic arteries.
3. As a familial entity, where it is usually unassociated with other congenital abnormalities except peripheral pulmonary-artery branch stenoses.

The specific physical signs include a tendency for the innominate artery to receive the jet through the supravalvular stenosis. Therefore pulses in the right arm and right carotids are full volume and jerky, whereas pulses in the left carotids, left arm and distal segments are small and slow rising.

Hypertrophic Obstructive Cardiomyopathy (HOCM)

This is probably more correctly regarded as an acquired than a truly congenital heart disorder, but the condition is occasionally recognized in the neonate. One infant exhibited congestive failure due to a large left-to-right shunt at atrial level secondary to a high left atrial pressure and the development of incompetence of valvular foramen ovale. More often, HOCM is first seen in early or even late adult life.[62] When HOCM is diagnosed in childhood, the condition is often particularly severe and carries a bad prognosis. Since the adults with HOCM have also been children in their time, either most children with HOCM are not recognized or the disease itself develops rapidly beyond the childhood years. The latter seems unlikely, since stability and slow progression are usually noteworthy;[116] therefore, it must be assumed that there is a very low incidence of recognition of HOCM in the childhood years.

Only 21 children with HOCM have been seen at the Royal Postgraduate Medical

School during the past 12 years, compared with well over 100 cases in adult life. The differences between children and adults are worth emphasizing. Only five of the children had significant left ventricular outflow-tract gradients or mitral regurgitation; the rest had either no gradient or only a small gradient. The children with outflow-tract obstruction were usually symptom free, and three had normal electrocardiograms and chest roentgenograms. In this group a false diagnosis of an innocent murmur, small VSD or trivial pulmonary stenosis may be made, with consequent failure to pursue the problem further. In contrast, the children without outflow-tract obstruction often had significant symptoms, five died suddenly and one developed congestive heart failure. These children tended to have insignificant or no murmurs but often grossly abnormal ECGs and considerably enlarged hearts radiographically.

A family history was common in the children without outflow-tract obstruction, and some family members had pronounced "classical" signs of HOCM. The hearts at autopsy showed typical features of the disease.

The difference between the patients with and without outflow-tract obstruction in HOCM can be explained by the following hypothesis. Patients with outflow-tract obstruction have hypertrophy which is gross but focal, being largely confined to the septum. In these patients the normal performance of the free wall muscle enables the left ventricle both to fill normally and to provide a normal external performance for a relatively long period. Equally, the presence of a large amount of normal free wall muscle permits the changes in the septal "hypertrophe" to progress until marked replacement fibrosis and loss of contractile ability occur. This is compensated for (as in ischemic heart disease with focal dysfunction) by increased contractile activity of the free wall muscle. The long axis of the cavity becomes bent around the immobile septum and increased shortening of the free wall in systole brings the anterior cusp of the mitral valve and papillary muscle into contact with the projecting septal hypertrophe, thereby giving rise to outflow-tract obstruction. The excessive contraction of the free wall and mitral-valve apparatus, together with its situation on the convexity of the bent cavity, fully accounts for the anterior dislocation of the mitral-valve cusps in systole which results in mitral regurgitation. This explains the coexistence of outflow-tract obstruction with mitral regurgitation in many patients.

By contrast, the patients with childhood symptoms have generalized hypertrophy involving all parts of the left ventricle. Diminished left ventricular distensibility accounts for slow filling and the reduction in stroke volume which accompanies tachycardia. Thus exercise-induced tachycardia may be associated with a critical fall in stroke volume, blood pressure and coronary flow, leading to sudden death.

This hypothesis does not mean that some patients with diffuse rather than focal hypertrophy may not be seen in adult life. Such patients are likely to have a smaller but more scattered population of abnormal myocardial cells, and many such patients are probably never recognized. It has been shown under blind conditions that it is possible to distinguish HOCM myocardium from the myocardium in organic left ventricular outflow-tract obstruction; the proportion and disposition of abnormal cells in the HOCM heart can be recognized by their histological features and mapped out.[153]

No biochemical fault has been found, and the link with skeletal dystrophy first suggested by Meerschwam has not yet been confirmed in the experience of others.[98] The disorder probably owes its origin to some abnormal response to a stimulus to hypertrophy: the "whorled" arrangement of the myocardial fibers noted by Olsen[153] may set up isometric stresses during contraction which generate further hypertrophy. At ultrastructural level a "crossover" of myofibrils noted by Ferrans[49a] may account for the development of isometric stresses at fibrillar level. This explanation also allows for the development of myocardial changes indistinguishable from those in HOCM in a small proportion of patients (particularly children) with organic left ventricular outflow-tract obstruction. One such patient with a patent ductus arteriosus, ligated in childhood, and discrete subaortic stenosis died of noncardiac causes and was found to have gross left ventricular hypertrophy out of all proportion to the severity of the discrete subaortic stenosis (Fig. 22). The histological appearances were typical of HOCM. This patient's mother had high blood pressure and died suddenly. At autopsy she too was found to have HOCM but without any structural abnormality of the outflow tract; the histological changes of HOCM were verified also in her case.

Surgical treatment of left ventricular outflow-tract obstruction in HOCM is on the whole disappointing, and in any case the patients with outflow-tract obstruction tend to be those with a relatively good medical prognosis. Surgical treatment is not appli-

cable to those with the diffuse form of the disease.

Treatment with beta-adrenergic blocking drugs helps to protect the patient from the dangers of exercise-induced tachycardia. It may also delay the genesis of arrhythmias and replacement fibrosis by reducing the gap between metabolic demand and coronary blood supply. The best subjective benefit is usually found in patients with angina.

Inheritance of HOCM is probably by a dominant gene, although a recent survey has suggested also a recessive mode.[48] (A relatively high incidence of asymptomatic carriers with mild forms of the disorder which are clinically undiagnosable has to be considered when assessing the significance of the latter finding.) In advising parents, it seems wise to suggest adoption if the family has a high incidence of the disease in its most severe form. It is likely that so-called sporadic cases are familial ones where known relatives do not have the disease in sufficiently severe form to be recognized, and the possibility of transmission of the disorder is probably the same.

AORTIC REGURGITATION

Aortic regurgitation may be found in conjunction with:

1. Bicuspid aortic valve
2. Congenital aortic-left ventricular tunnel
3. Ruptured sinus of Valsalva into the left ventricle
4. Complicating Marfan's syndrome[158]
5. Complicating other disorders of the aortic wall:
   Ehlers-Danlos syndrome
   Morquio's osteochondrodystrophy[94]
   Osteogenesis imperfecta[32]
   Collagen diseases
   Oriental arteritis
6. Rheumatic disorders
7. Postendocarditic (infective) disorders
8. Ventricular septal defect.

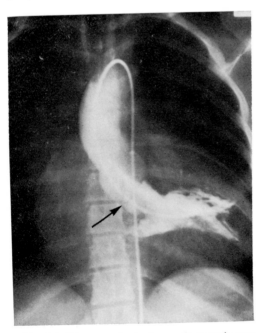

Fig. 22. Discrete subvalvular aortic stenosis complicated by HOCM (see text). LV angiogram. The obstruction is visible as a line below the aortic valve cusps (arrow). The gross LV hypertrophy is obvious.

A bicuspid aortic valve is rarely the seat of severe reflux unless it has been infected. *Postinfective aortic regurgitation* is by far the most common cause of aortic regurgitation in childhood. Infection on a bicuspid aortic valve is common and singularly lethal, probably because of lack of awareness that the heart was previously abnormal, because the acute onset of severe regurgitation was not immediately recognized and because the need for emergency valve replacement may not be appreciated.[163] Severe aortic regurgitation may follow infection on a discrete subaortic stenosis and infection may aggravate aortic regurgitation associated with VSD.

When aortic regurgitation is severe and has been present from birth, the cause is likely to be a congenital *aortic-left ventricular tunnel*.[15] In this rare (although still most common) cause of truly congenital "aortic regurgitation," there is an endothelialized connection between the aortic root and left ventricle. In the neonate it must be distinguished from truncus arteriosus with leaking truncal valve. Most cases are recog-

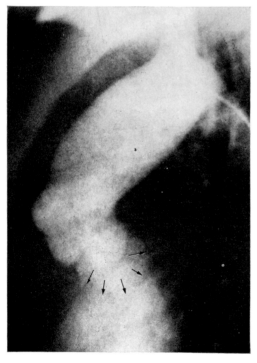

Fig. 23. Retrograde aortogram in aorto-left ventricular tunnel, left lateral view. The extreme dilation of the ascending aorta and the deformity of its root are well shown. The distinctive feature is the bulge at the commencement of the tunnel (arrows) which gives an appearance suggestive of a fourth sinus of Valsalva.

nized at or shortly after birth because of the florid physical signs and bounding pulses, hyperkinetic precordium and loud murmurs. Both the left ventricle and the aorta are greatly dilated, and pulsation under the right clavicle may be caused by the dilated ascending aorta. Despite the severity of the regurgitation, heart failure seems to be rare. In the absence of symptoms or signs of impending failure, there is much to be said for deferring operative intervention until the dilated aortic root will accept an adult-sized prosthesis. Of four children with the condition seen at the Royal Postgraduate Medical School, only one has been operated upon to date; she is left with severe aortic reflux.

The pathology of the condition is not the same as in *ruptured sinus of Valsalva* into the left ventricle (which is an even rarer cause of aortic regurgitation). It was well described by Levy[87] and is thought to represent a fistulous connection of a supernumerary coronary artery with the left ventricle. The channel lies anteriorly and usually enters through the upper part of the ventricular septum. The aortographic features are characteristic, the anterior site of the tunnel distinguishing it from a ruptured sinus of Valsalva while the presence of two normal coronary arteries distinguishes it from a coronary-cameral fistula.

Although theoretically an aortic-left ventricular tunnel should be amenable to simple repair, in practice the whole aortic root tends to become so distorted and dilated that replacement of the aortic valve is almost certain to be required. Perhaps repair in the neonate as soon as the condition is recognized would preserve the function of the aortic valve.

Aortic regurgitation *associated with severe forms of Marfan's syndrome* may develop soon after birth; when it does it may take a malignant form with the rapid onset of mitral regurgitation. Less severe forms may occur at any age and the typical physical stigmata of Marfan's syndrome need not be present. Aortography may show either generalized aortic dilatation or a localized aneurysm involving the first position of the ascending aorta and the sinuses of Valsalva. In such cases replacement with a rigid prosthesis may need to be considered, with graft replacement of the aneurysmal portion of aorta.[144]

REFERENCES

1. Aberdeen, E., et al: Successful "correction" of transposed great arteries by Mustard's operation. Lancet, *1*:1233, 1965.
2. Anderson, R. A., et al.: Rapidly progressing pulmonary vascular obstructive disease. Association with ventricular septal defects during early childhood. Amer. J. Cardiol., *19*:854, 1967.
3. Agustsson, M. H., et al.: Spontaneous functional closure of ventricular septal defects in 14 children demonstrated by serial cardiac catheterization and angiocardiography. Pediatrics, *31*:958, 1963.
4. Arcilla, R. A., et al.: Further observations on the natural history of isolated ventricular septal defects in infancy and childhood. Serial catheterization studies in 75 patients. Circulation, *28*:560, 1963.
5. Ash, R.: Natural history of ventricular septal defects in childhood; lesions with predominant arteriovenous shunts. J. Pediat., *64*:45, 1964.
6. Azevedo, de C. A., et al.: Ventricular septal defect: An example of its relative diminution. Acta Cardiol., *13*:513, 1958.
7. Baron, M. G., et al.: Endocardial cushion defects: Specific diagnosis by angiocardiography. Amer. J. Cardiol., *13*:162, 1964.
8. Baron, M. G.: Abnormalities of the mitral valve in endocardial cushion defects. Circulation, *45*:672, 1972.
9. Barratt-Boyes, B. G.: Cardiac surgery in neonates and infants. Circulation, *44*:924, 1971.
10. Barratt-Boyes, B. G., Simpson, M. H., and Neutze, J. M.: Intracardiac surgery in neonates and infants using deep hypothermia with surface cooling and limited cardiopulmonary bypass. Circulation, *43* (Suppl. 1): 1, 1971.
11. Black, J. A., and Bonham-Carter, R. E.: Association between aortic stenosis and facies of severe infantile hypercalcaemia. Lancet, *2*:745, 1963.
12. Black, J. A., Butler, N. R., and Schlesinger, B. E.: Aortic stenosis and hypercalcaemia. Lancet, *2*:547, 1965.
13. Bloomfield, D. K.: The natural history of ventricular septal defect in patients surviving infancy. Circulation, *29*:914, 1964.
14. Bonham-Carter, R. E., Capriles, M., and Noe, Y.: Total anomalous pulmonary venous drainage. A clinical and anatomical study of 75 children. Brit. Heart J., *31*:45, 1969.
15. Bove, K. E., and Schwartz, D. C.: Aortico-left ventricular tunnel. A new concept. Amer. J. Cardiol., *19*:696, 1967.
16. Braunwald, E., et al.: Congenital aortic stenosis. I. Clinical and haemodynamic findings in 100 patients. II. Surgical treatment and the results of operation. Circulation, *27*: 426, 1963.
17. Brotmacher, L., and Campbell, M.: Natural history of ventricular septal defect. Brit. Heart J., *20*:97, 1958.
18. Burnell, R. H., et al.: Management of critical valvular outflow obstruction in neonates. Thorax, *25*:116, 1970.
19. Burrough, J. T., and Edwards, J. E.: Total anomalous pulmonary venous connection. Amer. Heart J., *59*:913, 1960.
20. Campbell, M.: The natural history of congenital aortic stenosis. Brit. Heart J., *30*:514, 1968.
21. Campbell, M.: Natural history of ventricular septal defect. Brit. Heart. J., *33*:246, 1971.
22. Carlgren, L. E.: Incidence of congenital heart disease in children born in Gothenburg. Brit. Heart J., *27*:40, 1959.
23. Cartmill, T. B., et al.: Results of repair of ventricular septal defect. J. Thorac. Cardiov. Surg., *52*:486, 1966.
24. Celermajer, J. M., Venables, A. W., and Bowdler, J. D.: Catheterization of the pulmonary artery in transposition of the great arteries. Circulation, *41*:1053, 1970.
25. Chesler, E., et al.: Ultrasound cardiography in single ventricle and the hypoplastic left and right heart syndromes. Circulation, *42*:123, 1970.
26. Ching, E., et al.: Total correction of cardiac anomalies in infancy using extracorporeal circulation. J. Thorac. Cardiov. Surg., *62*:118, 1971.
27. Cleland, W. P., et al.: A decade of open heart surgery. Lancet, *1*:191, 1968.
28. Coleman, E. N., et al.: Ventricular septal defect repair after pulmonary artery banding. Brit. Heart J., *34*:134, 1972.
29. Collett, R. W., and Edwards, J. E.: Persistent truncus arteriosus: A classification according to anatomic types. Surg. Clin. N. Amer., *29*:1245, 1949.
30. Cooley, D. A., Hallman, G. L., and Leachman, R. D.: Total anomalous pulmonary venous drainage: Correction with the use of cardiopulmonary bypass in 62 cases. J. Thorac. Cardiov. Surg., *51*:88, 1966.
31. Crews, T. L., et al.: Auscultatory and phonocardiographic findings in Ebstein's anomaly: Correlation of first heart sound with ultrasonic records of tricuspid valve movement. Brit. Heart J., *34*:681, 1972.
32. Criscitiello, M. G., et al.: Cardiovascular abnormalities in osteogenesis imperfecta. Circulation, *31*:255, 1965.

33. Daicoff, G. R., Brandenburg, R. O., and Kirklin, J. W.: Results of operation for atrial septal defect in patients forty-five years of age and older. Circulation, 35 (Suppl. I): 143, 1967.

34. Daicoff, G. R., et al.: Surgical repair of complete transposition of the great arteries with pulmonary stenosis. Ann. Thorac. Surg., 7:529, 1969.

35. Daicoff, G. R., and Miller, R. H.: Congestive heart failure in infancy treated by early repair of ventricular septal defect. Circulation, 41 (Suppl. II):111, 1970.

36. Danielson, G. K., et al.: Repair of transposition of the great arteries by transposition of venous return. Surgical considerations and results of operation. J. Thorac. Cardiov. Surg., 61:96, 1971.

37. De la Cruz, M. V., and Rocha, J. P. D.: An ontogenetic theory for the explanation of congenital malformations involving the truncus and conus. Amer. Heart J., 51:782, 1956.

38. De la Cruz, M. V., et al.: Systematization and embryological and anatomical study of mirror image dextrocardias, dextroversions and laevoversions. Brit. Heart J., 33:841, 1971.

39. Diamond, M. A., et al.: Echocardiographic features of atrial septal defect. Circulation, 43:129, 1971.

40. Dillard, D. H., et al.: Correction of total anomalous pulmonary venous drainage in infancy utilizing deep hypothermia with total circulatory arrest. Circulation, 35 (Suppl. I):105, 1967.

41. Dollery, C. T, et al.: Regional pulmonary blood flow in patients with circulatory shunts. Brit. Heart J., 23:225, 1961.

42. Dollery, C. T., Hugh-Jones, P., and Matthews, C. M. E.: Use of radioactive xenon for studies of regional lung function. A comparison with oxygen. Brit. Med. J., 2:1006, 1962.

43. DuShane, J. W.: Total anomalous pulmonary venous connection: Clinical aspects. Mayo Clin. Proc., 31:167, 1956.

44. Edgett, J. W., et al.: Spontaneous closure of a ventricular septal defect after banding of the pulmonary artery. Amer. J. Cardiol., 22:729, 1968.

45. Edwards, J. E.: Ventricular septal defect: unresolved problems. Amer. J. Cardiol., 19: 832, 1967.

46. Elliott, C. P., et al.: Complete transposition of the great vessels. I. An anatomic study of sixty cases. Circulation, 27:1105, 1963.

47. Ellis, F., Ongley, P. A., and Kirklin, J. W.: Ventricular septal defect with aortic valvular incompetence: Surgical considerations. Circulation, 27:789, 1963.

48. Emanuel, R., Withers, R., and O'Brien, K.: Dominant and recessive modes of inheritance in idiopathic cardiomyopathy. Lancet, 2:1065, 1971.

49. Evans, J. R., Rowe, A. B., and Keith, J. D.: Spontaneous closure of ventricular septal defects. Circulation, 22:1044, 1960.

49a.Ferrans, V.: In: Cardiomyopathies. Vol. 2. Baltimore, University Park Press, 1972.

50. French, H.: The possibility of a loud congenital heart murmur disappearing when a child grows up. Guy Hosp. Gaz., 32:87, 1918.

51. Friedman, W. F., and Roberts, W. C.: Vitamin D and the supravalvar aortic stenosis syndrome. Circulation, 34:77, 1966.

52. Frye, R. L., et al.: Partial anomalous pulmonary venous connection without atrial septal defect. Amer. J. Cardiol., 22:242, 1968.

53. Garcia, R. E., et al.: Idiopathic hypercalcaemia and supravalvular aortic stenosis: Documentation of a new syndrome. New Eng. J. Med., 271:117, 1964.

54. Gasul, B. M., et al.: Ventricular septal defects: Their natural transformation into those with infundibular stenosis or with cyanotic or noncyanotic tetralogy of Fallot. JAMA, 164: 847, 1957.

55. Gathman, G. E., and Nadas, A. S.: Total anomalous pulmonary venous connection. Clinical and physiologic observations on 75 paediatric patients. Circulation, 42:143, 1970.

56. Gault, J. H., et al.: Atrial septal defect in patients over the age of forty years. Circulation, 37:261, 1968.

57. Gelband, H., Van Meter, S., and Gersony, W. M.: Truncal valve abnormalities in infants with persistent truncus arteriosus. Circulation, 45; 397, 1972.

58. Glew, R. H., et al.: Sudden death in congenital aortic stenosis. Amer. Heart J., 78:615, 1969.

59. Goldblatt, A., et al.: Pulmonary artery banding: indications and results in infants and children. Circulation, 32:172, 1965.

60. Gomes, M. M. R., et al.: Total anomalous pulmonary venous connection. Surgical considerations and results of operation. J. Thorac. Cardiov. Surg., 60:116, 1970.

61. Gomes, M. M. R., et al.: Double outlet right ventricle with pulmonic stenosis. Surgical considerations and results of operation. Circulation, 43:889, 1971.

62. Goodwin, J. F.: Congestive and hypertrophic cardiomyopathy: A decade of study. Lancet, 1:731, 1970.

63. Graham, T. P., Jr., et al.: Scintiangiocardiography in children. Amer. J. Cardiol., 25:385, 1970.

64. Hagan, A. D., et al.: Further applications of scintillation scanning techniques to the diagnosis and management of infants and children with congenital heart disease. Circulation, 45:858, 1972.

65. Halasz, N. A., Halloran, K. K., and Liebow, A. A.: Bronchial and arterial anomalies with drainage of the right lung into the inferior vena cava. Circulation, 14:826, 1956.

66. Hallidie-Smith, K. A., et al.: Effects of surgical closure of ventricular septal defects upon pulmonary vascular disease. Brit. Heart. J., *31*: 246, 1969.

67. Hallidie-Smith, K. A., et al.: Ventricular septal defect and aortic regurgitation. Thorax, *24*:257, 1969.

68. Hastreiter, A. R., et al.: Congenital aortic stenosis syndrome in infancy. Circulation, *28*:1084, 1963.

69. Hay, J. D.: Population and clinic studies of congenital heart disease in Liverpool. Brit. Med. J., *2*:661, 1966.

70. Heath, D., and Edwards, J. E.: The pathology of hypertensive pulmonary vascular disease. A description of six grades of structural changes in the pulmonary arteries with special reference to congenital cardiac septal defects. Circulation, *18*:533, 1958.

71. Hightower, B. M., Wiedman, W. H., and Kirklin, J. W.: Open intracardiac repair for complete transposition of the great arteries. Circulation, *33* (Suppl. I):1, 1966.

72. Hoffman, J. I. E. and Rudolph, A. M.: The natural history of ventricular septal defects in infancy. Amer. J. Cardiol., *16*:634, 1965.

73. Hoffman, J. I. E.: Natural history of congenital heart disease: Problems in its assessment with special reference to ventricular septal defects. Circulation, *37*:97, 1963.

74. Hollman, A., et al.: Auscultatory and phonocardiographic findings in ventricular septal defect. Circulation, *28*:94, 1963.

75. Hollman, A., and Hamed, M.: Mitral valve disease with ventricular septal defect. Brit. Heart J., *27*:274, 1965.

76. Hunt, L. E., et al.: Banding of the pulmonary artery: Results in 111 children. Circulation, *43*:395, 1971.

77. Imamura, E. S., et al.: Surgical considerations of ventricular septal defect associated with complete transposition of the great arteries and pulmonary stenosis. Circulation, *44*:914, 1971.

78. Iverson, R. E., Linde, L. M., and Kegel, S.: The diagnosis of progressive pulmonary vascular disease in children with ventricular septal defects. Pediatrics, *68*:594, 1966.

79. Kanjuh, V. I., Sellers, R. D., and Edwards, J. E.: Pulmonary vascular plexiform lesion. Pathogenetic studies. Arch. Path. *78*:513, 1964.

80. Keck, E. W. O., et al.: Ventricular septal defect with aortic insufficiency: A clinical and haemodynamic study of 18 proved cases. Circulation, *27*:203, 1963.

81. Keith, J. D., et al.: Ventricular septal defect. Incidence, morbidity and mortality in various age groups. Brit. Heart J., *33*:81, 1971.

82. Kidd, L., et al.: Ventricular septal defect in infancy. Amer. Heart J., *69*:4, 1965.

83. Kidd, L., and Mustard, W. T.: Haemodynamic effects of a totally corrective procedure in transposition of the great vessels. Circulation, *33* (Suppl. I):28, 1966.

84. Kirklin, J. W.: Pulmonary arterial banding in babies with large ventricular septal defects. Circulation, *43*:321, 1971.

85. Kriss, J. P., et al.: Radioisotopic angiocardiography. Wide scope of applicability in diagnosis and evaluation of therapy in diseases of the heart and great vessels. Circulation, *43*:792, 1971.

86. Lavoie, R., Sestier, F., and Gilbert, G.: Double outlet right ventricle with left ventricular outflow tract obstruction due to small ventricular septal defect. Amer. Heart J., *82*:290, 1971.

87. Levy, M. J., et al.: Aortico-left ventricular tunnel. Circulation, *27*:841, 1963.

88. Levy, A. M., et al.: Far advanced internal proliferation and severe pulmonary hypertension secondary to total anomalous pulmonary venous drainage. Amer. J. Cardiol., *16*:280, 1965.

89. Li, M. D., et al.: Spontaneous closure of ventricular septal defect. Canad. Med. Assoc. J., *100*:737, 1969.

90. Lindesmith, G. G., et al.: Surgical treatment of transposition of the great vessels. Ann. Thorac. Surg., *8*:12, 1969.

91. Lundstrom, N-R.: Ultrasoundcardiographic studies of the mitral valve region in young infants with mitral atresia, mitral stenosis, hypoplasia of the left ventricle and cor triatriatum. Circulation, *45*:324, 1972.

92. McGoon, D. C., Wallace, R. B., and Danielson, G. K.: Homografts in reconstruction of congenital cardiac anomalies. Expanded operability in complex congenital heart disease. Mayo Clin. Proc., *47*:101, 1972.

93. McGoon, D. C., Rastelli, G. C., and Ongley, P. A.: An operation for the correction of truncus arteriosus. JAMA, *205*:69, 1968.

94. McKusick, V. A.: In: *Heritable Disorders of Connective Tissue*, 3rd ed. St. Louis, C. V. Mosby Co., 1966.

95. Mair, D. G., et al.: Haemodynamics and evaluation for surgery of patients with complete transposition of the great arteries and ventricular septal defect. Amer. J. Cardiol., *28*:632, 1971.

96. Markman, P., Howitt, G., and Wade, E. G.: Atrial septal defect in the middle aged and elderly. Quart. J. Med., *34*: 409, 1965.

97. Marshall, H. W., et al.: Effect of breathing oxygen on pulmonary artery pressure and pulmonary vascular resistance in patients with ventricular septal defect. Circulation, *23*: 241, 1961.

98. Meerschwamm, I. S.: Electromyographic findings. In: *Hypertrophic Obstructive Cardiomyopathy*. Amsterdam, Excerpta Medica Foundation, 1969.

99. Menahem, S., and Venables, A. W.: Pulmonary artery banding in isolated or complicated ventricular septal defects—results and effects on growth. Brit. Heart J., *34*:87, 1972.

100. Miller, W. W., et al.: Congenital pulmonary atresia with ventricular septal defect. Amer. J. Cardiol., 21:673, 1968.

101. Mitchell, S. C., Berendes, H. W., and Clark, W. M.: The normal closure of the ventricular septum. Amer. Heart J., 73:334, 1967.

102. Mitchell, S. C., Korones, S. B., and Berendes, H. W.: Congenital heart disease in 56,109 births. Incidence and natural history. Circulation, 43:323, 1971.

103. Morton, W. E., and Huhn, L. A.: Epidemiology of congenital heart disease. Observations in 17,366 Denver school children. JAMA, 195:1107, 1966.

104. Mudd, J. G., et al.: The natural and postoperative history of 252 patients with proved ventricular septal defects. Amer. J. Cardiol., 39:6, 1965.

105. Mustacchi, P., Sherins, R. S., and Miller, M. J.: Congenital malformations of the heart and great vessels: Prevalence, incidence and life expectancy in San Francisco. JAMA, 183: 241, 1963.

106. Mustard, W. T., et al.: The surgical management of transposition of the great vessels. J. Thorac. Cardiov. Surg., 48:953, 1964.

107. Mustard, W. T., Keon, W. J., and Trusler, G. A.: Transposition of the lesser veins (total anomalous pulmonary venous drainage). Progr. Cardiov. Dis., 11:145, 1968.

108. Nadas, A. S., et al.: Ventricular septal defect with aortic regurgitation. Circulation, 29: 862, 1964.

109. Nadas, A. S., and Fyler, D. C.: Ventricular septal defect. Arch. Dis. Child., 43:268, 1968.

110. Neill, C. A.: Development of the pulmonary veins with reference to the embryology of anomalies of pulmonary venous return. Pediatrics, 18:880, 1956.

111. Lutembacher, R.: De la stenose mitrale avec communication inter auriculaire. Arch. Mal. Coeur, 9:237, 1916.

112. Naeye, R. L.: The pulmonary arterial bed in ventricular septal defect. Circulation, 34:962, 1966.

113. Nellen, M., Schrire, V., and Vogelpoel, L.: Ventricular septal defect with aortic incompetence. S. Afr. Med. J., 33:91, 1959.

114. Oakley, C. M., and Hallidie-Smith, K. A.: Assessment of site and severity in congenital aortic stenosis. Brit. Heart J., 29:367, 1967.

115. Oakley, C. M., and Somerville, J.: Oral contraceptives and progressive pulmonary vascular disease. Lancet, 1:890, 1968.

116. Oakley, C. M.: Hypertrophic cardiomyopathy—Patterns of progression. In: Hypertrophic Obstructive Cardiomyopathy. Ciba Foundation Study Group, J. & A. Churchill, 1971.

117. Okamoto, Y.: Repair of ventricular septal defect in infancy. Pediatrics, 27:961, 1969.

118. Omeri, M., et al.: The mitral valve in endocardial cushion defects. Brit. Heart J., 27:161, 1965.

119. Ongley, P. A., et al.: Continuous murmurs in tetralogy of Fallot and pulmonary atresia with ventricular septal defect. Amer. J. Cardiol., 18:821, 1966.

120. Parkes Weber, F.: Can the clinical manifestations of congenital heart disease disappear with the general growth and development of the patient? Brit. J. Dis. Child., 15:113, 1918.

121. Plauth, W. H., et al.: Transposition of the great arteries. Clinical and physiological observations on 74 patients treated by palliative surgery. Circulation, 27:317, 1968.

122. Pomerance, A.: Cardiac pathology and systolic murmurs in the elderly. Brit. Heart J., 30: 687, 1968.

123. Pridie, R. B., and Oakley, C. M.: Mechanism of mitral regurgitation in hypertrophic obstructive cardiomyopathy. Brit. Heart J., 32:203, 1970.

123a. Shah, P. M., Gramiak, R., and Kramer, D. H.: Ultrasound localization of left ventricular outflow obstruction in hypertrophic obstructive cardiomyopathy. Circulation, 40:3, 1969.

124. Pridie, R. B., Benham, R., and Wild, J.: Ultrasound in cardiac diagnosis. Clin. Radiol., 23:160, 1972.

125. Rad, P. S., and Sissman, N. J.: Spontaneous closure of physiologically advantageous ventricular septal defects. Circulation, 43:83, 1971.

126. Rashkind, W. J., and Miller, W. W.: Creation of an atrial septal defect without thoracotomy: A palliative approach to complete transposition of the great arteries. JAMA, 196:941, 1966.

127. Rastelli, G. C., Kirklin, J. W., and Kincald, O. W.: Angiocardiography of persistent common atrioventricular canal. Mayo Clin. Proc., 42:200, 1967.

128. Rastelli, G. C., Wallace, R. B., and Ongley, P. A.: Complete repair of transposition of the great arteries with pulmonary stenosis: Review and report of a case corrected by using a new surgical technique. Circulation, 39:83, 1969.

129. Reynolds, J. L., et al.: Critical congenital aortic stenosis with minimal electrocardiographic changes. New Eng. J. Med., 262:3, 1960.

130. Ritter, D. G., et al.: Ventricular septal defect. Circulation, 32 (Suppl. III):42, 1965.

131. Rowe, R. D., and Mehrizi, A.: In: The Neonate with Congenital Heart Disease. Philadelphia, W. B. Saunders, 1968.

132. Schrire, V., et al.: Ventricular septal defect: The clinical spectrum. Brit. Heart J., 27:813, 1965.

133. Scott, R. C., et al.: The syndrome of ventricular septal defect with aortic insufficiency. Amer. J. Cardiol., 2:530, 1958.

134. Senning, A.: Surgical correction of transposition of the great vessels. Surgery, 45:966, 1959.

135. Serrato, M., et al.: Palliative balloon atrial septostomy for total anomalous pulmonary venous correction in infancy. Pediatrics, 73:734, 1968.

136. Shah, K. D., et al.: Radio-isotopic scanning of the liver and spleen in dextrocardia and in situs inversus with levocardia. Circulation, 29:231, 1964.

137. Shah, P. M., et al.: Incidence of bacterial endocarditis in ventricular septal defects. Circulation, 34:127, 1966.

138. Shaher, R. M., et al.: Complete transposition of the great vessels with anatomic obstruction of the outflow tract of the left ventricle: Surgical implications of anatomic findings. Amer. J. Cardiol., 19:658, 1967.

139. Shem-Tov, A., et al.: Corrected transposition of the great arteries. Amer. J. Cardiol., 27:99, 1971.

140. Sigmann, J. M., Stern, A. M., and Swan, H. E.: Early surgical correction of large ventricular septal defects. Pediatrics, 39:4, 1967.

141. Simmons, R. L., Moller, J. H., and Edwards, J. E.: Anatomic evidence for spontaneous closure of ventricular septal defect. Circulation, 34: 38, 1966.

142. Simon, A. L., and Reis, R. L.: The angiographic features of bicuspid and unicommissural aortic stenosis. Amer. J. Cardiol., 28:353, 1971.

143. Singh, M. P., Bentall, H. H., and Oakley, C. M.: Successful total correction of congenital interruption of the aortic arch and ventricular septal defect. Thorax, 25:615, 1970.

144. Singh, M. P., and Bentall, H. H.: Complete replacement of the ascending aorta and the aortic valve for the treatment of aortic aneurysm. J. Thorac. Cardiov. Surg., 63:218, 1972.

145. Smith, G. W., et al.: Use of the pulmonary artery banding procedure in treating type II truncus arteriosus. Circulation, 29:108, 1964.

146. Somerville, J.: Clinical assessment of the function of the mitral valve in atrioventricular defects related to the anatomy. Amer. Heart J., 71:701, 1966.

147. Somerville, J., Brandao, A., and Ross, D. N.: Aortic regurgitation with ventricular septal defect: Surgical management and clinical features. Circulation, 41:317, 1970.

148. Somerville, J.: Hypernatraemia—special problems with angiocardiography in total anomalous pulmonary venous drainage. Brit. Heart J., 32:320, 1970.

149. Starr, A., Menashe, V., and Dotter, C.: Aortic insufficiency with ventricular septal defect. Surg. Gynec. Obstet., 111:71, 1960.

150. Van Mierop, L. H. S., et al.: Pathogenesis of transposition complexes. I. Embryology of the ventricles and great arteries. Amer. J. Cardiol., 72:216, 1963.

151. Van Mierop, L. H. S., and Wiglesworth, F. W.: Pathogenesis of transposition complexes. II. Anomalies due to faulty transfer of the posterior great artery. Amer. J. Cardiol., 72:226, 1963.

152. Van Mierop, L. H. S., and Wiglesworth, F. W.: Pathogenesis of transposition complexes. III. True transposition of the great vessels. Amer. J. Cardiol., 72:233, 1963.

153. Van Noorden, S. V., Olsen, E. G. J., and Pearse, A. G. E.: Hypertrophic obstructive cardiomyopathy, a histological, histochemical and ultrastructural study of biopsy material. Cardiov. Res. 5:118, 1971.

154. Van Praagh, R., and Van Praagh, S.: The anatomy of common aorticopulmonary trunk (truncus arteriosus communis) and its embryologic implications. A study of 57 necropsy cases. Amer. J. Cardiol., 16:406, 1965.

155. Van Praagh, R., Vlad, P., and Keith, J. D.: Complete transposition of the great arteries. In: Heart Disease: Infancy, Childhood, 2nd ed. (Keith, J. D., Rowe, R. D., and Vlad, P., Eds.). New York, Macmillan, 1967.

156. Vogel, J. H. K., and Blount, S. G.: Clinical evaluation in localizing level of obstruction to outflow from left ventricle. Amer. J. Cardiol., 15:782, 1965.

157. Wade, G., and Wright, J. P.: Spontaneous closure of ventricular septal defects. Lancet, 1:737, 1963.

158. Wagenvoort, C. A., Neufeld, H. N., and Edwards, J. E.: Cardiovascular system in Marfan's syndrome and in idiopathic dilatation of the ascending aorta. Amer. J. Cardiol., 9:496, 1962.

159. Walker, W. J., et al.: Interventricular septal defect: Analysis of 415 catheterized cases, ninety with serial haemodynamic studies. Circulation, 31:54, 1965.

160. Verel, D., Chandrasekhar, K. P., and Taylor, D. G.: Spontaneous closure of ventricular septal defect after banding of pulmonary artery. Brit. Heart J., 33:854, 1965.

161. Wesselhoeft, H., et al.: Nuclear angiocardiography in the diagnosis of congenital heart disease in infants. Circulation, 45: 77, 1972.

162. Williams, G. R., et al.: Pulmonary artery banding in infants with congenital heart disease other than ventricular septal defect. Amer. Surg., 29:160, 1963.

163. Wise, J., et al.: Urgent aortic valve replacement for acute aortic regurgitation in infective endocarditis. Lancet, 2:115, 1971.

164. Zaver, A. G., and Nadas, A. S.: Atrial septal defect—secundum type. Circulation, 31,32 (Suppl. III): 24, 1965.

Chapter 5

CARDIAC DYSRHYTHMIAS AS A PEDIATRIC PROBLEM*

Mary Allen Engle, M.D., and Kathryn Hawes Ehlers, M.D.

EFFECTS OF AGE

Disturbances of cardiac rhythm and conduction are almost as frequently seen by the pediatric cardiologist as is congenital heart disease.[73,84,88,89] There is a similar challenge to analyze the situation, arrive at the correct diagnosis, and manage the patient optimally. Herein lies a major difficulty for the cardiologist who deals primarily with children, however. He may be thoroughly familiar with the most common congenital cardiac abnormalities, he understands the deranged anatomy and physiology, he skillfully applies the diagnostic techniques he has mastered and may even have devised, and then he chooses with confidence based on a sizable experience the appropriate medical or surgical therapy. When the problem involves a dysrhythmia, however, he is often in less familiar territory. His knowledge is less secure concerning the anatomy, electrophysiology, diagnostic tools, and pharmacological therapy involved. Pediatric cardiologists are much indebted not only

to those workers in other fields who laid the background for such understanding but also to the current investigators who have recently contributed to a great expansion of knowledge of cardiac rhythm and conduction through detailed studies of anatomy, electrophysiological mapping, microelectrode recording, cardiac monitoring and pacing, surgical observations and pharmacological testing.

Dysrhythmias in children, as in adults, are due to disturbances in impulse formation (automaticity) or conduction or both.[10,40,114] While the electrocardiographic abnormalities may be similar in the two age groups, there are differences in manifestations, frequency, etiology, and management of the dysrhythmias. For example, it is estimated that 50 per cent of adults are unaware of their abnormal cardiac rhythms but may notice secondary effects. Even fewer children are so aware, and it is up to the parent or doctor to notice the secondary effects, which may be slower to manifest themselves because, unlike the situation in the adult, the other systems, e.g. cerebral, coronary, renal, mesenteric, and musculocutaneous circulation, are

* This work was supported in part by the Westchester Heart Association and by USPHS Training Grant #5T 12 HE 05789.

135

usually intact. Children are more prone to alterations in rhythm related to changes in vagal tone than the adult. Cholinergic stimulation is a commonly successful maneuver to terminate paroxysmal tachycardia in the adult, and is usually the treatment of first choice, but in infants it is rarely if ever successful. Children are much less likely to demonstrate dysrhythmias due to digitalis toxicity or myocardial infarction, so that the most common causes of dysrhythmias in adults are the rarest in the pediatric population. Hypertension, hyperthyroidism, and excesses of alcohol or nicotine also have little to do with etiology and management of dysrhythmias in the young.

Detection of Abnormality

Symptoms

The infant or child with a dysrhythmia is usually unaware of it unless the ventricular rate is either remarkably fast or unusually slow. Under either of these circumstances, syncope or cardiac failure may be the presenting symptom. Syncope or the related sensations of dizziness and light-headedness can occur with the sudden decrease in cerebral blood flow which accompanies the onset of either paroxysmal tachycardia or sudden bradycardia. Abrupt slowing of the sinus pacemaker or, in the case of heart block, of a lower center, or the transient slowing which follows the offset of a rapid heart action, can cause fainting. Especially in infancy, sustained tachycardia around 250 to 300 beats per minute, or ventricular bradycardia around 40 to 50 per minute, can decrease cardiac output sufficiently that cardiac failure occurs. Children old enough to verbalize may complain of pain over the precordium when they have paroxysms of tachycardia. Decrease in coronary arterial flow with the drop in systemic pressure which accompanies paroxysmal tachycardia is responsible for that symptom and its electrocardiographic corollary, depression of S-T segments and abnormalities of T waves (Fig. 1). Older children may notice and complain of palpitations when the ventricular rate accelerates

Examination

Since symptoms are unusual, most of the dysrhythmias are detected at the time of a physical examination of a healthy child or one being evaluated for another suspected cardiac abnormality. Cannon waves may be seen in the jugular veins when the atrium contracts against a closed atrioventricular valve, as in complete heart block or when a ventricular premature beat reciprocally stimulates an atrial contraction which occurs against a closed tricuspid valve. Usually, however, the dysrhythmia is suspected because the heart rate is irregular or unusually slow or fast.

Electrocardiogram

The electrocardiogram at rest and after exercise usually documents the dysrhythmia, but for those individuals with a history suggestive of paroxysmal tachycardia the tracing between attacks may be quite normal. We have found it helpful to ask the family to count the pulse if there is a recurrence and to take the child immediately to the nearest emergency room or doctor's office to try to "catch" the abnormality on an electrocardiogram.

Monitoring

Another useful method is the continuously recorded tape monitor (Holter apparatus) that an ambulatory child can wear for up to 10 hours during rest and activity.[10] Situations which in the past have provoked an attack can be simulated. The tape is then scanned at high speed (60 times real time) for irregularities, which are written out and analyzed at standard speed. Bedside monitoring of the hospitalized pediatric patient who has a rhythm disorder, or is a candidate for one, is helpful, just as it is with older subjects in a coronary-care unit.[68] We employ such monitoring regularly in the cardiac-catheterization laboratory, in postoperative cardiac

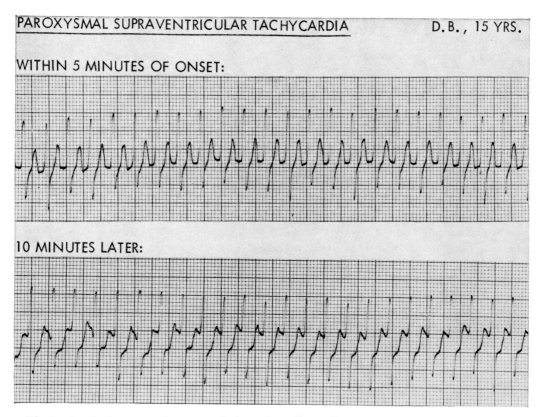

Fig. 1. Attack of paroxysmal supraventricular tachycardia at 250 beats per minute observed during continuous tape monitoring with Holter recorder. Note depression of S–T segments which appeared 10 minutes after onset of rapid rate.

surgical intensive-care areas, and in pediatric intensive-care units for high-risk neonates and sick children.

Etiology

Most episodes of paroxysmal rapid heart action occur in the absence of heart disease or detectable electrolyte imbalance. They are found more commonly in males than in females, and especially in the first few months of life; they have even been detected in utero.[5,19] It is likely that the instability produced by continued molding and development of the pacemakers and specialized conduction system that James described,[47] and the delay into the postnatal period of completion of sympathetic cardiac innervation reported by Friedman,[24] are responsible for these supraventricular and ventricular dys-

rhythmias in otherwise healthy newborns. They may even account for unexplained sudden death in babies.[14,46]

The other common time for dysrhythmias in otherwise healthy children is the pre-adolescent period from 8 to 12 years.[19] Perhaps the explanation lies in some autonomic imbalance during this phase of maturation also.

Certain children with heart disease are more prone to dysrhythmias than their normal counterparts. For example, those with atrial abnormality (such as that which occurs with mitral insufficiency, Ebstein's anomaly of the tricuspid valve, or following repair of an atrial septal defect or a Mustard procedure for transposition of the great arteries) tend to experience supraventricular dysrhythmias. Ventricular ectopic beats sometimes follow ventriculotomy for repair of a ventricular septal defect. Ectopic beats and tachyrhythmias are common in cardiomyopathies, especially in the terminal phase.[21,108] Arrhythmias can occur during periods of inadequate respiratory function and of hypoxia,[1] especially during anesthesia.[52,53] Emotions such as fright or anxiety may precipitate dysrhythmias,[4] as may serious electrolyte imbalance.[106]

Complete heart block is usually congenital[72,73,82] and the heart is otherwise normally formed, but it may occur in association with another congenital cardiac anomaly, the most common of which is "corrected" transposition of the great arteries with ventricular inversion. In this anomaly, the block may progress from partial to complete as the child grows. Temporary first-degree heart block in children is most often found in acute rheumatic fever.

Drugs, especially digitalis, are often responsible in adults for disturbance of rhythm or conduction, but this situation is unusual in the pediatric group, most of whom are taking no medication when the arrhythmia is detected. Furthermore, a digitalis-toxic rhythm is not often encountered in an infant or child taking digitalis under proper treatment.

Before reviewing the disorders of rhythm and conduction in the young, it may be helpful first to consider present concepts of arrangement and interaction of the conduction system of the heart.

ANATOMY AND FUNCTION OF CARDIAC CONDUCTION SYSTEM

Anatomy

The meticulous studies of James,[42-45,47,49] Lev,[57-62] Rosenbaum,[92,93] Hoffman[36-39] and others show that the human cardiac conduction system includes the following important components. The principal pacemaker is the *sinus node*, located at the junction of the superior vena cava and right atrium. It is supplied by the centrally placed sinus-node artery and although it contains no ganglia, it is innervated by parasympathetic and sympathetic fibers. Both the size of the sinus-node artery and its sympathetic innervation continue to develop postnatally.[24,47] Their relative immaturity in the newborn may be responsible for the high incidence of dysrhythmias and even sudden death in this age group.[46]

From the pacemaker cells in the sinus node, the impulse travels nonradially through the atria and atrial septum via three special tracts: the *anterior, middle, and posterior internodal pathways*. Knowledge of these fiber tracts is important not only for the cardiologist but also for the surgeon, who wishes to prevent supraventricular dysrhythmias when, for example, the atrial septum is excised and adjacent tissues are affected during the Mustard procedure for transposition of the great arteries.[80,100]

Fibers from the three pathways converge and interconnect at different areas on the *atrioventricular node*, which is located beneath the right atrial endocardium just anterior to the mouth of the coronary sinus and above the insertion of the tricuspid valve. Its concave surface rests on the central fibrous body or mitral annulus. Since some fibers enter lower on the A-V node than others, they may serve as bypass routes. There are no ganglia within the node but it too is richly innervated. Its blood supply is from a branch of the right coronary artery. At the anterior inferior margin of the A-V node, the fibers orient longitudinally and converge through the central fibrous body to form the *bundle of His*. The region of the A-V node and His bundle is critical as the chief region for delay in antegrade atrioventricular conduction and also as the point of reentry of *retrograde* impulse conduction. Enhanced automaticity of this junctional tissue or reentrant conduction through it is now considered to be the basis for most supraventricular tachycardias.[34,35,55] Bypass of the junctional region is the explanation for the Wolff-Parkinson-White syndrome.[6,67,113]

After the His bundle penetrates the central

fibrous body, it reaches the muscular ventricular septum and continues anteriorly into the inferior margin of the membranous ventricular septum. There a large band of fibers branches into what Rosenbaum designates as two fascicles of the left bundle branch: the broad *posterior fascicle of the left bundle branch* first and then the slender *anterior fascicle*.[92,93] The left bundle fans out over the septal surface of the left ventricle and the two divisions insert, one into the anterior and the other into the posterior papillary muscle. The right bundle branch continues directly from the main His bundle and courses beneath the endocardium of the right side of the ventricular septum. The distal portion traverses the moderator band to reach the papillary muscle of the right ventricle.

The anatomical locations of the junctional tissue and bundle branches are significant to the understanding of certain curious electrocardiographic patterns, for instance that associated with endocardial cushion defects, and are critical for the surgical avoidance of induced complete heart block when a ventricular septal defect is closed. Rosenbaum's concept of the three fascicles of the bundle branch system has opened up a new way to interpret certain physiological electrocardiographic problems.

The *Purkinje networks* of the left and right ventricles enter the *myocardial fibers*, the end points of the conduction system.

Electrophysiology

Transmembrane Potentials

In studies of isolated fibers from the sinus node, atria, and His-Purkinje system, Hoffman, among other investigators, clarified the intracellular events during depolarization and repolarization and the principles of automaticity and conductance.[36-39] He recorded transmembrane potentials from a single cell and described the resting potential (phase 4) and action potential with a rapid phase of depolarization (phase 0) and slower repolarization (phases 1,2,3). He compared these phases for the various kinds of specialized conducting tissue and defined the changes that account for normal automaticity and change in rate. As slow diastolic depolarization in phase 4 reduces membrane potential to the threshold potential, excitation of the cell occurs and an action potential results. Such spontaneous depolarization is the normal automatic mechanism, and it is present only in true and latent pacemaker cells: the sinus node, ectopic supraventricular pacemakers, and cells of the His-Purkinje system. The cell which first attains threshold and generates an action potential is the pacemaker. Under normal circumstances, this is the sinus node. Changes in rate come about through factors which change the time required for phase-4 depolarization to lower membrane potential to the threshold potential. In nonpacemaker cells of atrium and ventricle, the diastolic potential is steady.

Conduction of the cardiac impulse from the pacemaker through the conduction system involves sequential depolarization of adjacent areas of cell membrane by currents arising between active (or depolarized) and resting (or normally polarized) cells. Conduction velocity depends not only on the magnitude of the stimulus but also on threshold and membrane potentials and on fiber diameter. Slowing of velocity of conduction or a block occurs when the impulse arrives at cells which have not yet attained full repolarization after the preceding beat. Normal conduction is antegrade, but under certain conditions can be retrograde.

Refractory Periods

The responsiveness of the heart changes during the phases of de- and repolarization. In the absolute refractory period, from the QRS to and including the rise of T in the electrocardiogram, the cell does not respond to any stimulus. A strong stimulus will elicit a response during the relative partially refractory period (peak of T and its decline). A weaker-than-normal stimulus will induce a response in the brief supernormal phase of responsiveness (end of T wave). The rest of the time the conduction system is normally responsive. These fluctuations in refractoriness correlate with the duration of the action potential, which is progressively lengthened at lower levels of the conduction system. The refractory period is shorter in atrial than in ventricular fibers.

IONIC EFFECTS[30,104,105,110]

The cell membrane is permeable to potassium and chloride but relatively impermeable to sodium and calcium. Slow diastolic *depolarization* (phase 4) is a function of the interplay of conductance of K and Na. The cell becomes more excitable and the threshold lower as Na moves inward. Conversely, the threshold for excitation is raised as more K shifts outward and less Na inward. Some of the pharmacological agents which act as stabilizers (e.g. procainamide and quinidine) prevent or retard excitation by blocking the entry of Na into the cell. Calcium is also a membrane stabilizer; while it has no effect on the resting or action potentials, it shifts the firing threshold lower and so reduces cellular excitability. Calcium and sodium compete at the membrane surface. If calcium is reduced, the inward current of sodium is enhanced and excitability is increased.

During *repolarization*, Na conductance decreases rapidly but then levels off slightly above the diastolic resting plane, and the outward flow of K is retarded. When the outflow of K exceeds the inflow of Na, diastolic resting potential is achieved. Imbalance in these ionic changes can restore the resting potential prematurely and can either shorten or lengthen the plateau. Anoxia and digitalis, for example, shorten the action potential, while quinidine lengthens the plateau.

NERVOUS SYSTEM CONTROL

Cardiac rhythm and conduction are under the control of the autonomic nervous system.[11,38] In general, the actions of the parasympathetic and sympathetic nervous systems

are opposite in their effects on initiation and conduction of impulses.

On pacemaker cells in the sinus node, atrium, or A-V node, the *parasympathetics* by vagal stimulation and release of acetylcholine depress automaticity by decreasing the slope of the diastolic potential and hyperpolarizing the membrane. The sinus node is more affected than the A-V node and, in high concentration, may arrest; the pacemaker then shifts to a lower center. The His-Purkinje system is the least affected by acetylcholine. The effect on pacemaker cells throughout the heart of *sympathetic* stimulation or administration of catecholamines (norepinephrine and epinephrine) is to accelerate the rate by increasing the slope of diastolic depolarization. Conduction in the A-V node is delayed by vagal influence and accelerated by catecholamines. The denervated heart still beats, as animal experiments on denervation[18,109] and the experience in man with cardiac transplants have shown. The slow changes in rate which occur are probably in response to humoral agents.

The importance to cardiac rhythm of a coordinated patterning of impulses from the sympathetic and parasympathetic nervous systems has been stressed by Stewart, who emphasizes afferent, higher integrative, and efferent levels.[116]

Electrocardiographic Correlates of Conduction System

While the anatomy and function of the conduction system were being updated, a major advance occurred in the recording of the electrical activity of the human heart. In 1969 Scherlag and co-workers[94] developed an electrode catheter technique for intracardiac recording of His-bundle potentials and opened a new approach to clarification of cardiac conduction and rhythm, both normal and abnormal.[7,13,98,102]

The method consists of the transvenous passage of an electrode catheter under fluoroscopic control into the right heart across the tricuspid valve. Recordings made from the surface and intracardiac ECGs permit analysis of the electrical potentials generated in the various parts of the conduction system as they are explored and allow the identification of the point of delay and the direction of impulse conduction. Not only disturbances of rhythm and conduction but also the effects of cardio-active drugs can be studied in this way.

The well-known PQRS-T sequence of the ECG can be broken down into its component parts by correlation with the intracardiac ECG. The interval from onset of P to onset of QRS is composed of identifiable waves in the intracavitary ECG: the atrial electrogram (A), the A-V nodal potential (N), the His-bundle potential (H), and the right bundle potential (RB), in that order. The QRS complex correlates with the ventricular electrogram (V). Intervals can be measured between each of these waves so that delay or acceleration at any point of the system can be identified. In complete atrioventricular block, for example, it can be determined whether the disruption of conduction occurs prior to or following His-bundle depolarization. Simple and complex arrhythmias can similarly be analyzed as to origin of impulse

formation and its spread. This new technique has to date been employed chiefly in adults. The information derived therefrom has already clarified some problems in interpretation of standard electrocardiograms with complex arrhythmias.

TYPES OF DISORDERS

Disturbances of rhythm are more common than those of conduction, and mild degrees of abnormality are more often found than severe. Since a fast pulse rate is a common problem to evaluate, this range of rates may be helpful at the bedside or with the ECG to distinguish one tachycardia from another (Table 1). Usually the dysrhythmia occurs in pure form, but some children have problems of both rhythm and conduction. We shall first consider these disturbances in turn, proceeding from the sinus node downward.

Supraventricular Dysrhythmias

Supraventricular rhythm with normal conduction is characterized on the ECG by a narrow QRS of normal form. The origin of the impulse is indicated by the form of the P wave and by the P-R interval as well as by the rate. The supraventricular pace-

Table 1.   Tachyrhythmias

Rhythm	Pulse	Ventricular Rate	Atrial Rate
Sinus tachycardia	Regular	120–200	Same
Supraventricular tachycardia	Regular	150–300	Same
SV tachycardia with block	Irregular if varying block	120–200	Faster
Atrial flutter usually with block 2:1, 3:2	Irregular if varying block	125–300	300 or > 300
Atrial fibrillation with varying block	Grossly irregular	140–200	> 300
Ventricular tachycardia	Slightly irregular	150–250	Usually slower, or the same if reentry
Ventricular flutter	Regular	300	No relation unless reentry

maker is normally the sinus node but may be in atrial tissue (in which case the form of the P wave is abnormal and the P-R interval is longer than during sinus rhythm) or in the junctional region of the A-V node and His bundle (in which case the P wave is abnormal but the P-R interval is shorter than normal). With some supraventricular dysrhythmias, the form of the QRS is abnormal due to aberrant conduction below the His bundle.[97]

SINUS NODE

Sinus Arrhythmia

This is a periodic slowing and accelerating of the rate related to the phase of respiration under vagal control, and is the most common cause of irregular heartbeat in a child. Sometimes it is so exaggerated that dropped beats may be suspected and an ECG is needed for clarification of the normal P-QRS relation as the rate changes. Excessive sinus slowing with sinus arrhythmia may be a sign of digitalis excess (Fig. 2), hypoxia, or hypervagism.

Sinus Tachycardia

This condition is normal on exercise but at rest and in the absence of fever or cardiac

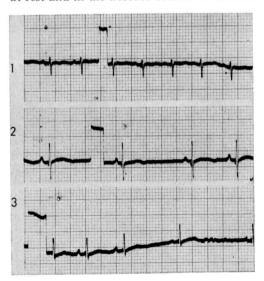

Fig. 2. Excessive sinus slowing during sinus arrhythmia in premature infant treated with digitalis for cardiac failure.

failure suggests the possibility of hyperthyroidism, ingestion of an atropine-like agent, or myocarditis. The smaller the baby, the higher is the normal heart rate at rest. The usual range for a newborn is 110 to 150; for a toddler, 85 to 125; for a preschool child, 75 to 115; and after the age of six years the range is 60 to 100 beats per minute.[87]

Sinus Bradycardia

This is normal for the trained athlete but sufficiently unusual otherwise in children that possibilities such as hypothyroidism or increased intracranial pressure are considered. Drugs such as propranolol produce sinus bradycardia by depressing the sinus pacemaker.

Shifting or Wandering Pacemaker

In children with sinus arrhythmias, at the times of marked slowing a lower center (usually junctional) may not uncommonly escape and become the pacemaker until the sinus node becomes dominant again (Fig. 3).

Sinus Pause

There is an abrupt cessation of sinus-node activity, characterized on the ECG by absence of P and QRS. It is uncommon as an isolated event but may occur with sinus-node depression, as for example from digitalis excess.

Sick Sinus-node Syndrome

In this unusual disorder the sinus node is quite undependable as a pacemaker. During long sinus pauses, a lower center escapes at its inherent slow rate or with bursts of rapid heart action. Either with the period of asystole or at the onset or offset of the tachycardia, the patient may faint. Illustrative strips of this dysrhythmia and its temporary modification by atropine and isoproterenol (Isuprel) are shown in Figure 4, from a young boy who was referred because of episodes of fainting on the school playground. No cause may be found to account for this abnormal sinus mechanism; however, unusually high

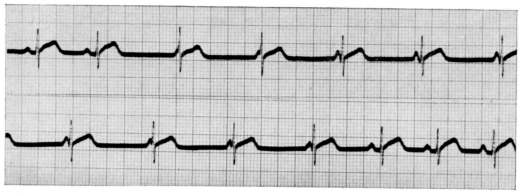

Fig. 3. Shifting pacemaker in child taking no medication. Sinus beats occur as the first two beats of top row and last three beats of bottom row. As sinus rate slows slightly from 90 beats/min, a lower junctional pacemaker escapes and junctional rhythm occurs at a rate of 65/min until sinus node accelerates again.

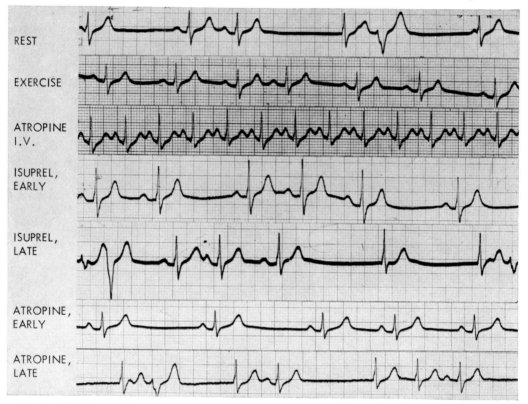

Fig. 4. "Sick sinus-node syndrome" in a 10-year-old boy with attacks of syncope on playground and with anomalous high insertion of inferior vena cava near mouth of superior cava. Top strip is representative of his usual resting electrocardiogram. The second and third QRS are preceded by P waves and normal P–R interval. The first, fourth, and sixth beats are junctional escape beats and the next-to-last beat is a premature contraction of aberrant QRS form (ventricular or supraventricular with aberration). Similar aberrant complexes are seen at the end of strip 5 and as the second beat of strip 7, when drugs were ineffective. Note the fixed coupling time of this premature beat.

Strips 2 and 4 show the effects of exercise and isoproterenol in producing a temporary acceleration of rate which is catecholamine induced, while strips 3 and 6 show the vagal-blocking effect of atropine intravenously (third strip) and orally (sixth strip). Neither isoproterenol nor oral atropine was effective as chronic therapy (fifth and seventh strips).

insertion of the inferior vena cava (as found in the boy just mentioned) and surgical trauma to the region (as might occur with caval cannulation for open-heart surgery) may be responsible. In children there are not many situations in which the fault is due to compromise of the sinus-node artery.

Sinus Arrest

When this occurs with no escape by a lower pacemaker, it is a mechanism of death. Whether it is one explanation for "crib death" in presumedly healthy babies is unknown. It may also be the final event in the unusual syndrome in which congenital deafness and a prolonged Q-T interval are associated with sudden death in families.[23,27,28,79,85,103] Marked hyperkalemia causes arrest of the sinus node.

ATRIUM, JUNCTIONAL REGION
(A-V NODE, HIS BUNDLE)

These regions possess latent pacemaker properties and may become active for isolated beats or runs of ectopic rhythm when the sinus node fails in its pacemaker function or when the latent pacemakers acquire enhanced automaticity. Formerly, supraventricular rhythm with a short P-R was referred to as "nodal rhythm," and when the P wave was inverted in leads II, III, and aVF the term "coronary sinus rhythm" was used. Recently it has been shown that the A-V node itself has no inherent rhythmicity and does not function as a pacemaker. Furthermore, stimulation of certain regions of the atria near the A-V node and His bundle can produce

negative P waves in leads II, III, and aVF, such as those which occur when the region of the coronary sinus is stimulated. The current term for these supraventricular rhythms in and about the A-V node and His bundle is "junctional rhythm."[23]

Supraventricular (atrial, junctional) Rhythm

Most of our concern is for the patient with supraventricular tachyrhythmia, for he may be symptomatic, even in shock or cardiac failure, especially if he is a newborn or has some compromise of cardiac function, e.g. associated congenital heart disease or that following open-heart surgery. Sometimes, however, the ectopic supraventricular pacemaker is dominant but at a rate only slightly faster or slower than the normal sinus rate. Then the dysrhythmia is usually detected only because an ECG is obtained (Fig. 3).

When the rate of the lower pacemaker is near that of the sinus node, the two pacemakers may both function and alternate or compete. If the lower one is more rapid, then the ventricle is unresponsive when the normal sinus impulse comes through. The atria and ventricles are dissociated and beat independently because the higher rate of the lower center interferes with the normal antegrade conduction from the sinus node. It usurps the role of pacemaker. As soon as the lower center slows or the sinus node accelerates to exceed the junctional rate, the sinus response can capture the ventricle, which at that time is not refractory. This set of circumstances is a form of atrioventricular dissociation called *interference dissociation*. It

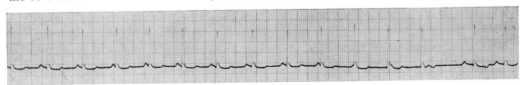

Fig. 5. Interference dissociation of atria and ventricles in child with rheumatic fever. Sinus rhythm of first two beats changes to junctional rhythm at slightly faster rate of 92/min. Both pacemakers function and the P–R becomes progressively shorter and then disappears (third to fifth beats from end) as junctional pacemaker overtakes sinus pacemaker, interfering with antegrade conduction until the P following the third-from-last QRS finds the ventricle refractory. After a pause, the sinus node resumes as pacemaker with a prolonged P–R, which once again begins progressively to shorten as the junctional region accelerates to usurp that pacemaker role.

is recognized by the more rapid rate for QRS than for P waves so that the P-R interval measures progressively shorter. If the tracing is recorded long enough, sinus capture can be demonstrated (Fig. 5).

Ectopic Contractions

Arising in atrial muscle or junctional tissue, the impulse is conducted along normal paths beyond. With atrial ectopic beats, the P-R interval is longer than for normal sinus beats and the P wave is abnormal: low and wide from a left atrial focus; high and peaked from the right atrium; or negative in leads II, III, and aVF if from the atrial region near the coronary sinus (Figs. 6, 7). Junctional ectopic beats show no P wave or a P wave with short PR or RP'. The ectopic beats may occur as escape beats when the sinus node slows or they may occur prematurely (Figs. 6–8). Then they may not be significant

or they may be the precursors of a more serious atrial dysrhythmia, especially in the newborn (Figs. 8, 9) or in someone with atrial enlargement. An early premature systole may find some areas of tissue ahead partly or completely refractory. In the presence of this unidirectional block, the impulse may turn back and reenter atrial tissue which may be in different stages of responsiveness. Unidirectional block and reentry favor circus movement and establishment of tachycardia. The reentrant P wave, designated P^1 when it follows the QRS, is often visible within the S-T segment of that QRS (Figs. 7–9). It may be blocked in returning through the junctional tissue and depolarizing the ventricle, in which case a pause will be recorded until the next sinus beat comes through (Figs. 7, 8), or the atrial echo (P^1) may find the junctional tissue sufficiently recovered (particularly if the last normally conducted

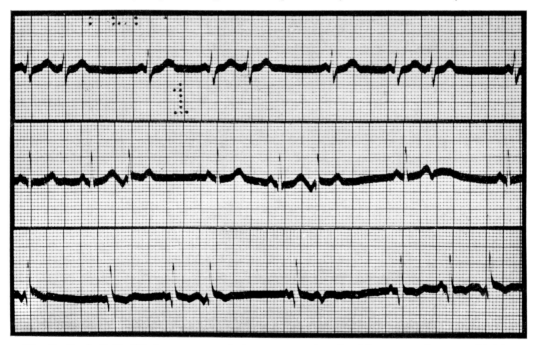

Fig. 6. Leads I, II, III show supraventricular premature junctional beats occurring every third beat through lead I and the first part of lead II. A negative P precedes these premature beats, which arise from atrial or junctional tissue near the coronary sinus. In lead II, after the next-to-last QRS, and again in the middle of lead III the abnormal P occurs at the same fixed coupling time as for the other premature beats, but the QRS response is blocked. The premature beats probably represent reentry beats with retrograde conduction through the A–V node and His bundle to stimulate the atrium and then turn in antegrade fashion to capture the ventricle, unless that impulse is blocked.

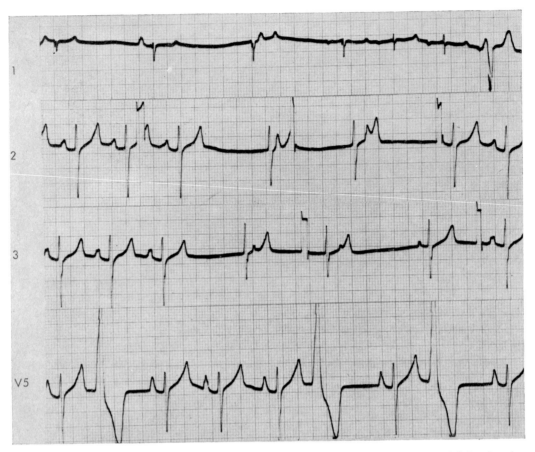

Fig. 7. Shifting pacemaker and junctional escape beats with P¹ following those beats and deforming the S–T segments. In the middle beats of leads I, II, and III, these reentrant P waves find the ventricle refractory. and so there is exit block and no ventricular capture, but in V₅ the ventricle is captured and a QRS–T of aberrant form, resembling a ventricular premature beat, is recorded (the second, sixth and eighth beats of V₅). Record from a boy with "corrected" transposition of the great arteries.

beat had a long P-R as evidence of some A-V conduction delay) to be responsive again, and a circus movement is set up and will continue so long as the wave front finds an excitable gap ahead (Fig. 9).

Supraventricular Tachyrhythmias

Even in the absence of bypass tracts there can be longitudinal dissociation within the junctional tissue so that reentry, atrial echo, and reciprocating tachycardia with circus movement occur. This is currently considered to be the chief mechanism for supraventricular tachycardias. An early extrasystole is more likely than a late premature beat to trigger a run of tachycardia. Most such episodes occur acutely, in paroxysms, for no apparent reason or sometimes during periods of excitement, such as a sporting event. Some are chronic and of years in duration.[79,103]

Supraventricular tachyrhythmias may be only slightly or considerably faster than the sinus rhythm. They occur in three chief forms: supraventricular tachycardia (Figs. 1, 10, 11, 13–16), atrial flutter (Figs. 10, 20, 21), and atrial fibrillation (Fig. 12).

Supraventricular tachycardia, sustained or in paroxysms, is the most common tachyrhythmia in the pediatric group. In a

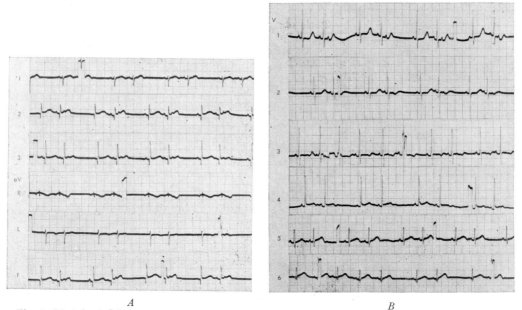

A   B

Fig. 8. Limb leads (*A*) and precordial leads (*B*) from an otherwise healthy newborn male on the first day of life. Note after every second QRS a P^1 is visible, deforming the S–T segment. The reentrant impulse captured the atrium, producing a P^1, but ventricular capture in antegrade fashion did not occur because the A–V node and His bundle area or the His-Purkinje system was refractory. In lead V_3 and for the first several beats of V_6, normal sinus rhythm with no reentrant activity or exit block occurred.

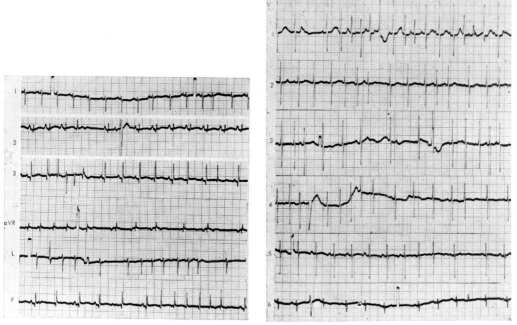

Fig. 9. Another newborn male on first day of life with dysrhythmia. Runs of supraventricular premature beats are seen in most leads, and there are frequent pauses as rhythm changes. Occasional QRS complexes are of aberrant form and may represent ventricular aberration or ectopic beats. A reentrant beat (atrial echo) with blocked QRS response to the P^1 is seen after the first QRS in lead aVF. Form of P waves preceding QRS complexes varies in same lead as supraventricular pacemaker shifts out of the sinus node.

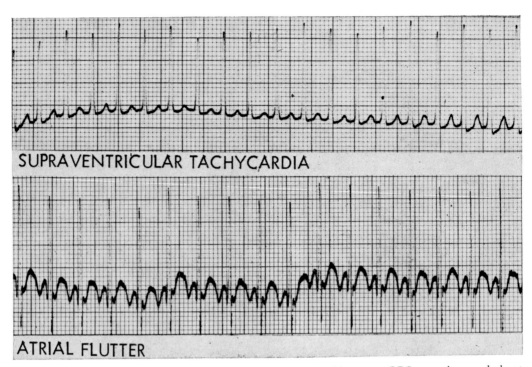

Fig. 10. *Top strip:* Paroxysmal supraventricular tachycardia with narrow QRS occurring regularly at rate of 240/min. T and P are probably superimposed. *Lower strip:* Atrial flutter with base line deformed by big, saw-toothed flutter waves, twice as fast as the ventricular rate, which is regular at 220/min.

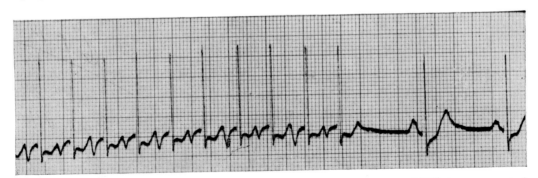

Fig. 11. Paroxysmal supraventricular (junctional or atrial) tachycardia at rate of 170/min at moment of conversion on digitalization to normal sinus rhythm (last two beats of strip). Note normal contour of sinus beats and inverted P waves of ectopic tachycardia.

survey of 50 patients with spontaneous occurrence of this condition, in the absence of medication or cardiac surgery, we found 34 under one year of age. Most were males. Fifteen patients had some form of congenital heart disease; the others were normal.

The pacemaker may be in atrial muscle, in which case the ECG shows an abnormal P wave and prolonged P-R, or in junctional tissue (Fig. 11). Then if the P wave is visible, it precedes or follows the QRS by an unusually short interval (Fig. 16). Sometimes the P and T are superimposed (Figs. 1, 10) so that P waves and P-R time cannot be judged; occasionally, by exploring the chest wall in the region of, above, and below leads V_{3R}–V_1, and by spreading out the waves through recording the ECG at double speed or double standardization, P waves can be identified (Fig. 22). Rarely is an esophageal lead considered necessary for this in babies. From point of view of management, it does not matter whether the patient has *paroxysmal atrial tachycardia* or *paroxysmal junctional tachycardia.* What is significant is that the pace-

maker is *supraventricular*. Then if the patient requires treatment, because the rate is rapid or the attack is sustained or recurrent, digitalization is the treatment of first choice under most circumstances (Fig. 11). Therapy will be discussed in a later section. With paroxysmal tachycardia, the infant's heart rate is usually perfectly regular and too fast to count, in the region of 240 to 280/min, and all leads of the ECG record this regular P-R interval at a rapid rate (Figs. 1, 10, 11, 16). A-V block with a slower ventricular rate is unusual (Fig. 13). Depression of S-T segments and inversion of T waves accompany sustained paroxysms (Fig. 1).

While the QRS is usually narrow in supraventricular tachycardia, it may be wide during the paroxysm so that the tracing resembles ventricular tachycardia. This can occur if there is ventricular aberration or bundle branch block (Figs. 14, 15). An example of the latter is seen in Figure 14, from a teen-aged boy who had undergone surgery to repair a ventricular septal defect and thereafter had a complete right bundle branch block. When he later experienced the sudden onset of rapid heart action, the ECG recorded a regular tachycardia with bizarre and wide QRS complexes (Fig. 14). Under sedation, a single DC countershock converted the tachyrhythmia to sinus rhythm with right bundle branch block (Fig. 15). Some patients with Wolff-Parkinson-White syndrome display the wide QRS form during paroxysms of tachyrhythmia.[32] In all these

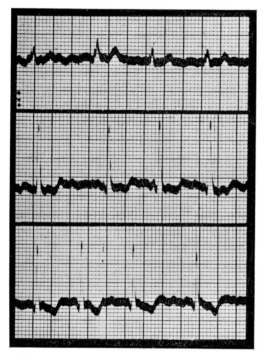

Fig. 12. Leads I, II, and III show atrial fibrillation in a child with rheumatic heart disease and mitral regurgitation. The QRS varies irregularly, a phenomenon attributed to concealed conduction.

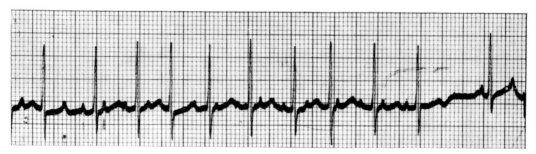

Fig. 13. Atrial tachycardia with variable A–V block, usually 2:1 but occasionally 1:1 (fourth QRS complex). The atrial rate is 280 and the ventricular rate is 160 until a pause occurs and the dysrhythmia converts to normal sinus mechanism. Record from a 3-week-old boy treated by digitalization to convert the tachycardia. On maintenance digitalis the rest of the first year, he had no recurrence of the tachycardia.

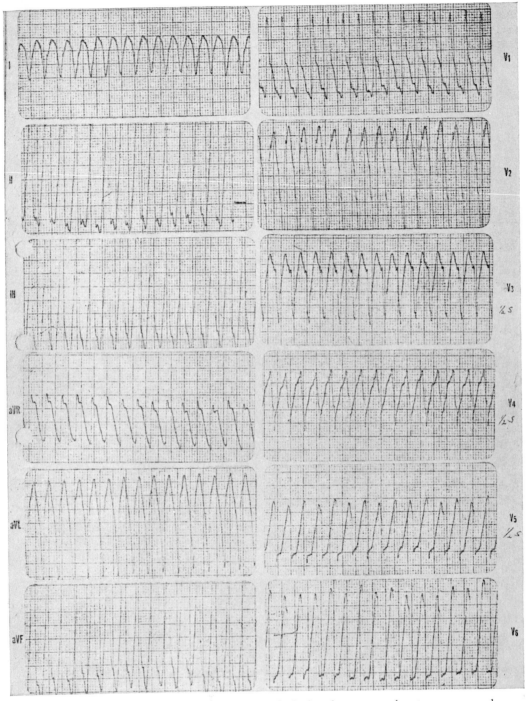

Fig. 14. Attacks of paroxysmal tachycardia in boy who had undergone open-heart surgery several years earlier to close a ventricular septal defect and relieve pulmonary stenosis. Note the absolute regularity of the rapidly occurring, abnormally wide QRS complexes at the rate of 260/min. The wide, bizarre complexes suggest ventricular tachycardia, but the rate and regularity, and what appears to be a P^1 deflection immediately following the QRS in leads II, aVF, V_1 and V_6, suggest supraventricular origin with ventricular aberration or RBBB. "Pseudoventricular tachycardia" was converted under sedation with one DC shock at 50 watt-sec to sinus rhythm with RBBB (Fig. 15).

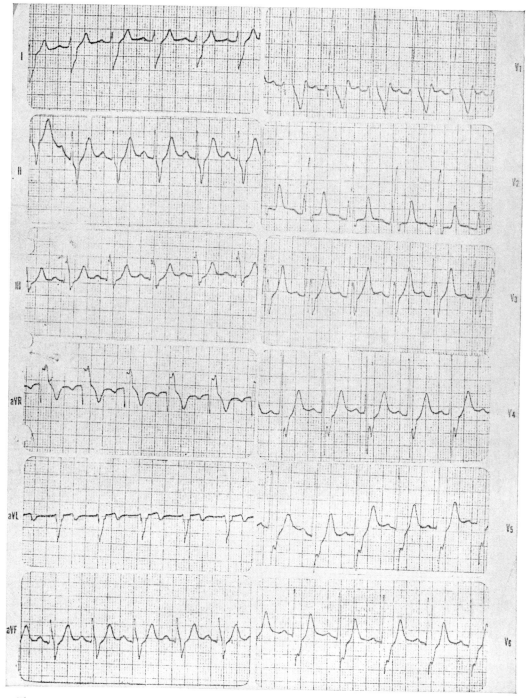

Fig. 15. Sinus rhythm with complete right bundle branch block in boy whose episode of paroxysmal tachycardia was supraventricular with wide QRS (Fig. 14).

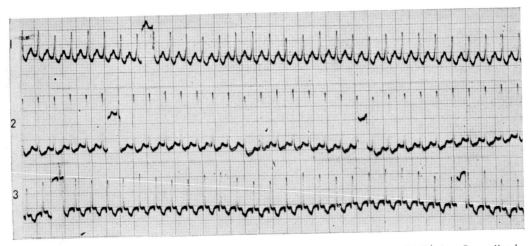

Fig. 16. Limb leads show paroxysmal supraventricular tachycardia at a rate of 250/min. Immediately following each QRS and deforming the S–T segment of each lead is a P¹ complex. The reentrant tachycardia converted on digitalization of this infant girl, whose electrocardiogram on conversion showed Wolff-Parkinson-White syndrome (Fig. 17).

situations of *pseudoventricular tachycardia*, a helpful distinguishing feature is that paroxysmal supraventricular tachycardia tends to be at a faster rate than ventricular tachycardia, e.g. around 250 in the former and 150 in the latter. If a distinction cannot be made, we believe that DC conversion of the tachycardia is preferable to drug therapy.

About one fourth of the infants and children with paroxysmal supraventricular tachycardia are found on conversion to have the *Wolff-Parkinson-White syndrome* (WPW) (Figs. 16–19). This electrocardiographic abnormality consists of the combination of short P-R and prolonged QRS with a delta wave initiating the QRS. Two chief types have been recognized: type A has initial positive forces in lead V_1 (Fig. 18) and type B has initial negative forces (Fig. 17). The QRS during attacks of tachycardia is usually normal in duration. The syndrome may occur intermittently[71] (Fig. 19) and it may be detected in the newborn period as a transient phenomenon.[32,48]

Anatomical dissection, surface mapping, and His-bundle recording have shown that the syndrome is due to a bypass of the usual junctional tissue.[48] Normal antegrade con-

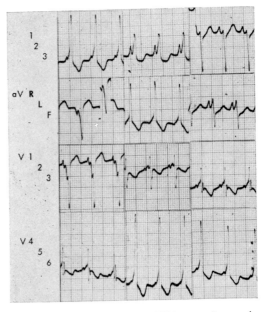

Fig. 17. Wolff-Parkinson-White syndrome in infant whose tachycardia is shown in Figure 16. The P–R is short and the QRS wide because of the delta wave. The initial forces are negative in V_1, so this is classified as type B Wolff-Parkinson-White syndrome. There is left axis deviation and the pattern resembles a left bundle branch block. Note short P–R, long QRS, and delta waves.

duction through the A-V node and His bundle might reenter the atrium in retrograde fashion via the nonrefractory bypass tracts, causing an atrial echo. A P[1] wave following the QRS indicates such an event (Fig. 16). Reciprocating rhythm and reciprocating tachycardia can become established when the atrial echo finds the distal conduction system and ventricles responsive and sets up a circus motion.

We have recently reviewed our long-term experience with 62 infants and children with this syndrome.[32]   Of the 29 infants and 6 children treated for attacks of paroxysmal tachycardia, all but one responded to digitalization for termination of attack and prevention of recurrence. Twenty had some form of congenital heart disease, the most frequent being a ventricular septal defect (10 cases), sometimes with pulmonary stensosis (in 5 of them).   Ebstein's anomaly of the tricuspid valve was present in two children, both of

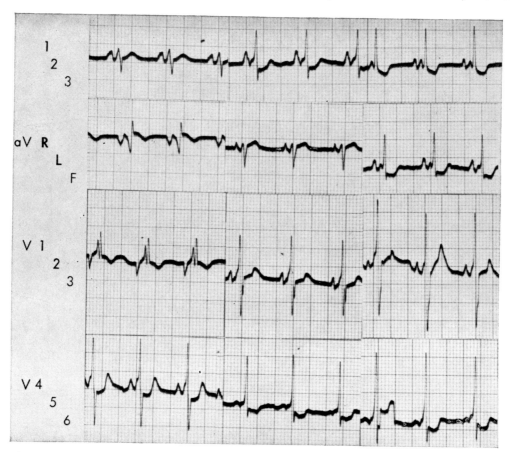

Fig. 18. Wolff-Parkinson-White syndrome, type A, with delta waves, short P–R, long QRS and initial positive forces in V₁ (resembles RBBB).

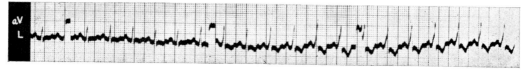

Fig. 19. Change from sinus rhythm with normal P–R, QRS and T waves to WPW syndrome with short P–R, long QRS and negative T waves with no change in rate.

whom had paroxysmal rapid heart action. While three fourths of the 42 babies had such episodes, only 4 of the 46 followed into childhood and adolescence were symptomatic. We concluded that the prognosis into adult life for infants and children with WPW was good.

Atrial Flutter

This is a combination of very rapid atrial activity, usually in the range of 280 to 300 beats per minute or more, and of atrioventricular block such that the ventricle responds to only a portion of the atrial impulses (Figs. 10, 20, 21). The block may vary but is often 2:1 to 4:1. It is sometimes difficult to determine whether the rhythm is atrial flutter or atrial tachycardia with block (Fig. 22). The atrial rate with flutter is often 280 or more but with tachycardia is usually less than 280. Flutter is thought to represent a circus movement with blocking of the im-

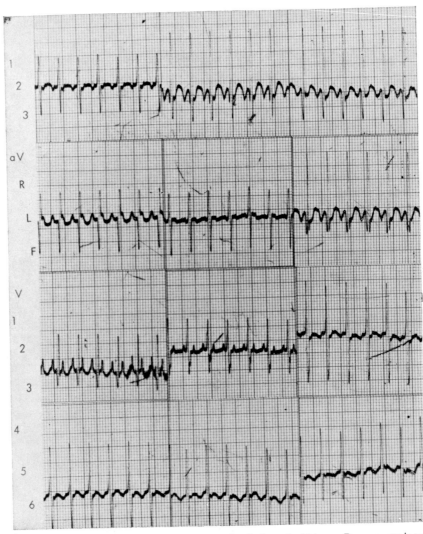

Fig. 20. Supraventricular paroxysmal rapid heart action in 3-week-old boy. P wave rate is twice as fast as ventricular rate; P waves are best seen in V₁ and II as high, peaked waves. In lead II they appear sawtoothed, as in atrial flutter. Ventricular rate is 220, atrial rate 440. Interpretation: atrial flutter with regular 2:1 block.

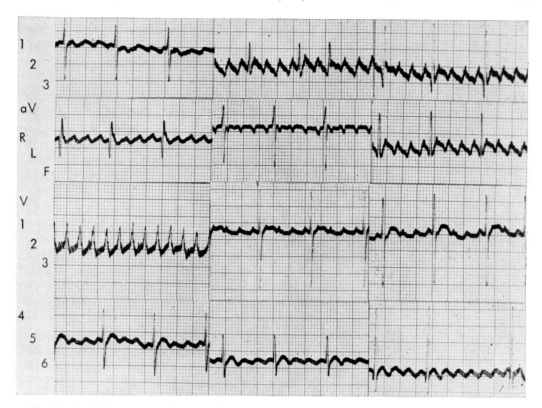

Fig. 21. Atrial flutter, probably congenital, in a 6-week-old boy with cardiac failure. Note saw-toothed waves of atrial flutter, easily visible in all leads but especially in II, III, aVF, V_1 and V_6. Flutter rate is 400/min; ventricular rate is 90 to 100/min, and the A–V block varies from 2:1 (lead II) to 7:1 (lead V_6). Flutter did not convert on digitalization. Ventricular rate slowed and then atrial fibrillation appeared. Conversion accomplished with one DC shock. Cardiac failure and cardiomegaly regressed, and child now has no evidence of heart disease.

pulse in one direction but propagation in the other to reach excitable tissue and restart the sequence. In the ECG typical large saw-toothed flutter waves undulate along the base line and are seen best in leads II and V_1 (Figs. 20, 21). The R-R interval is irregular if there is variable block. In our experience, this tachyrhythmia is unusual but when encountered is chiefly in children rather than in newborns. Most have had abnormal hearts with considerably enlarged atria, as with gross mitral insufficiency. Patients following atrial surgery such as the Mustard procedure have an anatomical basis for non-uniform unidirectional block and circus movement and they not infrequently have atrial flutter postoperatively (Fig. 22).

Atrial Fibrillation

This totally disordered rapid atrial activity with slower ventricular rate because of varying A-V block is the least common type of the supraventricular tachyrhythmias in pediatric practice. It occurs in seemingly normal newborns and also in children with atrial enlargement from mitral insufficiency or a cardiomyopathy. In the electrocardiogram no P wave is visible, but the base line may show small, irregular, rapid fibrillary waves (Fig. 12) and an irregular R-R interval. The irregularity of the ventricular response is because of concealed conduction when some supraventricular beats are blocked in manifest response and yet influence subsequent beats.[107]

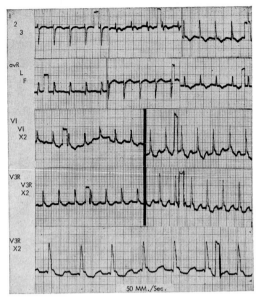

Fig. 22. Atrial flutter or atrial tachycardia with 2:1 A–V block in child following Mustard procedure for transposition of the great arteries. Increasing the sensitivity (V1 and V3R × 2) and increasing the paper speed to 50 mm/sec helped to identify P waves just following the QRS and another preceding the next QRS with a P–R interval of 0.14 sec. Conversion accomplished with digitalization, which was continued to prevent recurrences.

Ventricular Dysrhythmias

Until recently ventricular dysrhythmias have received little attention in pediatric cardiology aside from the feeling that ventricular ectopic beats are probably common and of little consequence. Our experience has convinced us that ventricular dysrhythmias are almost as common as those of supraventricular origin and that some "benign" ventricular premature beats may be the forerunners of more severe disturbance.[19] Continuous tape monitoring of the patient during rest and exercise has been helpful in eliciting those arrhythmias which are transient and in following the patient's response to treatment. Like the supraventricular disorders, the ventricular dysrhythmias occur chiefly in the first few months of life or in the preadolescent years, and then usually in boys with apparently normal hearts.[19] Among 50 patients we have studied with spontaneous occurrence of ventricular dysrhythmias sufficiently severe to cause symptoms or to require treatment, 30 had no evidence of heart disease. Six of these were infants, and seven

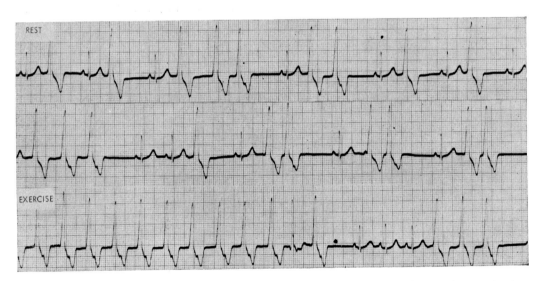

Fig. 23. Lead II of healthy 8-year-old boy whose irregular heart rate was detected on routine examination prior to elective surgery for strabismus. At rest, unifocal ventricular ectopic beats with wide QRS and abnormal T occur singly, in doublets and triplets. In the downstroke of the S–T segment of every second ectopic beat is a P[1], representing a ventriculoatrial echo. On exercise a paroxysm of ventricular tachycardia at a rate of 120/min occurred and spontaneously terminated, to be followed after a pause by a few sinus beats. His-bundle recording confirmed that these were ventricular ectopic beats.

of the 20 with heart disease were babies. Among the 20 with heart disease, we found cardiac failure, myocardiopathies including hemochromatosis, ventricular tumor, and cardiac surgery involving the ventricles.

VENTRICULAR ECTOPIC BEATS

Beats arising from the ventricle because of enhanced automaticity in the His-Purkinje system are more often premature than escape beats and are usually unifocal (Figs. 23 and 24) rather than multifocal (Fig. 25). Typically the QRS is wide and bizarre and the S-T segments and T waves of the repolarization phase are abnormal. If the ventricular ectopic focus is in the right ventricle, for example, the QRS-T form in the electrocardiogram resembles left bundle branch

block, since the left bundle has in effect been bypassed (Fig. 24). The ectopic ventricular beat may stimulate the junctional tissue and atrium in a retrograde fashion in which case a P^1 deflection may be identified following the abnormal QRS (Fig. 23). *Fusion beats* occur when the normal sinus impulse activates the atrium producing a P wave, but before the ventricle can be activated in normal fashion the ectopic ventricular focus fires, captures the ventricles, and produces the abnormal QRS that follows the P wave by a short and variable interval (Fig. 24). Narrow QRS complexes of a form different from normal are an unusual kind of ectopic ventricular beat, said by Rosenbaum to arise high in the three fascicles of the bundle branch system.[92,93] Since the impulse tra-

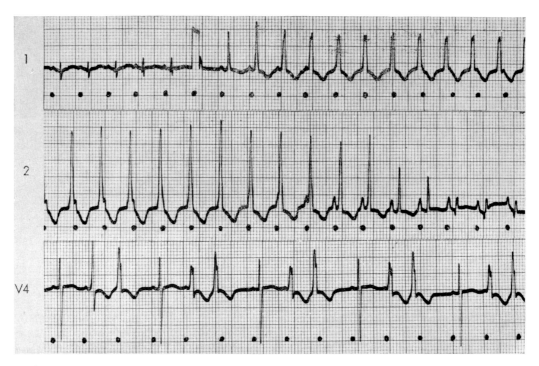

Fig. 24. Baby girl 5 days old whose irregular heartbeat was detected on routine examination. Note that occurrence of P waves is indicated by a dot, and that in lead I ventricular fusion beats with P-R shorter than normal and QRS of intermediate form initiate paroxysm of ventricular tachycardia. Lead II shows offset of ventricular dysrhythmia as sinus node overtakes ventricular rhythm. Fusion beats are again seen. Ventricular rate of 160 is little different from the sinus rhythm of this newborn, so this represents a form of interference dissociation. In lead V_4 a trigeminal rhythm occurs with one sinus beat, a fusion beat with P-R and QRS of intermediate form, and a ventricular premature beat. The coupling times in that lead are constant. Dysrhythmia converted on intravenous lidocaine, but infant required the combination of quinidine and propranolol for the first six months to maintain a normal rhythm.

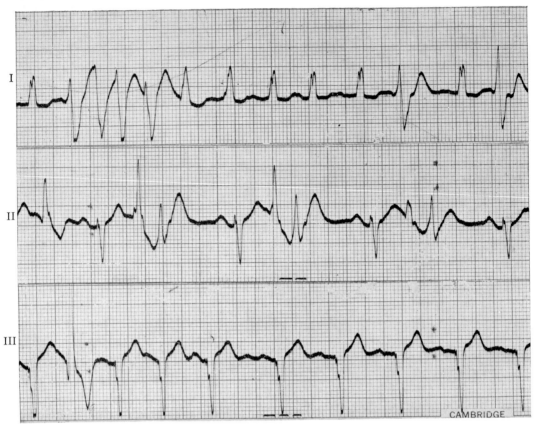

Fig. 25. Leads I, II and III from a 14-year-old boy with no known previous cardiac abnormality and receiving no medication. Several abnormalities of rhythm and conduction are evident. There is left-axis deviation of —50° and the QRS complexes, which are preceded by a P wave, are abnormally wide and notched. The QRS occurs irregularly. In lead II, trigeminal rhythm is present with the QRS sequence in three different forms. In lead I is a short run of four beats of ventricular tachycardia or flutter. The abnormal first and third beats of this run resemble each other, and the second and fourth beats are alike. After the dysrhythmia was controlled in the hospital on procainamide every 6 hours, cardiac diagnostic studies showed "corrected" transposition of the great arteries, ventricular inversion and mitral downward displacement. While receiving maintenance procainamide, the boy died suddenly at home a few months later.

verses fast-conduction pathways beyond, the QRS is not wide.

Aberrant forms of ventricular beats following a supraventricular impulse must be differentiated from ventricular ectopic beats[97] (Fig. 27). His-bundle recording clearly distinguishes them, for with a ventricular ectopic beat there is no His-bundle spike preceding V of the ectopic beat. Useful clues in the surface electrocardiogram are that aberrant beats: (1) often resemble a pattern of right bundle branch block, (2) are triphasic, in that they occur in relation to shortening

or lengthening of the cycle (as in an escape beat after a long pause), and (3) are preceded by a P wave.

When a rhythmic pattern of occurrence of the ectopic ventricular beats is established, the designation of bi-, tri, or quadrigeminy is made depending on whether that beat follows every second, third, or fourth sinus beat. A supernormal phase of responsiveness is important for bigeminy (Fig. 23). The ectopic beats can occur two or three together, in doublets or triplets (Figs. 23–25), but if four or more occur in sequence that represents a

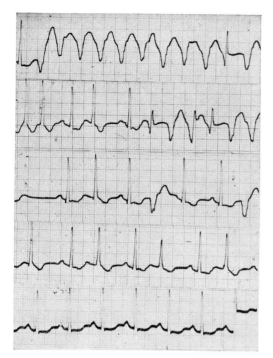

Fig. 26. Selected strips during pharmacological conversion of ventricular tachycardia (top strip) in a 12-year-old girl with thalassemia major and hemachromatosis, who was brought to the emergency room after she had fainted. The electrocardiogram showed ventricular tachycardia at a rate of 170/min. Intravenous procainamide was used, although today lidocaine would be administered. In the second strip the QRS form changes markedly. The first five complexes resemble her more normal supraventricular beats (bottom strip); then the ventricular dysrhythmia resumes. In the third strip there is sinus rhythm with isolated ventricular ectopic beats of same form as ventricular tachycardia. Strip 4 shows sinus beats interrupted by premature beats with narrow QRS, and the fifth strip shows normal sinus rhythm. At the end is the standardization mark.

run of ventricular tachycardia (Figs. 23–26). Herein lies the chief significance of ventricular ectopic beats: they may predispose to more serious ventricular tachyrhythmias. The vulnerable phase of supernormal responsiveness is near the peak of the T wave in the electrocardiogram. This is the dangerous period when the R-on-T phenomenon (Fig. 25) can induce ventricular fibrillation if the stimulus of the ectopic impulse is strong enough.

Ventricular Tachycardia

Four or more ectopic beats occur in sequence (Figs. 23–26). The tachyrhythmia may come and go in bursts (repetitive tachycardia) or may be sustained, usually at a rate around 150 to 180/min. While the rate is less rapid than that with paroxysmal supraventricular tachycardia, a child may notice palpitations, faint, or become hypotensive and in shock. The slower rate is less likely to cause cardiac failure than the rapid rate of supraventricular tachyrhythmias, but ventricular tachycardia is much more life threatening because of the possibility of progression to ventricular flutter or fibrillation.

Electrocardiographic diagnosis of this rhythm with wide, bizarre QRS complexes (QRS greater than 0.09 sec in infants and children) is based on the absence of P waves preceding each QRS (though a P[1] may follow by retrograde activation of the atria) (Fig. 23), and on the form of the QRS during paroxysms being the same as that of isolated premature ventricular contractions (PVC) (Fig. 23). Ventricular fusion beats in the tracing also confirm the ventricular ectopy (Fig. 24). The first beat at the onset of a paroxysm usually has the same or a shorter coupling time as the PVCs (Fig. 23).

Idioventricular Rhythm

A slow escape rhythm originates in the ventricle when higher centers fail to initiate an impulse or when these impulses are blocked from reaching the ventricle. An example of the former is severe hyperkalemia with depression of higher pacemakers (Fig. 28). Complete heart block with interruption distal to the His bundle is an example of the latter.

Ventricular Flutter

This refers to the rapid occurrence, at a rate around 300 per minute, of wide QRS complexes with little variation in form. It is rarely recorded as a spontaneous event, although we documented it by continuous tape monitoring of one boy with episodes of chest pain and PVCs in bigeminy on the

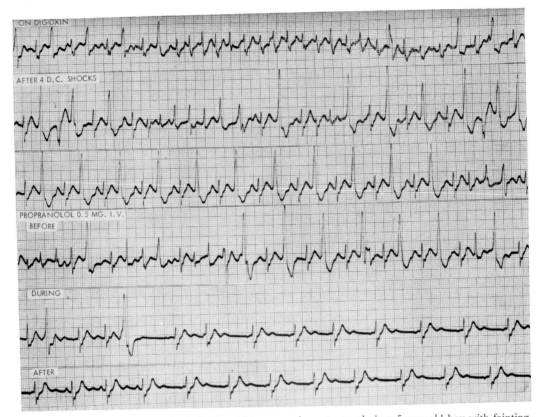

Fig. 27. Rapid, irregular tachyrhythmia which occurred spontaneously in a 5-year-old boy with fainting spells. Initial tracing resembled the first strip, which shows a recurrence of the arrhythmia while on maintenance digoxin at a measured, adequate therapeutic level. The recurrence was probably catecholamine induced because it occurred during crying prior to anesthesia for a urological procedure. Electrolytes were normal. Under anesthesia, four precordial shocks, to a maximum of 250 watt-sec, did not convert the tachycardia, but 0.5 mg of intravenous propranolol did. Oral propranolol was then added to therapeutic regimen with maintenance digitalis. The tachyrhythmia is irregular and the QRS complexes vary in form. Most are of the same form as his normal beats (see bottom strip) but some are of aberrant QRS–T form, so that the distinction between ventricular ectopy and aberrancy is difficult. His-bundle recording might have clarified the point, but therapy was considered indicated at once, and two modalities that would be effective against both supraventricular and ventricular tachyrhythmias were chosen: first DC countershock and then propranolol for what was probably a catecholamine-induced recurrence of tachyrhythmia on what had seemed to be adequate control by digitalis maintenance therapy.

standard electrocardiogram. It is a near-lethal rhythm and differs little from ventricular fibrillation.

VENTRICULAR FIBRILLATION

This is a chaotic, disorganized, ineffectual ventricular rhythm incompatible with life for more than a few minutes.[107] It is electrically induced regularly at open-heart surgery with the patient on cardiopulmonary bypass and usually is readily converted by DC counter-shock when the fibrillation is fine and fast. It is a terminal rhythm in many deaths from heart disease or other conditions.[75]

Parasystole[8]

Parasystole is a rare disturbance in rhythm in which a pacemaker different from the normal one exists and discharges at its inherent rhythmicity, capturing the ventricles when they are not refractory and being concealed when the normal pathway of conduc-

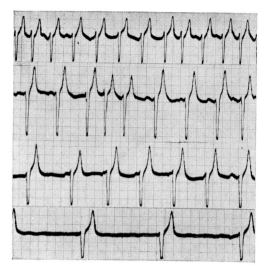

Fig. 28. Hyperkalemia, progressive and terminal, in child in renal failure. Note high, peaked T waves, then widening of QRS as His-Purkinje conduction is delayed, and disappearance of P waves as sinus-node activity is blocked. Idioventricular rhythm at slow rate was preterminal event.

tion renders the heart unresponsive to the parasystolic stimulus. The parasystolic focus is protected from influence of the normal pacemaker-conduction system. The condition is recognized when the electrocardiogram shows an abnormal beat at some multiple of a regular interval. If a long pause exists between these beats, because the parasystolic focus has found the system refractory, that interval will be some multiple of the minimal interparasystolic time. A long electrocardiographic recording is needed to map out the parasystolic firing and capture or concealment.

Disturbances of Conduction

Development of conduction disturbances is usually due to reduced levels of membrane potential at the time of excitation. The action potential is normally increasingly prolonged as the impulse advances distally in the system. *Decremental conduction* occurs when the action potential becomes a progressively less effective stimulus to propagation of the impulse to unexcited cells ahead. This is a mechanism for prolonged P-R interval after premature atrial beats, for ventricular aberration of premature supraventricular beats (see above) and of atrioventricular delay and block. An exaggeration of the normally decremental propagation accounts for most instances of partial heart block (first and second degree). During very rapid supraventricular rhythms, such as atrial flutter and fibrillation, many impulses enter the junctional tissue but do not emerge because of complete decrement. This is known as *concealed conduction*.[76] Decremental conduction is usually *unidirectional*. If an antegrade impulse is blocked at some point in the region of the A-V node and His bundle or in the His-Purkinje system, because of some inhomogeneity of conduction or because of longitudinal dissociation in the node, that impulse could turn around and initiate a retrograde conduction if the more proximal regions were responsive. Thus *reentry* would occur and a reciprocating rhythm or tachycardia could result, because the node was functionally longitudinally dissociated into two pathways with different refractory periods or because of accessory

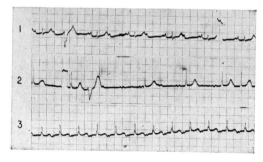

Fig. 29. Sequential recording of leads I, II, and III in a 2-year-old girl, receiving no medication, admitted for evaluation of cardiac enlargement. Diagnostic studies pointed to rhabdomyomatosis of heart. Six years later, this diagnosis was confirmed at autopsy. Wide, notched P waves, best seen in leads II and III, denote left atrial abnormality. Atrioventricular conduction delay causes first-degree A-V block (lead III) and also second-degree A-V block, 2:1 in leads I and II, or 3:1 in lead II. In leads I and II two premature beats of abnormal QRS-T form are interpreted as ventricular ectopic beats. A supraventricular premature beat is the last QRS in lead II. On another occasion this child demonstrated paroxysmal atrial flutter and cardiac failure, both of which responded to digitalization.

bypass tracts as in the Wolff-Parkinson-White syndrome. His-bundle recordings have verified these occurrences. Thus disturbances chiefly of conduction may become problems of tachyrhythmias (Fig. 29). Delay or block of conduction occurs at the sinus node, in the A-V node and His bundle, and in the His-Purkinje system.

Sinus Block

Already mentioned, sinus block or sinus pause may occur for no obvious cause or when severe hyperkalemia exists and atrial muscle is completely refractory (Fig. 28). Though the sinus node continues as pacemaker, no P wave is recorded in the electrocardiogram.

A-V Node and His Bundle

Impaired conduction is common.

First-degree A-V Block

The impulse is abnormally delayed in junctional tissue so that the P-R interval is prolonged, but each impulse is conducted to the

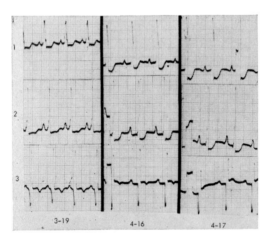

Fig. 30. Standard leads on admission, 3–19, of a child in cardiac failure due to rheumatic aortic regurgitation demonstrate two signs of digitalis excess on 4–16 and –17: prolongation of A–V conduction time and marked depression of S–T segments. In children, this degree of change may be the only forerunner of serious ventricular dysrhythmia (see also Fig. 41). We consider such a combination as an indication to withhold digitalis. Shortening of Q–T time is an effect of the drug related to decrease in activation time.

ventricles. Simple prolongation of the P-R interval is the most common electrocardiographic abnormality in acute rheumatic fever. It is present in some congenital anomalies, such as atrial septal defects, both of the secundum and primum varieties.[22] It is one of the effects of digitalis excess (Figs. 30, 31). A-V conduction is prolonged if the P-R exceeds 0.16 sec in an infant, 0.18 sec in a child, and 0.2 sec in an adolescent or adult.

Second-degree A-V Block

Partial heart block exists when some of the impulses fail to conduct to the ventricles (Figs. 29, 31, 32). Current terminology has revived the terms Mobitz type I and type II block.[74,101] The distinction of the two may have more significance in medical cardiology for patients with myocardial infarction and impending complete heart block than in pediatric cardiology. In children this partial heart block is usually in a setting of acute rheumatic fever, and the same child may show both types in a single electrocardiogram (Fig. 32). Congenital partial heart block is rare, but second-degree block may develop in that form of congenital heart disease in which there is corrected transposition of the great arteries with ventricular inversion. Partial A-V block may also occur with digitalis overdosage (Fig. 31). *Mobitz type I block* exhibits Wenckebach periodicity (Figs. 31, 32). The P-R interval gradually lengthens until a beat drops out. Junctional tissue then recovers and the same sequence repeats itself.

Mobitz type II block is an abrupt block, usually of every second beat (2:1 block) due to a disturbance in the conduction system distal to the A-V node (in or below the His bundle) (Fig. 32). When 2:1 block exists, its presence in the electrocardiogram may be masked because the P wave with blocked response is buried in the T wave of the conducted beat (Fig 32). When the ventricular rate is slow, such P waves should be sought; though hidden, they do usually deform the

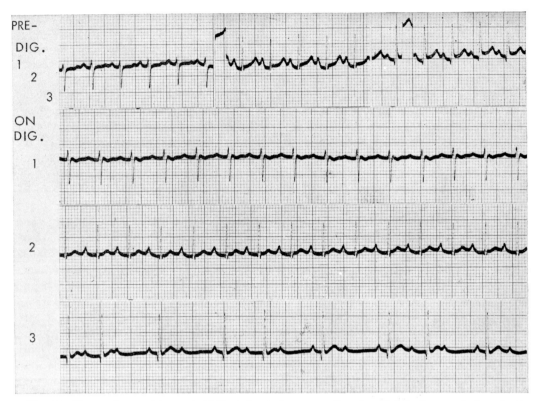

Fig. 31. First- and second-degree A–V block developing as manifestation of digitalis excess in 3-week-old baby in cardiac failure due to Taussig-Bing anomaly. First strip shows leads I, II and III on admission prior to therapy and the next three leads are recorded sequentially the following morning. Short Q–T and inversion of T_1 are digitalis effects. Digitalis excess is indicated in leads I and II by first-degree heart block with P–R interval of 0.20 seconds, and in lead III by second-degree A–V block with Wenckebach phenomenon and every third beat blocked (Mobitz type I).

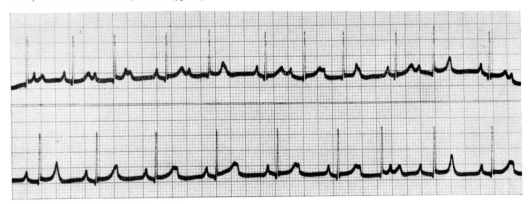

Fig. 32. Partial heart block, second degree, in a 6-year-old child with acute rheumatic fever. Wenckebach periodicity (Mobitz type I) is shown in top strip, where every third or fourth beat is blocked (3:2 or 4:3 A–V block). Partial and variable superimposition of P and T waves is well seen there and in strip below. When T and P are completely superimposed, as in the next-to-last T wave of top strip and first two beats of bottom strip, that T wave appears high and peaked. The presence of 2:1 A–V block (resembling Mobitz type II) at beginning of second strip could be overlooked unless other leads (such as V_1) are carefully searched for the hidden P with blocked response, or unless the rhythm changes, as in this record, to make the partial block obvious.

T wave sufficiently (especially in lead V_1) to be identified (Fig. 32).

Third-degree A-V Block

This is complete heart block. The atrial rate is faster than (or exceptionally the same rate as) the ventricular rate, and there are no captured beats. When the QRS duration is short, the block is usually proximal to the A-V node and His bundle. When the QRS is wide, the block may be proximal to His with a bundle branch block, there may be trifascicular block, or the interruption may be distal to the His bundle.[7,13,17,83,90,94] Congenital complete heart block usually shows a narrow QRS (Fig. 33), whereas surgically induced heart block usually has a wide QRS (Figs. 34, 35). His-bundle recordings localize

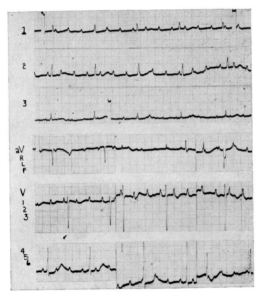

Fig. 33. Congenital complete heart block (third degree) recorded in a 1-hour-old boy who was subsequently shown to have no other cardiac abnormality. At three years, because of syncopal attacks, an epicardial pacemaker was implanted. In the subsequent four years he has been rehospitalized once or twice a year for a pacemaker-related procedure because of broken wires or pacemaker failure. This electrocardiogram shows complete dissociation of atria and ventricles with atrial rate of 180 and ventricular rate of 50 per minute. Narrow QRS indicates block is proximal to the His bundle. Ventricular ectopic contraction is seen at end of lead aVL and in middle of lead aVF.

the point of block.[7,13,17,83,90,94,101] A *ventriculophasic effect* can be demonstrated when the P-P interval surrounding a QRS is shorter than the P-P interval which does not enclose a QRS.

In an international cooperative study of 600 cases of congenital complete heart block,[72] 418 patients had no other evidence of heart disease. The period of greatest risk of dying was in the first few weeks of life, and cardiac failure was the chief cause of death. The babies at greatest risk were those with atrial tachycardia greater than 150 together with ventricular bradycardia less than 55 and with cardiomegaly. Cardiac failure was rare after early infancy. Stokes-Adams attacks caused death in 9 children. Of those without heart disease, 92 per cent were still alive and under long-term follow-up. The prognosis was much less good, however, for those with associated heart disease. Of the 53 deaths, 36 were in the first six months of life; 71 per cent were alive at last follow-up. The most common cardiovascular malformation was corrected transposition of the great arteries, usually in association with ventricular septal defect or single ventricle together with severe intracardiac anomalies; the next most common was patent ductus arteriosus. Simple ventricular septal defect was rarely associated with congenital complete heart block.

Permanent acquired complete heart block in the pediatric years is quite rare except for that surgically created by closing a ventricular septal defect.[56]

His-Purkinje System Block

This is manifest as aberration of premature supraventricular beats (see above) and as bundle branch block.

Right Bundle Branch Block

In pediatric cardiology right bundle branch block is differentiated into complete and incomplete forms, based on the prolonged or normal duration of QRS, respectively. Complete right bundle branch block is abnormal, but *incomplete right bundle branch block (IRBBB)*

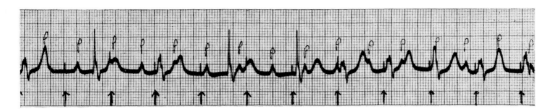

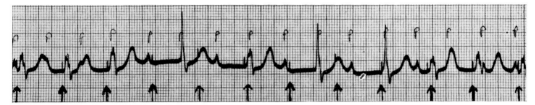

Fig. 34. Surgically induced, permanent complete heart block in child undergoing closure of ventricular septal defect. An artificial pacemaker has been implanted but only occasionally captures the ventricle (last half of first strip). This electrocardiogram shows three pacemakers all completely dissociated much of the time. The patient's atrial activity at a rate of 132/min is marked by the letter P. The pacemaker artefact at a rate of 94/min is indicated by an arrow. The wide QRS of idioventricular rhythm at 60/min is characteristic of damage to the conduction system distal to the His bundle. The pacemaker artefact is often superimposed on the T wave of an idioventricular beat, a potentially dangerous situation during the vulnerable or supernormal period after ventricular systole.

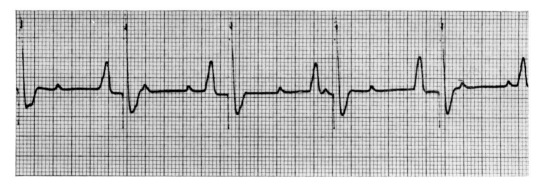

Fig. 35. Surgically induced, permanent complete heart block in child following repair of tetralogy of Fallot. Epicardial pacemaker was implanted but in this strip is malfunctioning. Three wave forms are seen: (1) the P wave of atrial activity at the rate of 130/min, (2) a wide R wave of independent ventricular activity at a rate of 55/min, and (3) the artificial pacemaker artefact and wide RS response at a rate of 57/min which occurs at the dangerous, vulnerable period of the idioventricular beat (R on top or near end of the T wave).

may be either abnormal or normal. The development of an rR′, rsR′ or rsr′ complex in lead V_1 is a normal phenomenon in the newborn as physiological right ventricular hypertrophy regresses postnatally. The same sequence of events occurs after a successful pulmonary valvotomy for severe valvular pulmonary stenosis when abnormal right ventricular hypertrophy regresses.[20] We consider such a pattern normal in a child if it is found only in leads V_{3R} and V_1 but abnormal if slurring of R or S is present in all leads of the electrocardiogram (Figs. 36, 37). This abnormal IRBBB is most often found in children with mild pulmonic stenosis or atrial septal defect. *Complete right bundle branch block (CRBBB)* is far less common and is most often seen following open-heart surgery to

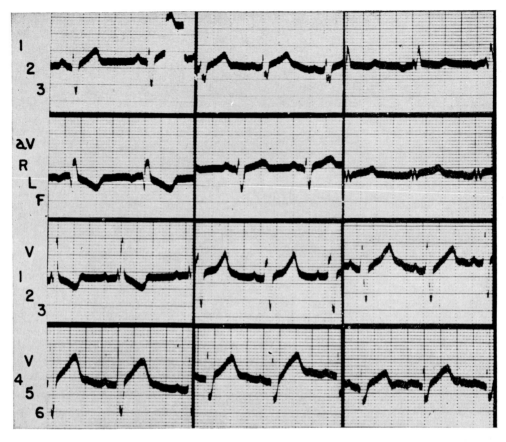

Fig. 36. Incomplete right bundle branch block (IRBBB) of abnormal proportions in a child with the secundum type of atrial septal defect. There is right-axis deviation around 110°. The rsR′ in lead V₁ represents the intraventricular delay. The QRS duration of 0.09 seconds makes the block incomplete rather than complete. The presence of slurred or notched R and S waves in all leads makes this an abnormal degree of IRBBB, greater than that seen in normal infants and young children. We do not read right ventricular hypertrophy, concentric, because the R′ deflection is less than 15 to 20 mm.

close a ventricular septal defect (Figs. 15, 38–40). Rarely, this postoperative RBBB may be intermittent (Fig. 39). Gelband and associates recently reported that the abnormally wide QRS occurs at the time of incision into the right ventricle and before the sutures are placed around the ventricular septal defect.[29] While this may be an explanation for some postoperative RBBB patterns, it is not the only one; we have observed some patients who have no such electrocardiographic abnormality following right ventriculotomy and others who do have RBBB but have not had an incision into the right ventricle, since closure of the ventricular septal defect was through an atriotomy.

Left Anterior Hemiblock (LAH)

As defined by Rosenbaum,[92,93] LAH or left anterior fascicular hemiblock can be diagnosed when there is left-axis deviation of −30° to −90° (axis superior and to the left) together with a QRS not so wide as 0.12 sec and a R₁-S₃ pattern in the electrocardiogram. RBBB and LAH may coexist. In children this pattern may follow surgery for ventricular septal defect[91] (Fig. 40). Whether this pattern will precede the development of

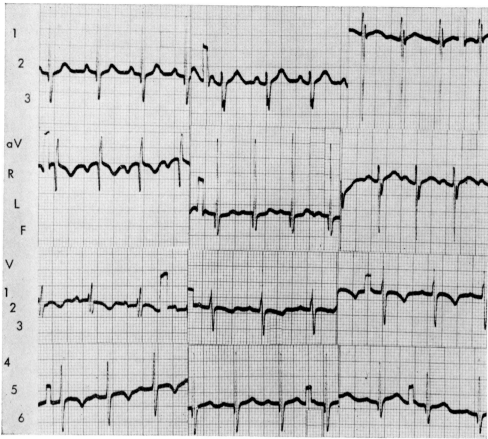

Fig. 37. IRBBB of abnormal proportions with left-axis deviation ($-60°$) in a boy with the ostium primum type of atrial septal defect and a cleft mitral valve. An rsr'S' of 0.08 seconds in lead V_1 indicates IRBBB, but the absence of a tall R' denies concentric right ventricular hypertrophy. A–V conduction time is normal.

complete heart block in these children is not known. It does not imply coronary artery disease, as in the adult.

Left Posterior Hemiblock (LPH)[92,93]

LPH or left posterior fascicular block is recognized when the electrical axis is 90° to 120° (inferior and to the right), the QRS is not prolonged, and there is an S_1-Q_3 pattern in the electrocardiogram. This pattern also occurs with right ventricular hypertrophy and in tall, slender people, a fact to be considered before diagnosing LPH. *RBBB with LPH* is suspected when ÂQRS is around 120°, there is an S_1-Q_3 pattern, the QRS is wide, and the conditions of right ventricular hypertrophy and vertical heart are excluded.

Bilateral Bundle Branch Block (BBBB)[95] and *Trifascicular Block*[92,93] (block of the right bundle and the two left fascicles)

These conditions have also been described but we have not encountered them in the pediatric group.

MANAGEMENT

Management of the infant or child with a disturbance of rhythm or conduction depends on: (1) accurate diagnosis, (2) assessment of the individual's condition and the situation in which the dysrhythmia occurred, (3) evaluation of the cumulative knowledge of the effects of the disorder and then, if intervention is indicated, (4) a knowledge of the agents available and their dosage.

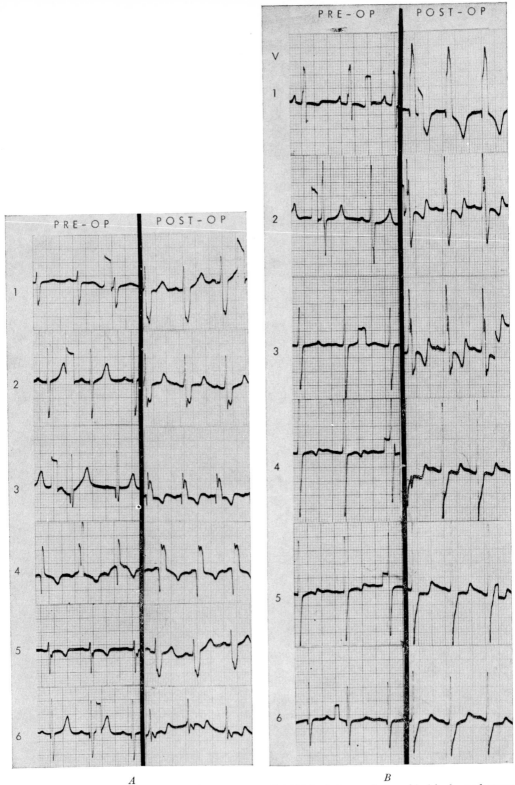

Fig. 38. Pre- and postoperative limb (*A*) and precordial (*B*) leads from a 5-year-old girl who underwent closure of a large ventricular septal defect through a right ventriculotomy. The numbers 4, 5 and 6 of limb leads denote the unipolar leads aVR, L and F. Note the change from preoperative incomplete right ventricular conduction delay (IRBBB with rR's in V_1 of 0.08-sec duration) to postoperative complete RBBB (qR in V_1 of 0.12-sec duration) without change in right-axis deviation.

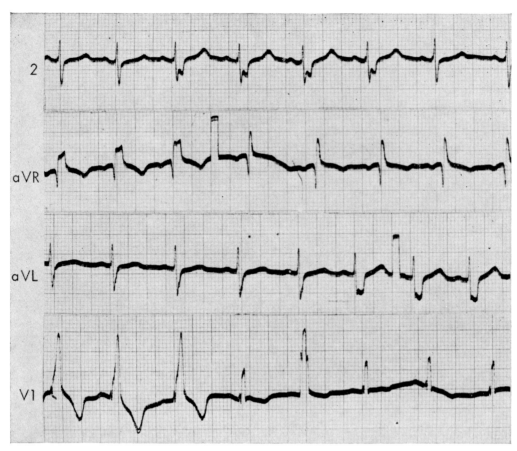

Fig. 39.   Intermittent complete and incomplete RBBB early postoperatively in child whose usual postoperative pattern of CRBBB is shown in Figure 38.   Note spontaneous change in form and duration of QRS without change in rate or A–V conduction as CRBBB for about four beats alternates with IRBBB for four to five beats.

Not every dysrhythmia needs treatment. Thus, no specific therapy is required for shifting pacemaker, escape rhythms, isolated premature contractions.   It is chiefly those situations of extremes of rate, too fast or too slow, and ventricular tachycardia even when the rate is not excessive, which require therapy.   Some dysrhythmias are true medical emergencies—the baby in shock or cardiac failure from sustained tachycardia, the child in the early postoperative period with supraventricular or ventricular tachycardia, the person with heart block and a Stokes-Adams attack, and the patient with cardiac arrest.   Such sick people may be hypotensive, hypoxic, acidotic, and hyper-

kalemic.   These derangements must be corrected by appropriate measures at the same time that the specific antiarrhythmic therapy is employed.   Indeed, such measures may be ineffective unless electrolytes are in balance. Table 2 summarizes the modalities, dosage, and toxic effects of the most commonly used drugs for infants and children with tachy- and bradycardia.

Tachyrhythmias

Available to the physician[41] are pharmacological antiarrhythmic agents, precordial shock, cholinergic maneuvers, cardiac pacing, and surgery.

ANTIARRHYTHMIC AGENTS[3,15,31,96]

These drugs exert their effect because they lessen excitability by decreasing automaticity and slowing conduction.

Digitalis

Digitalization is the treatment of first choice for infants and children with paroxysmal or chronic supraventricular, atrial, junctional tachycardia (SVT)[81] and atrial flutter and fibrillation, and for those with untreated cardiac failure who have frequent ectopic beats of supra- or ventricular origin. Digitalization converts SVT to normal sinus rhythm (Figs. 11, 13). It may convert atrial flutter or fibrillation but, if not, it increases the A-V

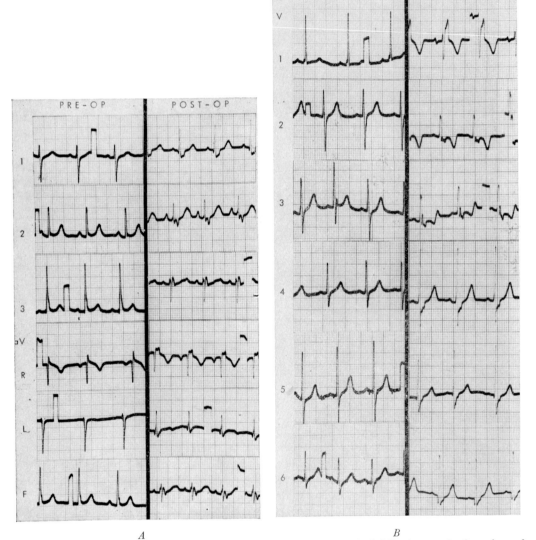

A   *B*

Fig. 40. Postoperative development of RBBB with left anterior hemiblock following repair of tetralogy of Fallot in a 6-year-old boy. Pre- and postoperative limb leads (*A*) and precordial leads (*B*) show change from preoperative right-axis deviation of 120° to postoperative left-axis deviation (about —45°), with $Q_1 S_3$ pattern. QRS duration increased from a preoperative normal 0.06 sec to a postoperative 0.12 sec. Preoperative right ventricular hypertrophy is indicated by tall rR′ in V_1 of 20 mm. Postoperative RBBB is shown by rSR′ in V_1.

Table 2. Common Antiarrhythmic Agents

Drug	Initial Therapy	Maintenance Therapy	Toxic Effects
For Tachyrhythmias			
Digitoxin	I.M. 0.035 mg/kg infants I.M. 0.025 mg/kg children	P.O. 1/10 digitalizing dose q.d.	Ventricular ectopic beats, tachycardia, fibrillation, atrial tachycardia with block. First-, second-, third-degree A-V block.
Digoxin	I.M. 0.035 mg/kg infants I.M. 0.025 mg/kg children	P.O. 1/8 digitalizing dose b.i.d.	
Quinidine	P.O. 2–3 mg/kg q 4–6 h	P.O. 2–3 mg/kg q 4–6 h	Rash, fever, GI symptoms, purpura, hemolytic anemia, hypotension.
Procainamide	I.V. 2 mg/kg of 1:10 dilution over 5 min	P.O. 10–15 mg/kg q 6 h	Lupus-like syndrome. Hypotension. Urticaria. GI symptoms.
Lidocaine	I.V. 1 mg/kg of 1:1000 dilution over 3–5 min; up to 2 mg/kg	I.V. 0.03 mg/kg/min of dilute solution of 5 mg/ml; decrease rate as arrhythmia continues controlled	Convulsions. Drowsiness. Euphoria. Muscle twitching.
Diphenylhydantoin	P.O. 2 mg/kg t.i.d.	P.O. 2 mg/kg t.i.d.	Hypotension. Ataxia.
Propranolol	I.V. 0.01–0.15 mg/kg over 3–5 min	P.O. 0.05–1 mg/kg/day in 4 divided doses.	Bradycardia. Hypotension. Cardiac failure. Asthma.
For Bradyrhythmias			
Isoproterenol	I.V. 1–3 μg/min of a solution containing 5 μg/ml	Same as initial therapy: drip rate adjusted to maintain stable rhythm and rate.	Ventricular ectopic beats, tachycardia.
Atropine	I.V. 0.01–0.03 mg/kg	P.O. 0.015 mg/kg q 6 h, 0–3 years P.O. 0.02 mg/kg q 6 h, 3–12 years	Mydriasis, dry mouth, flushing.
Epinephrine	Intracardiac 0.25 ml to 2 ml of 1:1000 solution.	I.V. 4–8 μg/min (about 20 mini drops/min of dilute solution: 2 ampules epinephrine in 500 ml dextrose in water)	Ventricular ectopic beats, tachycardia.

171

block and improves the patient's condition by decreasing the ventricular rate; then DC conversion can be undertaken (see below). Maintenance digitalis is continued in infants for the next 6 to 12 months to prevent recurrences during the period of greatest likelihood of another attack. Usually there is no further problem in those with normal hearts, unless the Wolff-Parkinson-White syndrome is present. Even then it has been our experience that recurrences of tachycardia are uncommon after the first year of life.[32] For those who have their first attacks in childhood, it is our impression that the attacks tend to recur and that digitalization may need to be reinstituted after it has been stopped. Figure 27 is from a 5-year-old boy with recurrent attacks who fainted on three occasions and was found to have an irregular tachycardia of supraventricular form with occasional aberration. The arrhythmia responded to digitalization, but while it was being maintained under control on therapy he was anesthetized for a urological procedure. During crying

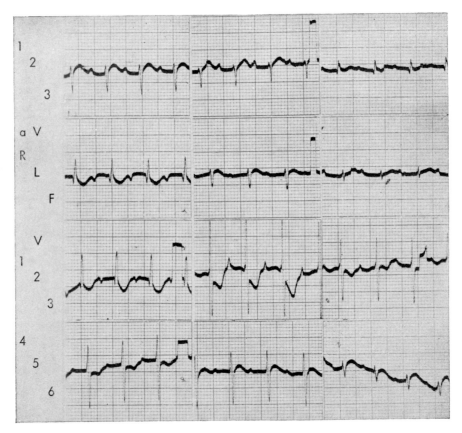

Fig. 41. Electrocardiographic signs of digitalis excess on admission in a 2-week-old infant transferred because cardiac failure, shown later to be due to coarctation of the aorta, had not responded to digitalization. Toxicity is indicated by the first-degree A–V block (P–R of 0.22 to 0.24 sec) and the marked depression of S–T segment in lead V_2. Within about an hour of recording this electrocardiogram and without isolated ventricular premature beats, ventricular fibrillation occurred. The baby was promptly defibrillated and resuscitated, and a few hours later the coarctation was successfully excised. He is now healthy and normally active at eight years.

Especially in infants being monitored by electrocardiogram for signs of digitalis effect or excess, we recommend that a full 12-lead electrocardiogram be recorded, not just a "rhythm strip" of a single lead II, for abnormally deep S–T segment depression may not be seen except in V leads. (Contrast with Figure 30 from a child with left ventricular hypertrophy and with evidence of deep depression of S–T in limb leads.)

prior to anesthesia, the tachycardia recurred and did not respond to DC conversion but did to intravenous propranolol.

Digitalis acts[69,70,99,115] through its inotropic effect and by prolonging A-V conduction (the A-to-His interval), probably a vagotonic effect. In excess dosage it can become an arrhythmogenic agent because it then increases automaticity of atrial and ventricular muscle; it depresses conduction velocity in the atria, specialized conduction tissue, and ventricles, and it prolongs A-V conduction. It shortens the refractory period, the effect of which in the electrocardiogram is to shorten the Q-T time, but the excess effect of which is to promote ectopic beats. In infants and children, marked depression of S-T segments in limb or precordial leads and prolongation of A-V conduction usually precede these arrhythmogenic actions (Figs. 30, 41). Radioimmunoassay of digoxin and digitoxin levels should provide a laboratory guide for therapeutic or toxic levels of the drug. It is most important that the physician treating any baby with digitalis because of cardiac failure or SVT use caution in calculating and administering the drug and in checking a 12-lead electrocardiogram for early signs of digitalis excess (Figs. 30, 31, 41). Toxicity would not have occurred in the babies shown in Figures 31 and 41 had not their pediatricians administered digoxin *parenterally* in the larger dose recommended for *oral* digitalization.

Myocardial Depressants

Several drugs are included in this category, the prototype of which is quinidine. Their pharmacological effects are similar and yet there are certain differences, so that one agent may succeed when another has failed to control the dysrhythmia. They depress automaticity of pacemakers and potential pacemaker fibers by inhibiting phase-4 depolarization. We employ these agents for patients with ventricular tachycardia to convert the dysrhythmia and as maintenance therapy for the next 6 to 12 months to prevent recurrences. Although they are also effective against atrial and junctional dysrhythmias, we rarely need to use them for supraventricular tachyrhythmias in infants and children except in the unusual situation when atrial flutter or fibrillation tends to recur.

Quinidine, in addition to reducing automaticity by inhibiting diastolic depolarization, decreases conduction velocity by lowering the resting membrane potential and decreasing the maximum rate of depolarization. It prolongs the refractory period by altering the duration of the action potential. In the electrocardiogram the evidence of this effect is prolongation of the Q-T or Q-U interval.

Procainamide increases the refractory period and conduction time in atrium, ventricle and in the junctional region by increasing the His-ventricle or in retrograde fashion the His-sinus interval. In some patients Damato found that the atrium-His interval was also lengthened, while in others there was no change.[13]

Lidocaine has become the drug of first choice in the initial treatment intravenously of the patient with ventricular tachycardia, to convert the rhythm to normal and to maintain it that way temporarily until the cause can be corrected or until maintenance therapy with another drug in this group of myocardial depressants is instituted. Its antiarrhythmic effect is transitory, but is superior to procainamide and quinidine in the emergency situation, as for instance after open-heart surgery. Unlike procainamide, it does not alter A-V conduction.[13]

Propranolol is a beta-adrenergic blocking agent[33,66,77,78,86] which affects intracellular potentials as quinidine does but also has local anesthetic properties. It reduces the heart rate and also the contractile force of the heart, so that the drug is contraindicated in patients with cardiac failure. Like digitalis, propranolol lengthens the A-H interval. Propranolol is effective against ventricular and supraventricular tachyrhythmias, but its special usefulness is in situations where there is

(1) a central nervous system component to the dysrhythmia (Fig. 27), (2) a digitalis-toxic rhythm, and (3) recurrent tachycardia with the Wolff-Parkinson-White syndrome. The agent may be used effectively in combination with another antiarrhythmic agent, e.g. digitalis, when an arrhythmia is difficult to control by either drug alone.

Diphenylhydantoin (Dilantin) is useful in the treatment of digitalis-toxic rhythms, both ventricular and supraventricular, and may counteract the depressant effect of procainamide.[12] It depresses ventricular automaticity, and it enhances A-V conduction by shortening the A-H interval. Its effect is transient so its value as a prophylaxis against arrhythmias may be limited.

Cholinergic Stimulation

For children (but usually not infants) with repetitive or sustained supraventricular tachycardia, cholinergic stimulation, directly by drugs or reflexly by increasing vagal tone, may terminate the attack.

Cholinergic drugs, such as acetylcholine, neostigmine, or edrophonium (Tensilon) are rarely necessary in infants and children. If used, an antidote such as atropine should be drawn up in a syringe and available if needed.

Reflex vagal stimulation by such maneuvers as gagging, coughing, the Valsalva maneuver, emesis, or unilateral carotid-sinus massage may halt the eqisode. Older children and adolescents with infrequent attacks can be taught to manage their attacks themselves in this way and parents may be similarly instructed to help their children. We believe that pressure over the eyeball should not be employed.

DC CONVERSION

The technique of precordial shock by DC current[63,64,112] has added greatly to the physician's ability to treat cardiac emergencies such as ventricular fibrillation or tachyrhythmias of either ventricular or supraventricular origin in critically ill patients. The method may also be used when atrial

flutter and fibrillation have not been converted by drug therapy and for those tachyrhythmias with wide QRS complexes where it is difficult to determine whether the mechanism is ventricular or pseudoventricular tachycardia (Fig. 14). Cardioversion should be accomplished by a team familiar with the cardiovertor and with equipment that has been regularly checked for proper performance. The shock is delivered through paddles over the precordium and posterior chest wall. The electronic circuitry times the delivery of the shock according to the R wave

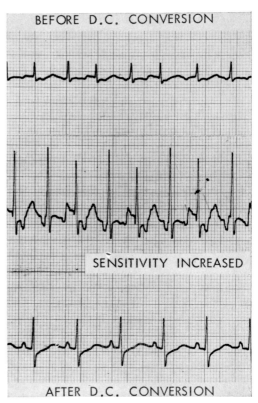

Fig. 42. DC conversion of a recurrent supraventricular tachyrhythmia in a 10-year-old girl following repair of an atrial septal defect. In the top strip, the R–R interval is irregular and rapid with a ventricular rate of 140/min. Increasing the sensitivity clarified the abnormal P waves as inverted at a rate of 260/min. There is variable A–V block, 2:1 alternating with 1:1. With the sensitivity increased, timing of the signal for DC countershock at 25 watt-sec was accomplished and the tachyrhythmia (paroxysmal supraventricular tachycardia with variable A–V block) was converted to normal sinus rhythm.

on the oscilloscope screen. It may be necessary to alter the gain to assure that the R wave is distinct from the P or T wave (Fig. 42). In infants a shock of 5 to 10 watt-sec and in children 20 to 30 watt-sec is used first and is usually effective. Rarely should the setting be increased above 200 to 250 watt-sec for fear of burning the skin. Once the tachyrhythmia has been converted, anti-arrhythmic medication must be initiated or continued to prevent recurrence.

CATHETER PACING[26,65]

A pacing catheter passed transvenously into the atrium has been utilized in adults to deliver an appropriately timed stimulus to terminate a tachyrhythmia or to pace at a rate faster than the refractory tachycardia to achieve overdrive suppression of the dys-rhythmia. We have not needed to utilize the method in our pediatric patients.

SURGERY

In patients with Wolff-Parkinson-White syndrome and serious recurrent episodes of tachycardia unresponsive to the usual methods of control, electrocardiographic surface map-ping to define the accessory tract and surgical incision of it have been reported with some success.[9] None of our patients has required this intervention.

Bradyrhythmias

When the patient is symptomatic and the ventricular rate is too slow because of sinus-node depression or complete heart block, acceleration of the heart rate may be accom-plished by drugs or pacemaker.

CARDIO-ACCELERATOR DRUGS

Sympathomimetics

Sympathetic stimulation or the administra-tion of catecholamines increases the heart rate by increasing the slope of diastolic depolarization and by shifting the pacemaker site to a higher and faster one. If the resting potential is abnormally decreased, these agents will increase the resting potential and improve excitability and responsiveness to an extent that conduction may return in areas of block. In the His-Purkinje system, they increase contractility of the myocardium but in large doses, as the rate increases, latent pacemakers may become active pacemakers or multiple pacemakers may appear.

We have found these drugs useful in the emergency or acute situation—after syncope with the sick sinus-node syndrome, after cardiac arrest, in the immediate postoperative period, or in a patient with heart block—for support until a pacemaker can be inserted. As chronic therapy, they are of limited value (Fig. 4).

In cardiopulmonary resuscitation from cardiac arrest, intracardiac injection of *epinephrine* in a 1:1000 dilution may restore cardiac action. Intravenous infusion of a dilute solution may be run in at a rate sufficient to maintain an adequate heart rate. More often, however, an infusion of iso-proterenol is used to maintain the rate.

A dilute infusion of 1 mg *isoproterenol* in 200 cc of 5 per cent dextrose in distilled water is given intravenously at a drip rate sufficient to maintain the heart rate and rhythm at an acceptable level.

Vagolytics

In those situations, especially in young infants, when increased vagal tone is con-sidered responsible for cardiac slowing, atropine may be administered parenterally to elevate the rate or to change a junctional pacemaker to a sinus pacemaker.[2] Atropine is of more value in the acute situation than for chronic use because of the other effects it produces in the body.

PACEMAKERS[26,65]

The symptomatic infant or child with too slow a ventricular rate because of sick sinus-node syndrome or complete heart block is a candidate for pacemaker therapy, by either intracardiac or epicardiac pacing.[16,25,111] The large size of the units and the need to replace batteries or repair broken wires at intervals of about 1 to $1\frac{1}{2}$ years make this form of treatment far from optimal in an active young child, but improvements should be forthcoming in these mechanical aspects of the problem. The patient is at great risk at the moment of pacemaker failure if his own cardiac pacemaker has been inhibited and fails to take over promptly. Two examples of pacemaker malfunction are shown in Figures 34 and 35. Artificial pacemaker arrhythmias may be serious,[50,51] especially if a pacemaker impulse occurs during the vulnerable period of the patient's own ventricular impulse (R-on-T phenomenon) (Fig. 35).

Pacemaker insertion is indicated for children with complete heart block, even though they have not been symptomatic, when some form of anesthesia and surgery may be planned.[72]

The best therapy for surgically induced complete heart block is the prevention of injury at the time of surgery. Appropriate techniques have been devised and are being successfully utilized by surgeons who undertake open-heart surgery in areas near the A-V node and His bundle.[54]

CONCLUSIONS

There is renewed interest in and awareness of problems of cardiac rhythm and conduction among pediatric cardiologists just as among medical cardiologists, cardiac surgeons, physiologists, and pharmacologists. This multidisciplinary involvement should improve the understanding and the management of dysrhythmias in patients of all ages.

ACKNOWLEDGMENTS

We wish especially to thank Ethel Longo, Chris Robinson, Angela Gilladoga, Andrea Giardina, Mira Frand and others of the pediatric cardiology fellows and technicians who have shared our interest and helped us in our work with infants and children with disturbances of cardiac rhythm and conduction.

REFERENCES

1. Ayres, S. M., and Grace, W. J.: Inappropriate ventilation and hypoxemia as causes of cardiac arrrhythmias. Amer. J. Med., 46: 495, 1969.
2. Bauer, C. H., Engle, M. A., and Mellins, R.: Hypervagism and cardiac arrest. Bull. N.Y. Acad. Med., 35:260, 1959.
3. Bellet, S.: Drug therapy in cardiac arrhythmias: I–IV. New Eng. J. Med., 262:769, 979, 1179; 263:85, 1960.
4. Bishop, L. F., and Reichert, P.: The interrelationship between anxiety and arrhythmias. Psychosomatics, 4:330, 1970.
5. Blumenthal, S., Jacobs, J. C., Steer, C. M., and Williamson, S. W.: Congenital atrial flutter: report of a case documented by intra-uterine electrocardiogram. Pediatrics, 41:659, 1968.
6. Boineau, J. P., and Moore, E. N.: Evidence for propagation of activation across an accessory atrio-ventricular connection in types A and B pre-excitation. Circulation, 41:375, 1970.
7. Castellanos, A., Castillo, C. A., and Agha, A. S.: Contribution of His bundle recordings to the understanding of clinical arrhythmias. Amer. J. Cardiol., 28:499, 1971.
8. Chung, E. K. Y.: Parasystole. Progr. Cardiov. Dis., 11:64, 1968.
9. Cobb, F. R., et al.: Successful surgical interruption of the bundle of Kent in a patient with the Wolff-Parkinson-White syndrome. Circulation, 38:1018, 1968.
10. Corday, E., et al.: Cardiac arrhythmias and conduction disturbances. In: The Heart (Hurst, J. W., and Logue, R. B., Eds.). New York, McGraw-Hill, 1966.
11. Daggett, W. M., and Wallace, A. G.: Vagal and sympathetic influences on ectopic impulse formation. In: Mechanisms and Therapy of Cardiac Arrhythmia (Dreifus, L. S., Likoff, W., and Moyer, J. H., Eds.). New York, Grune and Stratton, 1966.
12. Damato, A. N.: Diphenylhydantoin: pharmacologic and clinical use. Progr. Cardiov. Dis., 12:1, 1969.
13. Damato, A. N., and Lau, S. H.: Clinical value of the electrocardiogram of the conduction system. Progr. Cardiov. Dis., 13:119, 1970.
14. Dawes, G. S.: Sudden death in babies: Physiology of the fetus and newborn. Amer. J. Cardiol., 22:469, 1968.
15. Dreifus, L. S., and Watanabe, Y.: Antiarrhythmic drugs. In: Cardiovascular Disorders (Brest, A. N., and Moyer, J. H., Eds.). Philadelphia, F. A. Davis, 1968.
16. Dreifus, L. S., Morse, D., Watanabe, Y., and Flores, D.: The advantages of demand over fixed-rate pacing; report of clinical experience. Dis. Chest, 54:86, 1968.
17. Dreifus, L. S., Watanabe, Y., Haiat, R., and Kimbiris, D.: Atrioventricular block. Amer. J. Cardiol., 28:371, 1971.

18. Ebert, P. A., Vanderbeek, R. B., Allgood, R. J., and Sabiston, D. C.: Effect of chronic cardiac denervation on arrhythmias after coronary artery ligation. Cardiov. Res., 4:141, 1970.
19. Ehlers, K. H.: Supraventricular and ventricular dysrhythmias in infants and children. In: Cardiovascular Clinics: Pediatric Cardiology (Engle, M. A., Ed.). Philadelphia, F. A. Davis, 1972.
20. Engle, M. A., et al.: Regression after open valvulotomy of infundibular stenosis accompanying severe valvular pulmonic stenosis. Circulation, 17:862, 1958.
21. Engle, M. A., Erlandson, M., and Smith, C. H.: Late cardiac complications of chronic, severe refractory anemia with hemachromatosis. Circulation, 30:694, 1964.
22. Feldt, R. H., DuShane, J. W., and Titus, J. L.: The atrioventricular conduction system in persistent common atrioventricular canal defect: Correlations with electrocardiogram. Circulation, 42:437, 1970.
23. Fisch, C., and Knoebel, S. B.: Junctional rhythms. Progr. Cardiov. Dis., 8:141, 1970.
24. Friedman, W. F.: Neuropharmacologic studies of perinatal myocardium. In: Cardiovascular Clinics: Pediatric Cardiology (Engle, M. A., Ed.). Philadelphia, F. A. Davis, 1972.
25. Furman, S., Escher, D. J. W., and Solomon, N.: Experiences with myocardial and transvenous implanted cardiac pacemakers. Amer. J. Cardiol., 23:66, 1969.
26. Furman, S., and Escher, D.: Principles and Techniques of Cardiac Pacing. New York, Harper and Row, 1970.
27. Gale, G. E., Bosman, C. K., Tucker, R. B. K., and Barlow, J. B.: Hereditary prolongation of QT interval. Study of two families. Brit. Heart J., 32:505, 1970.
28. Garza, L. A., Vick, R. L., Nora, J. J., and McNamara, D. G.: Heritable Q-T prolongation without deafness. Circulation, 41:39, 1970.
29. Gelband, H., et al.: Etiology of right bundle branch block in patients undergoing total correction of tetralogy of Fallot. Circulation, 44:1022, 1971.
30. Gettes, L. S., Shabetai, R., Downs, T. A., and Surawicz, B.: Effects of changes in potassium and calcium concentrations on diastole threshold and strength-interval relationships of the human heart. Ann. N.Y. Acad. Sci., 167:693, 1969.
31. Gettes, L. S.: The electrophysiologic effects of anti-arrhythmic drugs. Amer. J. Cardiol., 28:526, 1971.
32. Giardina, A. C. V., Ehlers, K. H., and Engle, M. A.: The Wolff-Parkinson-White syndrome in infants and children: A long term follow-up study. Brit. Heart J., 34:839, 1972.
33. Gibson, D., and Sowton, E.: The use of beta-adrenergic receptor blocking drugs in dysrhythmias. Progr. Cardiov. Dis., 12:16, 1969.
34. Han, J.: The mechanism of paroxysmal atrial tachycardia. Amer. J. Cardiol., 26:329, 1970.
35. Han, J.: The concept of re-entrant activity responsible for ectopic rhythm. Amer. J. Cardiol., 28:253, 1972.
36. Hoffman, B. F., and Cranefield, P. F.: Electrophysiology of the Heart. New York, McGraw-Hill, 1960.
37. Hoffman, B. F., Cranefield, P. F., and Wallace, A. G.: Physiological basis of cardiac arrhythmias (II). Mod. Conc. Cardiov. Dis., 35:107, 1966.
38. Hoffman, B. F.: Autonomic control of cardiac rhythm. Bull. N.Y. Acad. Med., 43:1087, 1967.
39. Hoffman, B. F., Cranefield, P. F., and Wallace, A. G.: Physiological basis of cardiac arrhythmias (I). Mod. Conc. Cardiov. Dis., 35:103, 1966.
40. Hurst, J. W., and Myerburg, R. J.: Cardiac arrhythmias: Evolving concepts (I). Mod. Conc. Cardiov. Dis., 37:73, 1968.
41. Hurst, J. W., and Myerburg, R. J.: Cardiac arrhythmias: Evolving concepts (II). Mod. Conc. Cardiov. Dis., 37:79, 1968.
42. James, T. N.: Morphology of the human atrioventricular node, with remarks pertinent to its electrophysiology. Amer. Heart J., 62:756, 1961.
43. James, T. N.: Anatomy of the human sinus node. Anat. Rec., 141:101, 1961.
44. James, T. N.: The connecting pathways between the sinus node and the A–V node and between the right and left atrium in the human heart. Amer. Heart J., 66:498, 1963.
45. James, T. N.: Cardiac innervation; anatomic and pharmacologic relations. Bull. N.Y. Acad. Med., 43:1041, 1967.
46. James, T. N.: Sudden death in babies: new observations in the heart. Amer. J. Cardiol., 22:479, 1968.
47. James, T. N.: Cardiac conduction system: fetal and postnatal development. Amer. J. Cardiol., 25:213, 1970.
48. James, T. N.: The Wolff-Parkinson-White syndrome: evolving concepts of its pathogenesis. Progr. Cardiov. Dis., 13:159, 1970.
49. James, T. N., and Sherf, L.: Specialized tissues and preferential conduction in the atria of the heart. Amer. J. Cardiol., 28:414, 1971.
50. Kaiser, G. C.: Implantable pacemakers: detection and management of malfunction. Heart Bull., 18:50, 1969.
51. Kaster, J. A., and Leinbach, R. C.: Pacemakers and their arrhythmias. Progr. Cardiov. Dis., 13:240, 1970.
52. Katz, R.: Effects of alpha and beta adrenergic blocking agents on cyclopropane-catecholamine cardiac arrhythmias. Anesthesiology, 26:289, 1966.
53. Katz, R.: Clinical experience with neurogenic cardiac arrhythmias. Bull. N.Y. Acad. Med., 43:1106, 1967.
54. Kirklin, J. W., and Karp, R. B.: The Tetralogy of Fallot from a Surgical Viewpoint. Philadelphia, W. B. Saunders, 1970.

55. Kistin, A. D.: Atrial reciprocal rhythm. Circulation, 32:687, 1965.
56. Lauer, R. W., Ongley, P., DuShane, J. W., and Kirklin, J.: Heart block after repair of ventricular septal defect in children. Circulation, 22:526, 1960.
57. Lev, M.: The architecture of the conduction system in congenital heart disease. II. Tetralogy of Fallot. Arch. Path., 67:572, 1959.
58. Lev, M.: The architecture of the conduction system in congenital heart disease. III. Ventricular septal defect. Arch. Path., 13:529, 1960.
59. Lev, M.: Anatomic basis for complete A–V block. Amer. J. Med., 37:742, 1964.
60. Lev, M.: The pathology of complete atrioventricular block. Progr. Cardiov. Dis., 6:317, 1964.
61. Lev, M., et al.: Lack of connection between the atria and the more peripheral conduction system in congenital atrioventricular block. Amer. J Cardiol., 27:481, 1971.
62. Lev, M., Cuadros, H., and Paul, M.: Interruption of the atrioventricular bundle with congenital atrioventricular block. Circulation, 43:703, 1971.
63. Lown, B.: "Cardioversion" of arrhythmias (I). Mod. Conc. Cardiov. Dis., 33:863, 1964.
64. Lown, B.: Electrical reversion of cardiac arrhythmias. Brit. Heart J., 29:469, 1967.
65. Lown, B., and Kosowsky, B. D.: Medical progress: artificial cardiac pacemakers. New Eng. J. Med., 283:907, 971, 1023, 1970.
66. Lucchesi, B. R., and Whitsitt, L. S.: The pharmacology of beta-adrenergic blocking agents. Progr. Cardiov. Dis., 11:410, 1968.
67. Luria, M. H., and Hale, C. G.: Wolff-Parkinson-White syndrome in association with atrial reciprocal rhythm and reciprocating tachycardia. Brit. Heart J., 32:134, 1970.
68. Marriott, H. J., and Fogg, E.: Constant monitoring for cardiac dysrhythmias and blocks. Mod. Conc. Cardiov. Dis., 39:103, 1970.
69. Mason, D. T., and Braunwald, E.: Digitalis and related preparations. In: Cardiovascular Disorders (Brest, A. N., and Moyer, J. H., Eds.). Philadelphia, F. A. Davis, 1968.
70. Mason, D. T., Sann, J. F., Jr., and Zelis, R.: New developments in understanding of the actions of the digitalis glycosides. Progr. Cardiov. Dis., 11:443, 1969.
71. Massumi, R. A., and Zakauddin, V.: Patterns and mechanisms of QRS normalization in patients with Wolff-Parkinson-White syndrome. Amer. J. Cardiol., 28:541, 1971.
72. Michaëlsson, M., and Engle, M. A.: International cooperative study of congenital complete heart block. In: Cardiovascular Clinics: Pediatric Cardiology (Engle, M. A., Ed.). Philadelphia, F. A. Davis, 1972.
73. Miller, R. A., and Rodriquez-Coronel, A.: Congenital atrioventricular block. In: Heart Disease in Infants, Children and Adolescents (Moss, A. J., and Adams, F. N., Eds.); Baltimore, Williams and Wilkins, 1968.
74. Mobitz, W.: Uber die unvollstandige Storung der Erregungsuberleitung zwischen Vorhof und Kammer des menschlichen Herzens. Z. Ges Exp. Med., 41:180, 1924.
75. Molthan, M. E., Miller, R. A., Hastreiter, A. R., and Paul, M. H.: Congenital heart block with fatal Adams-Stokes attacks in childhood. Pediatrics, 30:32, 1962.
76. Moore, E. N., Knoebel, S. B., and Spear, J. F.: Concealed conduction. Amer. J. Cardiol., 28:406, 1971.
77. Moran, N. C.: Adrenergic receptors, drugs, and the cardiovascular system (I). Mod. Conc. Cardiov. Dis., 35:93, 1966.
78. Moran, N. C.: Adrenergic receptors, drugs, and the cardiovascular system (II). Mod. Conc. Cardiov. Dis., 35:99, 1966.
79. Morgan, C. L., and Nadas, A. S.: Chronic ectopic tachycardia in infancy and childhood. Amer. Heart J., 67:617, 1964.
80. Mustard, W. T.: Successful two-stage correction of transposition of great vessels. Surgery, 55:469, 1964.
81. Nadas, A. S.: Pediatric Cardiology, 2nd ed. Philadelphia, W. B. Saunders, 1963.
82. Nakamura, F. F., and Nadas, A. S.: Complete heart block in infants and children. New Eng. J. Med., 270:1261, 1964.
83. Narula, O. S., et al.: Localization of A–V conduction defects in man by recording of His bundle electrogram. Amer. J. Cardiol., 25:228, 1970.
84. Paul, M. H.: Cardiac arrhythmias in infants and children. Progr. Cardiov. Dis., 9:136, 1966.
85. Phillips, J., and Ichinose, H.: Clinical and pathologic studies in the hereditary syndrome of a long QT interval, syncopal spells and sudden death. Chest, 58:236, 1970.
86. Pitt, B., and Ross, R. S.: Beta adrenergic blockade in cardiovascular therapy. Mod. Conc. Cardiov. Dis., 38:47, 1969.
87. Robinson, S. J.: Treatment of cardiac arrhythmias. Pediat. Clin. N. Amer., 11:315, 1964.
88. Robinson, S. J.: Arrhythmias. In: Heart Disease in Infants, Children and Adolescents (Moss, A. J., and Adams, F. N., Eds.). Baltimore, Williams and Wilkins, 1968.
89. Robinson, S. J.: Disorders of rate and rhythm in infants and children. Heart Bull., 20:24, 1971.
90. Rosen, K., Mehta, A., Rahimtoola, S. H., and Miller, R.: Sites of congenital and surgical heart block as defined by His bundle electrocardiography. Circulation, 44:833, 1971.
91. Rosenbaum, M. B., et al: Right bundle branch block with left anterior hemiblock surgically induced in tetralogy of Fallot. Amer. J. Cardiol., 26:12, 1970.
92. Rosenbaum, M. B., Elizari, M. and Lazzari, J. O.: The hemiblocks. Tampa Tracings, 1970.

93. Rosenbaum, M. B.: The hemiblocks: diagnostic criteria and clinical significance. Mod. Conc. Cardiov. Dis., *39*:141, 1970.

94. Scherlag, B. J., et al.: Catheter techniques for recording His bundle activity in man. Circulation, *30*:13, 1969.

95. Schuilenburg, R. M., and Durrer, D.: Observations on atrioventricular conduction in patients with bilateral bundle branch block. Circulation, *41*:967, 1970.

96. Singer, D. H., and Ten Eick, R. E.: Pharmacology of cardiac arrhythmias. Progr. Cardiov. Dis., *11*:488, 1969.

97. Singer, D. H., and Ten Eick, R. E.: Aberrancy: Electrophysiologic aspects. Amer. J. Cardiol., *28*:381, 1971.

98. Smithen, C. S., and Sowton, E.: His bundle electrograms. Brit. Heart J., *33*:633, 1971.

99. Soyka, L. F.: Clinical pharmacology of digoxin. Pediat. Clin. N. Amer., *19*:241, 1972.

100. Spach, M. S., et al.: Excitation sequences of the atrial septum and the AV node in isolated hearts of the dog and rabbit. Circ. Res., *29*:156, 1971.

101. Spear, J. F., and Moore, E. N.: Electrophysiologic studies on Mobitz type II second degree heart block. Circulation, *44*:1087, 1971.

102. Stock, J. P. P.: New frontiers in arrhythmias. Brit. Heart J., *33*:809, 1971.

103. Strom, G., Zetterqvist, E., and Zetterqvist, P.: Chronic supraventricular tachycardia of continuous or repetitive type in children. Acta Paediat., *49*:827, 1960.

104. Surawicz, B., Lepeschkin, E., Herrlich, H. C., and Hoffman, B. F.: Effect of K and Ca deficiency in the monophasic action potential, ECG and contractility of isolated rabbit hearts. Amer. J. Physiol., *196*:1302, 1958.

105. Surawicz, B.: Role of electrolytes in etiology and management of cardiac arrhythmias. Progr. Cardiov. Dis., *8*:364, 1966.

106. Surawicz, B.: Arrhythmias and electrolyte disturbances. Bull. N.Y. Acad. Med., *43*:1160, 1967.

107. Surawicz, B.: Ventricular fibrillation. Amer. J. Cardiol., *28*:268, 1971.

108. Takao, A., Kusakawa, S., and Sekiguchi, M.: Arrhythmia in myocardial diseases in childhood. Cardiol. Pneumol., *9*:107, 1971.

109. Vanderbeek, R. B., and Ebert, P. A.: Potassium release in the denervated heart. Amer. J. Physiol., *218*:803, 1970.

110. Vassalle, M.: Automaticity and automatic rhythms. Amer. J. Cardiol., *28*:245, 1971.

111. Vellani, C. W., Tildesley, G., and Davies, L. G.: Endocardial pacing: a percutaneous method using the subclavian vein. Brit. Heart J., *31*:106, 1969.

112. Wagner, G. S., and McIntosh, J.: The use of drugs in achieving successful DC cardioversion. Progr. Cardiov. Dis., *11*:431, 1968.

113. Wallace, A. G., Boineau, J. P., Davidson, R. M., and Sealy, W. C.: Wolff-Parkinson-White syndrome: A new look. Amer. J. Cardiol., *28*:509, 1971.

114. Watanabe, Y., and Dreifus, L. S.: Genesis of cardiac arrhythmias. In: *Cardiovascular Disorders* (Brest, A. N., and Moyer, J. H., Eds.). Philadelphia, F. A. Davis, 1968.

115. Wilson, W. S.: Metabolism of digitalis. Progr. Cardiov. Dis., *11*:479, 1969.

116. Wolf, S.: Central autonomic influences on cardiac rate and rhythm. Mod. Conc. Cardiov. Dis., *38*:29, 1969.

Chapter 6

RECENT ADVANCES IN THE BUNDLE
OF HIS ELECTROGRAM*

Anthony N. Damato, M.D., Robert N. Schnitzler, M.D.,
and Sun H. Lau, M.D.

The A-V node, bundle of His (common bundle), right and left bundle branches and the Purkinje network constitute the specialized conducting fibers responsible for the transmission of atrial impulses to the ventricles. The recording of the electrical activity of these specialized conducting fibers by both intra- and extracellular techniques has enhanced our understanding of the atrioventricular and ventriculoatrial transmission process.[1,2,4,13,14,16,19,21,23–25,33,39,43,49,53–60,62,64,66] The bundle of His and the conducting fibers distal to it (right bundle branch, left bundle branch and the Purkinje network) have been designated the His-Purkinje system or the ventricular specialized system (VSCS).

Since the introduction of the microelectrode technique by Ling and Geraud in 1949, intracellular recordings of transmembrane action potentials have been obtained from all

portions of the A-V conducting system.[37] The different functional properties of the A-V conducting system are reflected in the different configurations of the transmembrane action potentials recorded at various sites.[21]

Extracellular recordings of the A-V conducting system have been obtained using various techniques. In 1953, Burchell and co-workers recorded activity from the distal specialized conducting system (either right bundle branch or Purkinje fiber) of the dog's ventricle, using plunge needle electrodes.[4]

In 1958, Alanis and co-workers obtained extracellular recordings from the bundle of His in the isolated perfused hearts of dogs and cats[1,2] by inserting steel needle electrodes into the anatomical region of the bundle of His. The bundle of His deflection, which they called the H potential, appeared as a biphasic spike between the atrial and ventricular electrograms. These investigators validated the H potential by noting its response to various physiological and pharmacological interventions (atrial pacing, vagal

* This work was supported in part by the Federal Health Program Service, USPHS Project Py 72-1 and National Heart and Lung Institute Grants HE-11829 and HE-12536.

stimulation, acetylcholine and epinephrine injections). Furthermore, they demonstrated that the H potential was an independent phenomenon belonging to neither the atrial nor the ventricular electrograms. The recording of H activity permitted the A-V interval to be divided into two subintervals—the A-H and H-V intervals.

In 1959, Sodi-Pallares and associates obtained extracellular recordings of right and left bundle branch activity using steel needle electrodes.[62] Hoffman and co-workers used endocardial plaque electrodes sewn over the ventricular specialized conducting system to obtain bipolar electrograms of the His bundle, right and left bundle branches and peripheral Purkinje fibers.[21] In 1967, Scherlag and associates described a plunge wire technique for recording His bundle activity in the intact dog heart.[59]

Reports of extracellular recordings of A-V nodal activity (N potential) have been less frequent than those of the ventricular specialized conducting system. Most reports indicate that the A-V nodal potential is a slow, notched, low-voltage wave contiguous with the atrial electrogram and extending to the His deflection.[16,49,56,57,62,64] Despite these similarities, there is lack of agreement as to what constitutes a true A-V nodal potential which stems primarily from the fact that there is, as yet, no acceptable way of validating the N potential. Unlike the bundle of His, it is extremely difficult, if not impossible, to stimulate the A-V node.

In 1960, Giraud, Peuch and Latour obtained recordings of bundle of His activity in a patient with trilogy of Fallot during cardiac catheterization with an electrode catheter.[19] Similar recordings of His activity were obtained by Watson and associates in 1967, who used an electrode catheter to study a patient with Ebstein's anomaly.[66] In both of these studies, the electrode catheter was introduced through an antecubital vein. In 1968, Scherlag and associates used a J-shaped electrode catheter introduced via a femoral vein; they obtained consistent recordings of

His bundle activity in the intact anesthetized dog.[58] One year later, this same technique was reported to be safe and reliable for the recording of His bundle activity in the human heart.[60] Damato and associates applied the technique to record the electrical activity of the human A-V node and right bundle branch,[13] and it has also been used to record

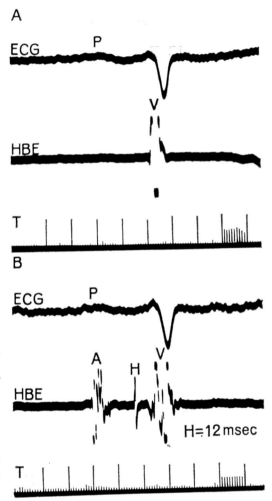

Fig. 1. Electrode catheter recording of His bundle activity. In each panel, ECG is lead II; HBE is the His bundle electrogram tracing, and T = time lines at 10 and 100 msec. A: The electrodes are situated in the right ventricular cavity and only record ventricular activity (V). B: As the catheter is withdrawn to the region of the tricuspid valve, atrial (A), His bundle (H) and ventricular (V) activities are recorded. The duration of the H deflection is 12 msec.

activity from the left bundle branch in man and dog.[14,33,43,53]

TECHNIQUE

The clinical technique of recording A-V nodal, bundle of His and proximal right bundle branch activity involves the percutaneous insertion of a J-shaped electrode catheter (bi-, tri- or multipolar) into a femoral vein. The catheter is fluoroscopically advanced across the tricuspid valve into the right ventricle, and the tip is directed toward the apex of the ventricle. The proximal terminals are formed into bipolar leads which are fed into an A-C input of the electrocardiographic preamplifier. In our laboratory we commonly use a #7 French tripolar catheter with ring electrodes 2 mm wide. Electrode 1 is located at the distal tip of the catheter and electrodes 2 and 3 are located 1 and 2 cm, respectively, from the tip. Thus, three bipolar intracardiac electrograms can be recorded simultaneously or sequentially. Castillo and co-workers have used ring electrodes of narrower width (1 mm).[6] One or more standard electrocardiographic leads are simultaneously recorded. As illustrated in Figure 1A a preponderance of intraventricular activity is recorded with the catheter in the right ventricle. As the catheter is slowly withdrawn across the tricuspid valve (Fig. 1B) atrial and ventricular activity is recorded.

The His potential appears as a bi- or triphasic spike between the atrial and ventricular electrograms. Bundle of His activity can be recorded at various filter frequency settings. In our laboratory we commonly use settings of 40 and 500 Hz. Figure 2 depicts simultaneous recordings from the same bipolar lead at filter frequency settings of 0.1 to 200 Hz (frequencies used for standard electrocardiographic recordings) and 40 to 500 Hz. It is to be noted that the onset and duration of the two His deflections are the same. We have also employed low-frequency filters to attenuate and distort low-frequency components and thereby facilitate the display of the His spike. Recent studies in our laboratory have shown that optimal His bundle potentials are recorded at 90 to 150 Hz.

In all of our studies a quadripolar electrode is also percutaneously inserted into an antecubital vein under local anesthesia and fluoroscopically positioned against the lateral wall of the right atrium. The distal pair of electrodes is used to stimulate the right atrium and the proximal pair to record a bipolar

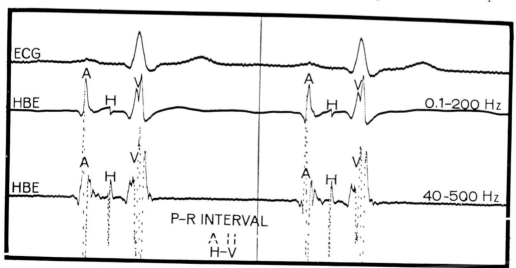

Fig. 2. Simultaneous His bundle activity recorded through the same electrode pair at two different frequency settings. Time lines 10 and 100 msec. (From Scherlag, et al.[60])

electrogram from a high position in the right atrium. When appropriate, a bipolar catheter is also positioned in the apex or outflow of the right ventricle for ventricular studies.

Figure 3 is representative of the usual type of recording. During sinus rhythm, the sequence of activation proceeds from the high right to the low right atrial region. The interval from the onset of the low atrial electrogram to the onset of the His deflection is designated as the A-H interval and is considered to approximate A-V nodal conduction time. The interval from the onset of the His deflection to the onset of ventricular depolarization has been designated the H-V interval and reflects His-Purkinje conduction time. The onset of ventricular activation is measured either from the intracardiac ventricular electrogram (V) or from the surface electrocardiogram (onset of the Q or R waves). In our laboratory, the normal A-H interval is between 60 to 140 msec and the normal H-V interval is 30 to 55 msec. The use of a time-mark generator from which time marks can be continuously recorded at various millisecond intervals (usually 10 and 100 msec) lends a higher degree of accuracy to the measurements. The His deflection is 15 to 20 msec in duration. The right bundle branch potential is 10 to 15 msec in duration.

Figure 4 depicts simultaneous recordings

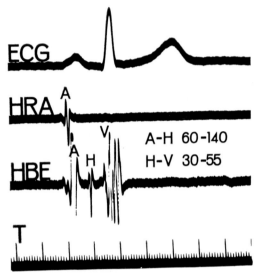

Fig. 3. Normal conduction times in our laboratory. HRA = high right atrial bipolar electrogram recording. The range of A–H intervals is 60 to 140 msec and the range for H–V intervals is 30 to 55 msec.

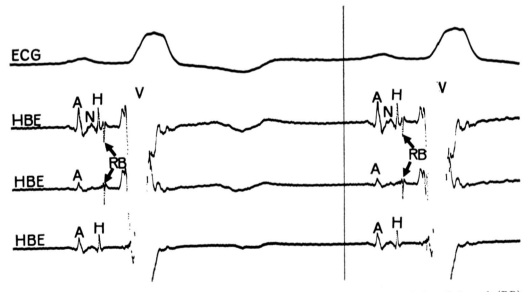

Fig. 4. Simultaneous recordings of A-V nodal (N), His bundle (H) and proximal right bundle branch (RB) potentials in a patient with LBBB. Three simultaneous bipolar electrograms were recorded using combinations of the three electrodes on the catheter. The N potential is a slow, notched wave extending from the A electrogram to the H potential.

of A-V nodal, His bundle and right bundle branch activity from a single catheter positioned in the region of the tricuspid valve. The A-V nodal potential appears as a slow, notched wave occurring between the atrial and His bundle electrograms.

The electrical activity of the A-V node, bundle of His and the proximal portion of the left bundle branch can be recorded by retrogradely advancing an electrode catheter into the posterior or noncoronary aortic cusp.[33] Figure 5 illustrates His and right bundle branch activity recorded from a catheter positioned in the tricuspid valve area and His and left bundle branch activity recorded from a separate catheter in the noncoronary aortic cusp. In addition, a His potential is simultaneously recorded from close bipolar wires plunged into the anatomical region of the common bundle.

ELECTRICAL STIMULATION OF THE HEART

Various stimulators are available to pace the atrium or ventricles in man, in conjunction with His bundle recordings, for diagnostic and physiological studies. In our laboratory, we use a programmed digital stimulator which permits the delivery of up to six independent stimuli within the cardiac cycle. The pulse duration and amplitude can be independently adjusted. We routinely use rectangular pulses of 1.5-msec duration and stimulate the heart at approximately twice diastolic threshold, i.e. <3 ma. For refractory period studies, an atrial electrogram is used as a sensing signal which triggers the stimulator to deliver an impulse after a preset delay. All stimuli delivered to the heart pass through a stimulus isolation unit. It is important that the patient and all equipment are maintained at an equipotential ground.

Generally, the human right atrium can be stimulated through an electrode catheter at 0.5 to 3.0 ma. Right ventricular stimulation is usually accomplished at 1.0 ma or less. Bundle of His stimulation has been used for verification of the recorded potential.[11,45,56] Since in our experience the current requirements for His stimulation through an electrode catheter are quite large (8 ma or

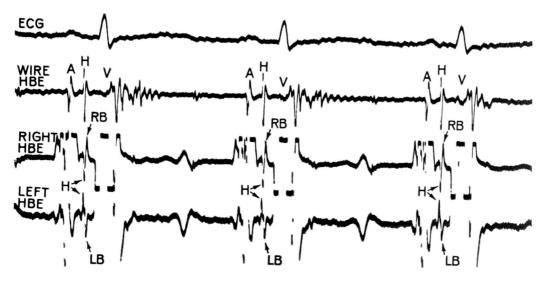

Fig. 5. Simultaneous recordings from the intact heart of a dog. The second tracing (wire HBE) was recorded using close bipolar plunge wire electrodes inserted into the region of the common bundle. The "right HBE" tracing was obtained from an electrode catheter in the region of the tricuspid valve. The "left HBE" tracing was recorded from an electrode catheter in the posterior or noncoronary-artery cusp. The three H deflections occur simultaneously. The proximal RB and LB potentials also occur simultaneously.

greater), we do not routinely use this procedure in our clinical studies. Figure 6 demonstrates His bundle recordings in a dog heart with validation by electrical stimulation.

P-R PROLONGATION

The division of the P-R interval into the A-H and H-V subintervals has provided a more precise way of localizing A-V conduction delays.[11,17,18,34,46,47] The most common cause of P-R prolongation is A-V nodal delay, an example of which is illustrated in Figure 7. A-V nodal conduction time, as indicated by the A-H interval, is prolonged at 310 msec, while the H-V interval is normal at 39 msec. When drugs such as digitalis and propranolol

cause P-R prolongation, they do so by prolonging the A-H interval. Figure 8 illustrates an example of P-R prolongation from simultaneous conduction delay in the A-V node and the His-Purkinje system.

In normal physiological situations, such as during exercise, there is a balance (mediated by the autonomic system) between the increase in heart rate and A-V nodal conduction time, so that the P-R interval remains normal or even decreases slightly. In contrast, when the patient is in a resting stage a progressive prolongation of the P-R interval results whenever the atrial rate is artificially increased by electrical stimulation.[38] This is illustrated in Figure 9, which shows that the progressive prolongation is due exclusively to

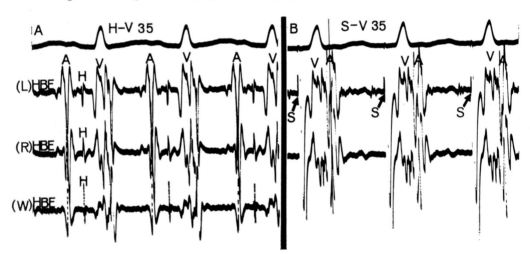

Fig. 6. Validation of His potentials. *A*: Three simultaneous H potentials recorded from the posterior aortic cusp (L HBE), tricuspid valve region (R HBE) and by plunge wire technique (W HBE). The H–V interval is 35 msec. *B*: Pacing the bundle of His through the wire electrodes results in a stimulus to V time of 35 msec and normal ventricular activation. (From Damato, et al.[11])

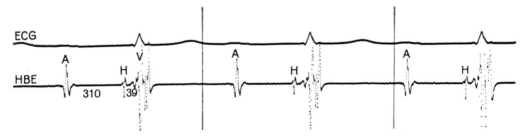

Fig. 7. Patient with a P-R interval of approximately 349 msec in which the conduction delay is due to prolonged A-V nodal conduction time (A-H 310 msec). (From Lau and Damato.[34])

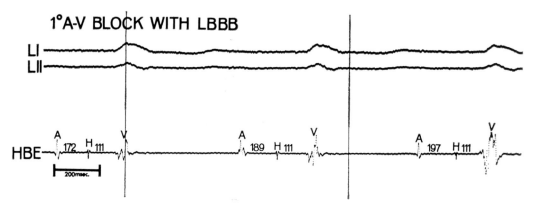

Fig. 8. Patient with first-degree heart block and LBBB. Conduction delay occurs at both the A-V nodal and His-Purkinje levels. (From Lau and Damato.[34])

progressive increases in the A-H intervals. At any given paced heart rate, exercise, isoproterenol or atropine will decrease the P-R interval by decreasing the A-H interval.

It has been demonstrated both clinically and experimentally that P-R prolongation can also be due to conduction delay occurring within the bundle of His.[10,11,44,50] Figures 10 and 11 are from a dog experiment in which plunge wires were inserted into the common bundle, whereupon a temporary intra-His delay occurred. In Figure 10 two His deflections are recorded (H and H') with an interval of 45 msec between them. A-V nodal conduction time as reflected in the A-H interval remains constant at 50 msec. The H'-V interval also remains constant at 30 msec. Figure 11, recorded a few minutes later, demonstrates that the P-R interval has shortened as a result of a lesser delay between the two His deflections. Ultimately, the two His deflections fused into one and the P-R interval returned to normal values. It is to be noted that the QRS complexes remained normal during the changes in intra-His conduction.

SECOND-DEGREE HEART BLOCK

Second-degree heart block has been classified into two types based upon electrocardiographic criteria.[27] As will be shown, these electrocardiographic criteria are generally but not entirely accurate in localizing the site of conduction delay and block in all clinical situations.

Type-I second-degree A-V block (commonly referred to as the A-V nodal Wenckebach phenomenon) is electrocardiographically characterized by a progressive prolongation in the P-R interval followed by a nonconducted atrial impulse. In its typical form, the greatest increment of delay occurs in the second beat of the cycle. The commonest causes of this electrocardiographic pattern are conduction delay and block occurring at the A-V nodal level. When this electrocardiographic pattern occurs in association with a normal QRS pattern, the conduction delay and block are almost certainly at the A-V nodal level. A typical example of type-I second-degree A-V block is illustrated in Figure 12. When, however, the electrocardiographic pattern (prolongation of P-R interval preceding a blocked impulse) occurs in association with intraventricular conduction delay or bundle branch block patterns, the localization of the delay and block is less certain (see below).

Clinical observations using His bundle recordings are in agreement with the experimental observations of Watanabe and Dreifus who demonstrated, using microelectrode techniques, that A-V nodal conduction delay and block were the most common

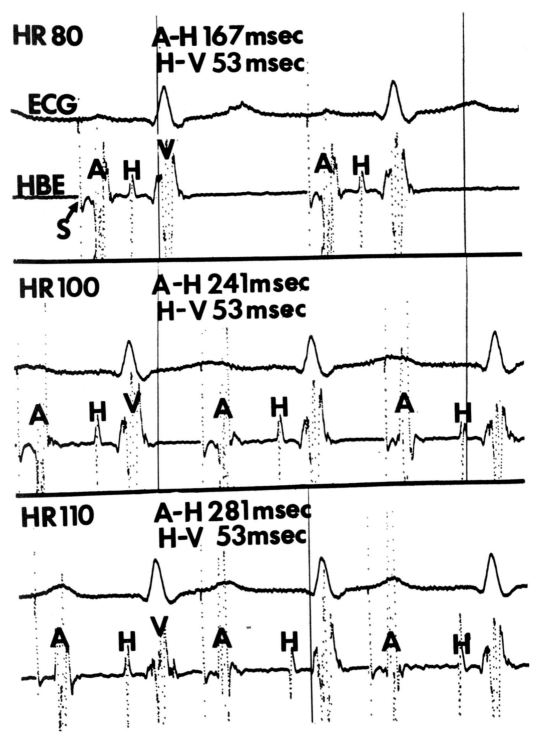

Fig. 9. Atrial pacing at increasing rates above the sinus rate produces, in the resting subject, a progressive increase in the A–H interval. (From Damato et al.[17a])

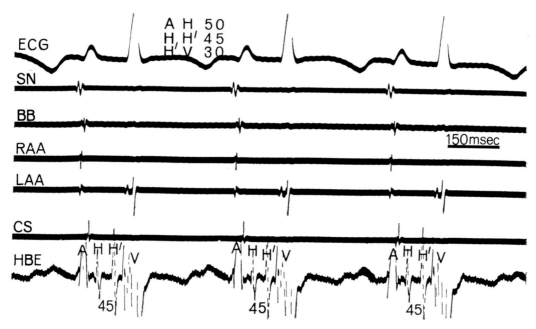

Fig. 10. P-R prolongation due to intra-His delay in the dog. Close bipolar electrogram recordings were obtained from the region of the sinus node (SN), Bachmann's bundle (BB), the right atrial appendage (RAA), the left atrial appendage (LAA), the coronary sinus (CS), and the bundle of His (HBE). ECG is lead II. The interval between the two His deflections (H and H') is 45 msec.

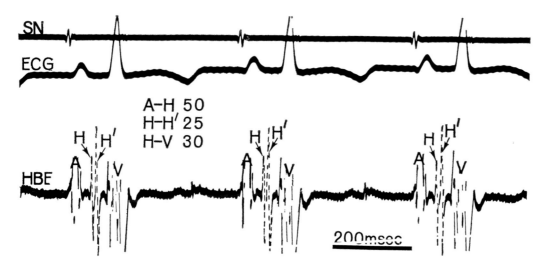

Fig. 11. Same animal experiment as shown in Figure 10. All atrial electrograms except the SN have been omitted. The P-R interval has shortened because the H-H' interval has decreased to 25 msec. No changes in the A-H or H'-V intervals have occurred. The QRS complexes have remained normal.

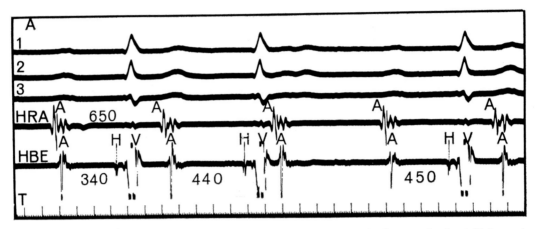

Fig. 12. Typical type-I second-degree A-V block. There is a progressive increase in the A-H interval (causing prolongation of the P-R interval) prior to the blocked P wave. The third atrial impulse is blocked proximal to the bundle of His.

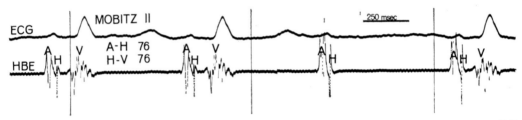

Fig. 13. Typical type-II second-degree A-V block. There is 3:2 A-V conduction with a constant P-R interval preceding the unexpected block of the third atrial impulse within the His-Purkinje system. A-V nodal conduction time (A-H 76 msec) is normal. The H-V interval of conducted beats is prolonged at 76 msec. (From Lau and Damato.[34])

causes of type-I second-degree A-V block.[65] Type-I second-degree A-V block may occur during inferior-wall myocardial infarctions or digitalis administration and in these situations the block is generally reversible.

Type II is the rarer form of second-degree A-V block and is electrocardiographically characterized by a constant P-R interval preceding an unexpected nonconducted atrial impulse. The constant P-R interval may be normal or prolonged. Generally, patients who manifest type-II block have an associated pattern of intraventricular conduction delay or bundle branch block. His bundle recordings have demonstrated that failure of conduction occurs within the His-Purkinje system. Figure 13 is a typical example of type-II block occurring in a patient with LBBB. The third atrial impulse is unexpectedly

blocked within the His-Purkinje system. Watanabe and Dreifus also demonstrated experimentally that block occurred in the His-Purkinje in type-II second-degree A-V block.[65]

Dizziness and syncope are common symptoms associated with type-II block. In our experience these symptoms result from the development of intermittent high-degree (2:1, 3:1, 4:1, etc.) or complete A-V block. The demonstration of type-II block requires that a permanent ventricular pacemaker be inserted, since such a block almost always leads to complete A-V block within a relatively short period of time.

Figure 13 also demonstrates that a significant conduction delay can exist in the presence of a normal P-R interval. For all conducted sinus beats, the P-R interval is approximately

0.156 sec. In the presence of this normal P-R interval the H-V interval is prolonged at 76 msec.

The application of the above-mentioned electrocardiographic criteria to types I and II second-degree A-V block will lead to the correct diagnosis in most cases.[30] However, in certain situations the electrocardiographic criteria are not adequate in localizing the site of conduction delay and block.

In Figure 14, a progressive increase in the P-R interval precedes a nonconducted atrial beat in a patient with RBBB. By electrocardiographic criteria this tracing would qualify as a type-I A-V block which according to traditional concepts would suggest that the conduction delay and block are at the A-V nodal level. However, as revealed by the His bundle recordings, the conduction delay responsible for the P-R prolongation is in the His-Purkinje system, and the nonconducted atrial beat is blocked distal to the His recording. Figure 14 represents a type-I block (Wenckebach phenomenon) occurring within the His-Purkinje system. The electrophysiological, pathophysiological and clinical characteristics of this type of conduction delay are more consistent with a conventional type-II second-degree A-V block.

Figure 15 is from a dog experiment and similarly demonstrates how conduction delay and block occurring within the His-Purkinje

system cause P-R prolongation and thereby simulate (according to electrocardiographic criteria) a type-I (A-V nodal) second-degree A-V block.

In both Figures 14 and 15, the electrocardiographic tracing gave no clue as to the site of conduction delay and block. In both instances there was a fixed bundle branch block pattern and consequently the morphology of the QRS complexes did not change as progressive conduction delay occurred down the contralateral bundle. Progressive conduction delay occurring within the His-Purkinje system is more easily recognized on the surface electrocardiogram when the QRS complexes are normal or nearly normal, as illustrated in Figure 16.

The electrocardiographic criteria of type I second-degree A-V block can also be produced by conduction delay and block occurring within the bundle of His. Figure 17 depicts tracings obtained from a dog in which the bundle of His was injured. A-V nodal conduction time and the QRS complexes remain normal as the P-R interval preceding a blocked atrial impulse increases. An intra-His Wenckebach phenomenon accounts for the electrocardiographic findings. This phenomenon has been documented to occur clinically.

The electrocardiographic patterns of type I and II second-degree A-V block can be

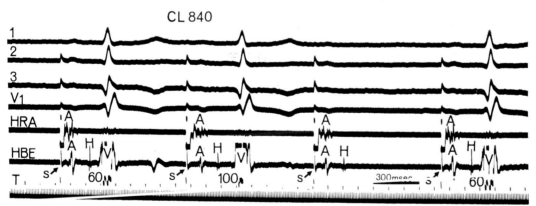

Fig. 14. Wenckebach type of conduction within the His-Purkinje system. During 3:2 A-V conduction in the presence of RBBB, the P-R interval increases prior to the nonconducted atrial impulse. Both the conduction delay and block occur within the His-Purkinje system.

produced by concealed His extrasystoles. Examples of this phenomenon will be demonstrated under the section on concealed conduction (see below).

COMPLETE HEART BLOCK

During complete A-V dissociation, the block may exist anywhere along the A-V conducting system and can be readily local-

ized using bundle of His recordings.[17a,46,47,61,63] In general, when complete A-V dissociation is associated with normal QRS complexes, the atrial impulses are blocked at the A-V nodal level. When the QRS complexes are wide (0.12 sec or greater), the block occurs within the His-Purkinje system. However, there are exceptions to these general rules.

Figure 18 shows complete A-V dissociation

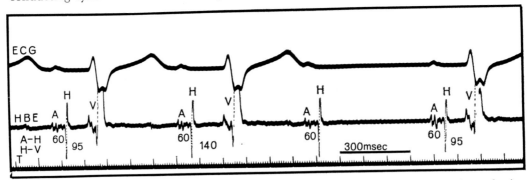

Fig. 15. Tracing is from a dog experiment. RBBB exists. The progressive increase in the P-R interval prior to the blocked beat is due to H-V prolongation from 95 to 140 msec.

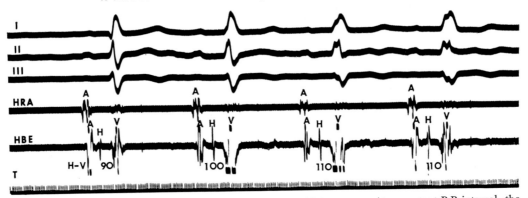

Fig. 16. Wenckebach type of conduction within the His-Purkinje system. At a constant P-P interval, the morphology of the QRS complexes progressively changes to an LBBB pattern. Concomitant with this change is a progressive increase in the H-V interval from 90 to 110 msec.

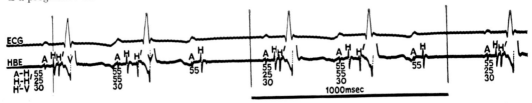

Fig. 17. Wenckebach type of conduction occurring within the bundle of His. During 3:2 A-V conduction in the presence of a normal QRS complex, the P-R interval preceding the nonconducted atrial impulse increases. A-V nodal conduction time remains constant (A-H 55 msec). Two His deflections (H and H') are recorded. The H'-V interval (30 msec) for all conducted beats remains constant. The increase in the P-R interval is due to an increase in the H-H' interval (25 to 55 msec.) The third atrial impulse is blocked within the bundle of His. (From Damato et al.[11])

with normal QRS complexes. The non-conducted atrial impulses are blocked proximal to the bundle of His. Each of the normal QRS complexes is preceded by a single His deflection with normal H-V intervals indicating that the pacemaker for the ventricles was in the bundle of His. It is to be noted that, if the patient had a wide QRS complex prior to the development of A-V nodal block, the morphology of the QRS complexes would remain the same if the pacemaker for the ventricles were in the bundle of His.

Figure 19 is an example of complete A-V dissociation with the block occurring within the His-Purkinje system. Each of the non-conducted atrial impulses is followed by a His deflection. The wide QRS complexes are not preceded by His deflections, indicating

that the pacemaker for the ventricles is subjunctional.

Another exception to the general rule relating the level of block to the morphology of the QRS complexes is illustrated in Figure 20. In this dog experiment complete A-V dissociation with normal QRS complexes is present. Since each of the nonconducted atrial impulses is followed by a His deflection, the block is not within the A-V node. The QRS complexes are normal and are preceded by a single His deflection. The findings of Figure 20 are compatible with an intra-His block in which the nonconducted atrial impulses are blocked within some portion of the bundle of His, and the pacemaker for the ventricles resides within the bundle of His but below the level of block. Similar findings

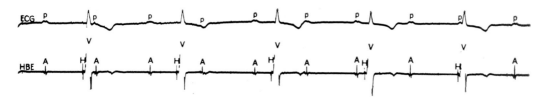

Fig. 18. Complete A-V dissociation due to A-V nodal block. The bundle of His is the pacemaker for the ventricles. (From Damato et al.[11])

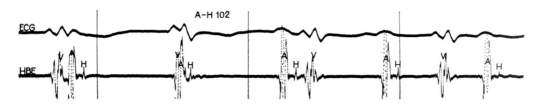

Fig. 19. Complete A-V dissociation due to block within the His-Purkinje system.

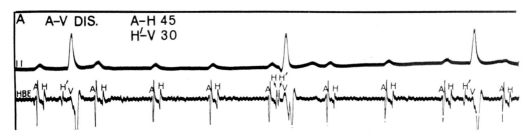

Fig. 20. Complete A-V dissociation with normal QRS complexes. Each nonconducted atrial impulse is followed by a His deflection (H). Each normal QRS complex is preceded by a single H′ deflection with a normal H′-V interval of 30 msec.

in clinical studies have been reported by Narula and associates and Schuilenberg and Durrer.[44,50]

Rosen and associates recently reported on the association of heart block and acute myocardial infarction.[51] In their patients heart block developing in the presence of a diaphragmatic myocardial infarction was at the A-V nodal level. Heart block occurring in association with an anterior myocardial infarction was due to block within the His-Purkinje system.

CONCEALED CONDUCTION

Impulses which fail to traverse the entire A-V conduction system are *concealed*. Impulses may be concealed within the A-V node or His-Purkinje system.[12,13,18] Lewis and Master were the first to demonstrate that premature stimuli blocked in the A-V conducting system could influence the conduction of subsequent beats.[36] The term *concealed conduction* was introduced into electrocardiography by Langendorf in 1948 and refers to the effect which concealed impulses have on the conduction of subsequent impulses.[28,32] The phenomenon has been invoked to explain (1) postextrasystolic prolongation of A-V conduction of one or more subsequent beats, (2) the irregularity of the ventricular response during atrial fibrillation,

(3) the slower ventricular response during atrial fibrillation as compared to atrial tachycardia or flutter in the same patient, (4) alternation of the P-R interval and (5) alteration of the discharge rate of junctional and subjunctional pacemakers.

A typical example of antegrade concealed conduction, in which a blocked premature atrial beat causes prolonged A-V conduction of a subsequent sinus beat, is illustrated in Figure 21. As indicated by the first beat in this figure, sinus impulses normally have an A-V nodal conduction time of 130 msec. The second atrial impulse is premature and fails to traverse the entire A-V conducting system (concealed beat). The partial penetration of this nonconducted atrial beat into the A-V node causes this structure to be in a relatively refractory state when the next sinus beat (third atrial impulse) occurs. Consequently, the second sinus impulse is conducted with a prolonged A-V nodal conduction time (180 msec).

Figure 22 is another example of antegrade concealed conduction and represents the clinical counterpart of earlier experiments by Lewis and Master.[36] During 1:1 A-V conduction at an atrial rate of 80/min, A-V nodal conduction time measures 110 msec. At an atrial rate of 160/min with 2:1 A-V block (ventricular rate 80) the A-V nodal conduc-

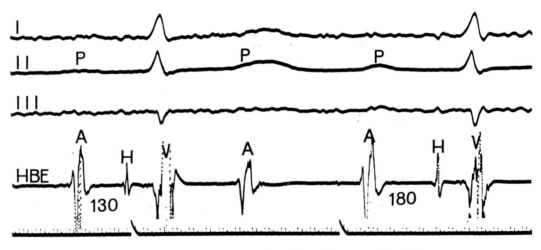

Fig. 21. Antegrade concealed conduction. (From Damato and Lau.[12])

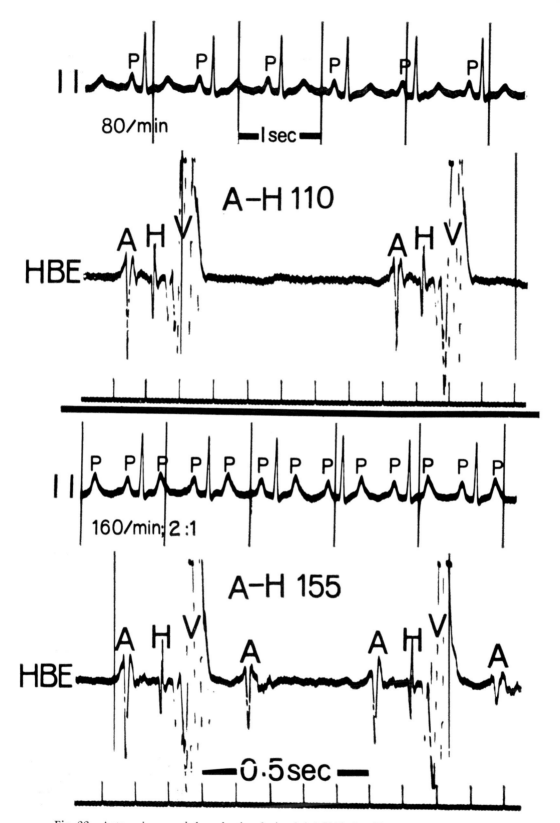

Fig. 22. Antegrade concealed conduction during 2:1 A-V block. (From Damato and Lau.[12])

tion time has increased to 155 msec. Thus, the blocked impulses caused A-V nodal conduction delay of the subsequent conducted atrial impulses. In Figures 21 and 22 both the regions of concealment and subsequent conduction delay were in the A-V node.

Retrograde impulses which conceal within the A-V node can also result in antegrade conduction delay of subsequent impulses. An example of retrograde concealed conduction produced by an interpolated premature ventricular beat is illustrated in Figure 23. The premature ventricular beat (second beat) retrogradely depolarizes the bundle of His (obscured within the ventricular electrogram) and is blocked within the A-V node. The next sinus impulse is antegradely conducted with a prolonged A-V nodal conduction time (145 msec) relative to other sinus beats (112 msec).

An example of a concealed beat altering the discharge rate of a junctional pacemaker is illustrated in Figure 24. There is complete A-V dissociation with an atrial cycle length of 580 msec. The junctional pacemaker is discharging at an H-H interval of 1080 to 1090 msec. The fourth QRS complex is a premature ventricular beat which retrogradely depolarizes the bundle of His and delays the next discharge of the junctional pacemaker.

CONCEALED HIS EXTRASYSTOLES

A variety of cardiac arrhythmias can be produced by concealed impulses arising within the bundle of His.[5,15,31,52] The mechanism for these interesting arrhythmias was first proposed by Langendorf and Mehlman from their analysis of clinical electrocardiograms.[31] Clinical and experimental confirmation of their hypothesis was sub-

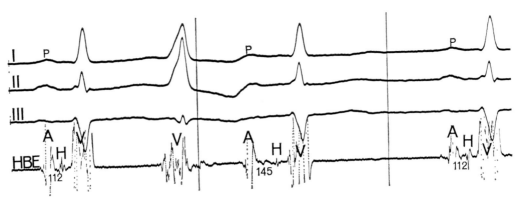

Fig. 23. Retrograde concealed conduction produced by an interpolated premature ventricular beat. (From Damato and Lau.[12])

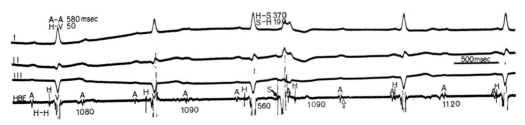

Fig. 24. Concealed retrograde conduction altering the discharge rate of a junctional pacemaker. The H-H interval denotes firing rate of the junctional pacemaker (1080 to 1090 msec). The fourth QRS complex is a premature ventricular beat which retrogradely depolarizes the bundle of His (4th H deflection). The open arrows indicate the expected time of the normal junctional pacemaker firing had the premature ventricular beat not occurred or had it not retrogradely depolarized the bundle of His. (From Damato and Lau.[12])

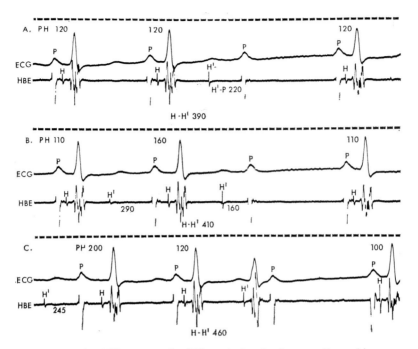

Fig. 25. Concealed bundle of His extrasystoles (H') producing the electrocardiographic patterns of type II (*A*) and type I (*B*) second-degree A-V block. *A*: A His extrasystole (H') occurring 390 msec after a sinus His deflection causes the third P wave to be blocked. *B*: Successive His extrasystoles retrogradely conceal in the A-V node, causing conduction delay of second P wave and block of the third P wave. *C*: A His extrasystole occurring at an H-H' interval of 460 msec is propagated along the distal conducting system and results in aberrant ventricular activation. (From Rosen, Rahimtoola and Gunnar.[52])

sequently obtained using His bundle recordings.[5,15,52]

Figure 25 is from a clinical report by Rosen and associates and illustrates how concealed His extrasystoles can produce the electrocardiographic pattern of types I and II second-degree A-V block.[52] The electrocardiographic tracing in Figure 25*A* shows an unexpected blocked P wave preceded by a constant P-P and P-R interval. The His bundle electrogram recording reveals that the blocked P wave is preceded by a bundle of His extrasystole (H') which occurred at a time in the cardiac cycle when the distal conducting system was refractory; there was no ventricular response. The extrasystolic impulse retrogradely penetrated the A-V node, causing this structure to be refractory to the third atrial impulse. Figure 25*B* illustrates that retrograde concealment within the A-V node of His extrasystoles (H') occur-

ring in successive cardiac cycles results in the electrocardiographic pattern of type-I second-degree A-V block. This phenomenon can be diagnosed from the clinical electrocardiographic tracing when it is noted (Fig. 25*C*) that there are also His extrasystoles occurring later in the cardiac cycle which do conduct to the ventricles with normal or aberrant ventricular activation.

The recognition that His extrasystoles simulate type-II A-V block is of more than academic interest, since this phenomenon does not require permanent ventricular pacemaker therapy while a true type-II block does.

Figure 26 is from a dog experiment in which the same phenomenon is demonstrated by prematurely stimulating the bundle of His (S).[15] Using this method, it has been demonstrated that concealed His extrasystoles can cause types I and II second-degree A-V block, 2:1 A-V block, alternation

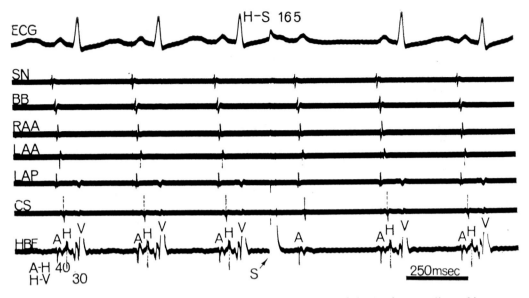

Fig. 26. Experimental demonstration that His extrasystoles can result in the electrocardiographic pattern of type-II second degree A-V block. ECG is lead II. Electrogram recordings were obtained from the region of the sinus node (SN), Bachmann's bundle (BB), the right atrial appendage (RAA), the left atrial appendage (LAA), the posterior left atrium (LAP), the coronary sinus (CS) and the bundle of His (HBE). Following the third sinus beat, the bundle of His was prematurely stimulated at an H-S coupling interval of 165 msec. Retrograde concealment into the A-V node caused block of the fourth P wave. (From Damato, Lau and Bobb.[15])

of the P-R interval and simulate nonconducted atrial bigeminal rhythms.[15]

ATRIAL FIBRILLATION AND FLUTTER

During atrial fibrillation, the atria are generating impulses, in a chaotic fashion, in excess of 400/min. The functional capacity of the A-V node is such that it cannot transmit all of these impulses to the ventricles and many impulses are blocked or concealed within the node. In addition, some of the atrial impulses do not even enter the A-V node. Thus, during atrial fibrillation, the irregular ventricular rate is predominately determined by the number of atrial impulses which enter the A-V node, the degree of penetrance and concealment within the A-V node and the speed of A-V nodal conduction. It is generally conceded that concealment within the A-V node is the major determinant of the irregular ventricular response in atrial fibrillation.[22,26,32,35,40,42]

Electrophysiological studies by Moore and associates, using microelectrode techniques, have demonstrated that during atrial fibrillation the major zone of concealment is the A-V node.[42] These investigators also noted that occasionally atrial impulses were concealed within the ventricular specialized conducting system.

Studies using His bundle recordings in five clinical cases of atrial fibrillation have confirmed that the A-V node is the major zone of concealment, regardless of whether or not the patients are taking digitalis. We have observed similar findings in the intact dog heart in which atrial fibrillation was acutely induced. In these studies it was demonstrated that each normal or aberrantly activated QRS complex was preceded by a single His deflection. His deflections which were not followed by QRS complexes were never observed. Despite the consistency of our results, it can be predicted that in clinical cases of atrial fibrillation concealment may occur within the His-Purkinje system. This is likely to occur in patients who (1) have a prolonged effective refractory period of the His-Purkinje system, or (2) have an underlying type-II second-degree A-V block and develop atrial fibrillation.

In atrial fibrillation, bundle of His recordings are especially useful in distinguishing aberrant ventricular conduction of supraventricular impulses from ventricular ectopic beats. In the former, the abnormal QRS complex is preceded by a His deflection with an H-V interval normal or greater than normal. In the latter, either the abnormal QRS complex is not preceded by a His deflection or else the H-V interval is significantly less than the normal value for that patient. A short H-V interval preceding a

ventricular ectopic beat may signify a fusion beat or a retrograde His deflection from the ventricular impulse. Figure 27 illustrates aberrant ventricular conduction during atrial fibrillation. Note the absence of P waves on the electrocardiographic and HBE tracings. A single His deflection with an H-V interval of 50 msec precedes the first three and last two QRS complexes. The fourth QRS complex has an RBBB pattern and results from aberrant activation of the ventricles by a supraventricular impulse. The H-V interval is prolonged at 70 msec. The aberrant beat terminates a short R-R cycle which is preceded by a longer R-R cycle. An example of ectopic ventricular activity during atrial fibrillation is shown in Figure 28.

Cohen and associates presented compara-

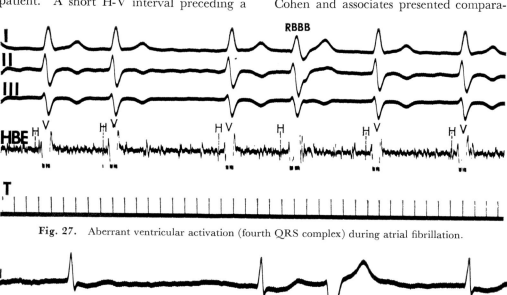

Fig. 27.   Aberrant ventricular activation (fourth QRS complex) during atrial fibrillation.

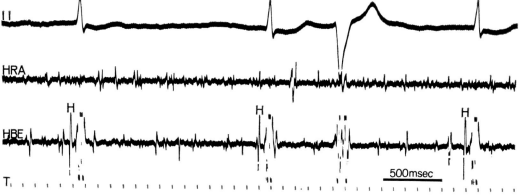

Fig. 28.   Ectopic ventricular activity during atrial fibrillation.

tive data on the transmission properties of the A-V conducting system before and during atrial fibrillation in both man and dogs.[26] In each instance, it was noted that the ventricular response during atrial fibrillation was slower than during atrial tachycardia. The results of five clinical studies showed that the average ventricular response during atrial tachycardia was 133 ± 40 while the average response during atrial fibrillation was 97 ± 19. These results provided additional evidence that concealed conduction within the A-V node plays a major role in determining the ventricular response during atrial fibrillation.

In 12 cases of atrial flutter which we have studied the area of block for the nonconducted atrial impulses was found to be proximal to the bundle of His.

ABERRATION

Ventricular aberration can be defined as an alteration in the sequence of ventricular activation which results whenever an impulse of supraventricular origin is asynchronously conducted within the His-Purkinje system. Most often, aberration results because the supraventricular impulse enters the His-Purkinje system at a time when a portion of this system is either relatively or effectively refractory.[3,7,8,20,29,41,48,67] For atrial impulses the determinants of aberration include (1) the degree of prematurity of the atrial impulse, (2) the cycle length (R-R interval) preceding the premature atrial impulse, (3) the speed of A-V nodal conduction, and (4) the state of recovery of excitability of the His-Purkinje system. For junctional beats (bundle of His), arising below the A-V node, determinant 3 is not a consideration in the production of ventricular aberration.

Clinically, the most common type of ventricular aberration is that of a right bundle branch block pattern. Cohen and associates studied in man the various aberration patterns which occurred when premature atrial depolarizations were introduced at progressively earlier times in the cardiac cycle. In a total

of 52 subjects, the frequencies of aberrant conduction patterns were as follows: RBBB without axis shift, 31; RBBB with left anterior hemiblock, 27; left anterior hemiblock, 14;

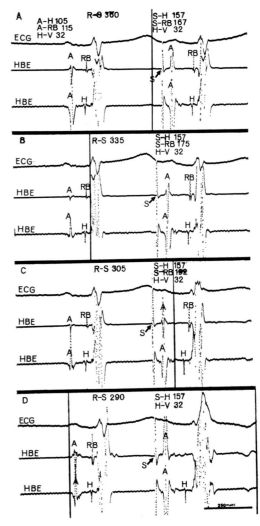

Fig. 29. Right bundle branch aberration resulting from proximal delay in the right bundle branch. The H-RB interval for all of the sinus beats (first beat in each panel) is 10 msec. From A to D, premature atrial beats (second beat in each panel) are introduced at progressively shorter R-S intervals. At an R-S coupling interval of 360 msec (A), the H-RB interval remains at 10 msec and normal ventricular activation occurs. As the R-S coupling interval is decreased to 335 and 305 msec (B and C), the H-RB intervals increase by 18 and 35 msec respectively and different degrees of RBBB aberration occur. A complete RBBB pattern results (D) when the H-RB interval exceeds 35 msec.

RBBB with inferior axis shift, 7; inferior axis shift, 6; LBBB, 6.

Figure 29 illustrates a clinical example of progressive RBBB aberration which results when premature atrial depolarizations encounter conduction delay in the proximal portion of the right bundle branch. In each panel, the first beat is a sinus beat in which H and proximal RB potentials were recorded. For all sinus beats the interval from the onset of the H deflection to the onset of the RB potential is 10 msec. The second beat in each panel results from a premature atrial depolarization which was introduced at progressively shorter R-S coupling intervals. Figure 29B shows that the H-RB intervals of the premature beats progressively increase and that this is associated with increasing degrees of RBBB aberration. It is presumed that (Fig. 29D) the RB potential is delayed to such an extent that it is obscured within the ventricular electrogram.

Figure 30 depicts alternating left (beat 2) and right (beat 4) bundle branch block aberration in a dog during premature atrial stimulation. Electrode catheter recordings of H, LB and RB potentials were recorded. Beats 1 and 3 are the sinus beats showing the normal H-LB-RB relationships. Conduction delay in either the left or right bundle branch produces a corresponding bundle branch block pattern.

Activation of the ventricular septum begins on the left side. Activation of the right side of the septum occurs either simultaneously with left-sided activation or follows the latter by only a few milliseconds (<5 msec). Thus, it would be expected that during isolated conduction delay in the right bundle branch the H-V interval should remain normal. Similarly, during isolated conduction delay in the main left bundle, or that portion of the left bundle which delivers the impulse to the septum, activation would be initiated from the right side and the H-V interval ought to be normal or increased by no greater than

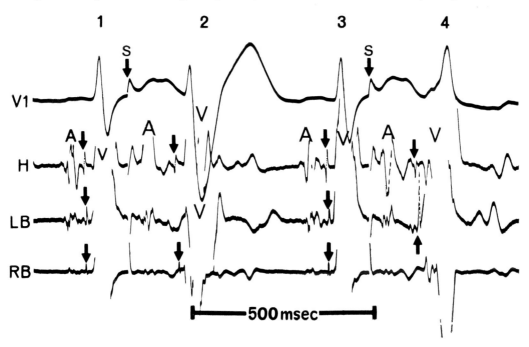

Fig. 30. Alternating left (beat 2) and right (beat 4) bundle branch block aberration during premature atrial stimulation. The first and third beats are the sinus beats showing the normal H-LB-RB relationships. During LBBB aberration there is a delay in activation of the LB potential and during RBBB aberration there is delay in activation of the RB potential. (From Lau, Bobb and Damato.[33])

5 msec above normal. As illustrated in Figure 29 the H-V interval remains normal (32 msec) during the development of all forms of RBBB aberration, indicating that the initiation of septal activation on the left side was unaffected.

In Figure 31, alternating right and left bundle branch block aberration results from successive premature stimulation of the right atrium at a constant coupling interval. The H-V interval of the normal sinus beats measures 35 msec. During RBBB aberration a modest conduction delay also occurs in the left bundle as reflected in an H-V interval of 47 msec. Similarly, during LBBB aberration a significant conduction delay occurs in

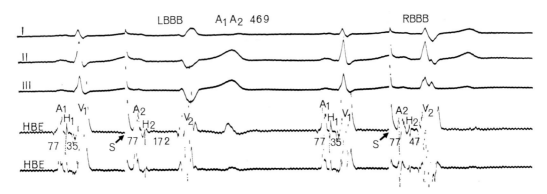

Fig. 31. The development of alternating LBBB and RBBB aberration during successive coupled stimulation of the right atrium. $A_1 A_2$ interval of 469 msec indicates the coupling interval of the premature atrial beat (A_2) after the sinus beat (A_1).

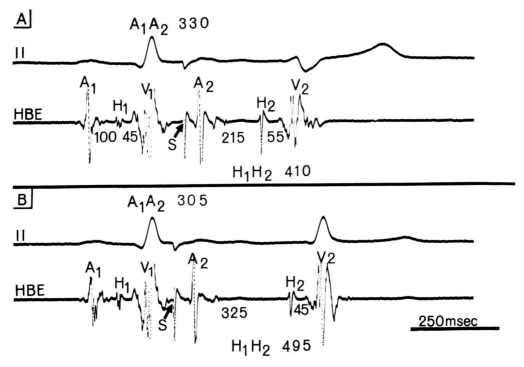

Fig. 32. The role of A-V nodal delay in preventing aberration.

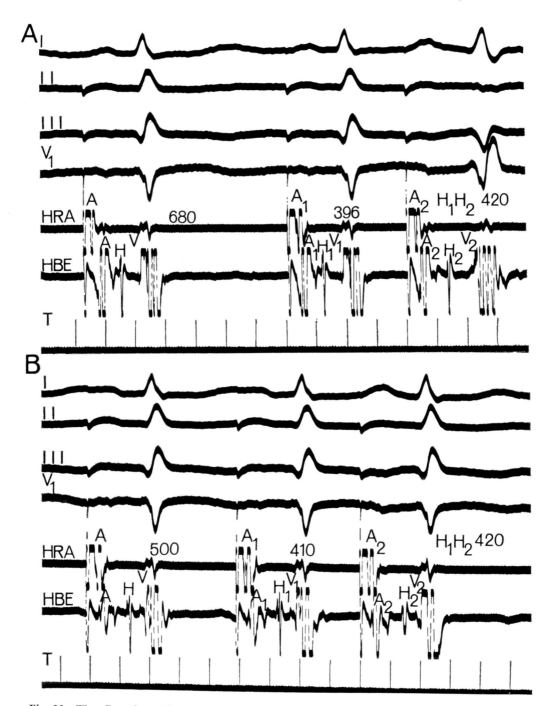

Fig. 33. The effect of preceding cycle length on ventricular aberration. A: The right atrium is driven at a basic cycle length of 680 msec ($A_1 - A_1$). A premature atrial depolarization, A_2, introduced after every eighth basic beat at an $A_1 A_2$ interval of 396 msec results in ventricular aberration. The corresponding $H_1 H_2$ interval is 420 msec. B: The basic cycle length was decreased to 500 msec. A premature atrial depolarization, induced at an $A_1 A_2$ interval of 410 msec, results in the same $H_1 H_2$ interval of 420 msec but no aberration occurs.

the right bundle branch as indicated by an
H-V interval of 172 msec. It is to be noted
in Figure 31 that the lack of significant A-H
interval delay (77 msec) for the premature
atrial beats enhances the probability that the
premature impulse will be delivered to the
His-Purkinje system prior to its full recovery
and that aberration will result.

The role of A-V nodal delay in preventing
aberration is illustrated in Figure 32. The
first beat is a sinus beat. The A-H and H-V
intervals are 100 and 45 msec respectively.
The cycle lengths preceding the sinus beats
are the same. In Figure 32A a premature atrial
depolarization occurring at an $A_1 A_2$ interval
of 330 msec results in ventricular aberration.
The $H_1 H_2$ interval is 410 msec. In Figure
32B an earlier premature atrial depolarization encounters greater A-V nodal delay
(A-H = 325 msec). The corresponding H_1
H_2 has increased to 495 msec. As a result of the longer $H_1 H_2$ interval, the premature impulse enters the His-Purkinje
system after it has recovered and aberration
does not occur.

Figure 33 demonstrates the effect of cycle
length on ventricular aberration. Figure 33A
shows a premature atrial impulse (A_2) resulting in ventricular aberration at an $H_1 H_2$
interval of 420 msec. The R-R cycle length
preceding A_2 is 680 msec. In Figure 33B,
when the preceding cycle length is decreased
to 500 msec, A_2 does not result in ventricular
aberration despite the fact that the $H_1 H_2$
remains the same at 420 msec. Shortening
the preceding cycle length shortens the
refractory period of the His-Purkinje system
and thereby lessens the likelihood of aberration.

REFERENCES

1. Alanis, J., Gonzales, H., and Lopez, E.: Electrical activity of the bundle of His. J. Physiol., 142:127, 1958.
2. Alanis, J., et al.: Propagation of impulses
   through the atrioventricular node. Amer. J.
   Physiol., 197:1171, 1959.
3. Ashman, R., and Byer, E.: Aberration in the
   conduction of premature ventricular impulses.
   J. Louisiana State Univ. School Med., 8:62,
   1946.
4. Burchell, H. B., Essex, H. F., and Lambert,
   E. H.: Action potentials of specialized conduction pathways in the dog's ventricle.
   Circ. Res., 1:186, 1953.
5. Cannom, D. S., et al.: Concealed bundle of His
   extrasystoles simulating nonconducted atrial
   premature beats. Amer. Heart J., 83:777,
   1972.
6. Castillo, C. A., and Castellanos, A.: Retrograde activation of the His bundle during
   intermittent paired ventricular stimulation in
   the human heart. Circulation, 42:1079, 1970.
7. Cohen, S. I., et al.: Experimental production
   of aberrant ventricular conduction in man.
   Circulation, 36:673, 1967.
8. Cohen, S. I., et al.: Variations of aberrant
   ventricular conduction in man. Evidence of
   isolated and combined block within the
   specialized conduction system. Circulation,
   38:899, 1968.
9. Cohen, S. I., et al.: Concealed conduction
   during atrial fibrillation. Amer. J. Cardiol.,
   25:416, 1970.
10. Damato, A. N., et al.: Subjunctional conduc-
    tion. In: 25th Hahnemann Symposium on
    Cardiac Arrhythmias, in press.
11. Damato, A. N., et al.: Use of His bundle re-
    cordings in understanding A-V conduction
    disturbances. Bull. N.Y. Acad. Med., 47:
    905, 1971.
12. Damato, A. N., and Lau, S. H.: Concealed
    and supernormal A-V conduction. Circula-
    tion, 43:967, 1971.
13. Damato, A. N., et al.: Recording of specialized
    conducting fibers (A-V nodal, His bundle and
    right bundle-branch) in man using an elec-
    trode catheter technic. Circulation, 39:435,
    1969.
14. Damato, A. N., Lau, S. H., and Bobb, G. A.:
    Studies on ventriculo-atrial conduction and
    the reentry phenomenon. Circulation, 41:
    423, 1970.
15. Damato, A. N., Lau, S. H., and Bobb, G. A.:
    Cardiac arrhythmias simulated by concealed
    bundle of His extrasystoles. Circ. Res., 28:
    316, 1971.
16. Damato, A. N., et al.: Recording of A-V nodal
    activity in the intact dog heart. Amer.
    Heart J., 80:353, 1970.
17. Damato, A. N., et al.: Study of atrioventricular
    conduction in man using electrode catheter
    recordings of His bundle activity. Circula-
    tion, 39:287, 1969.
17a.Damato, A. N., et al: A study of heart block
    in man using His bundle recordings. Circu-
    lation, 39:297, 1969.
18. Damato, A. N., et al.: A study of atrioventricu-
    lar conduction in man using premature atrial
    stimulation and His bundle recordings.
    Circulation, 40:61, 1969.
19. Giraud, G., Puech, P., and Latour, H.:
    L'activite electrique physiologique du noeud
    de Tawara et du faisceueau de His chez
    l'homme. Acad. Nat. Med., 144:363, 1960.

20. Gouaux, J. L., and Ashman, R.: Auricular fibrillation with aberration simulating ventricular tachycardia. Amer. Heart J., *34*:366, 1947.
21. Hoffman, B. F., and Cranefield, P. F.: *Electrophysiology of the Heart.* New York, McGraw-Hill, 1960.
22. Hoffman, B. F., Cranefield, P. F., and Stuckey, J. H.: Concealed conduction. Circ. Res., *9*: 194, 1961.
23. Hoffman, B. F., et al.: Electrical activity during the P–R interval. Circ. Res., *13*:1200, 1960.
24. Hoffman, B. F., Paes DeCarvalho, A., and Carlos DeMello, W.: Transmembrane potentials of single fibers of the atrioventricular node. Nature, *181*:66, 1958.
25. Hoffman, B. F., et al.: Electrical activity of single fibers of the A–V node. Circ. Res., *7*:11, 1959.
26. Horan, L. G., and Kistler, J. C.: Study of ventricular response in atrial fibrillation. Circ. Res., *9*:305, 1961.
27. Katz, L. N., and Pick, A.: *Clinical Electrocardiography: I. The Arrhythmias.* Philadelphia, Lea and Febiger, 1956.
28. Langendorf, R.: Concealed A–V conduction: The effect of blocked impulses on the formation of subsequent impulses. Amer. Heart J., *35*:542, 1948.
29. Langendorf, R.: Aberrant ventricular conduction. Amer. Heart J., *41*:700, 1951.
30. Langendorf, R., Cohen, H., and Gozo, E. G.: Observations on second degree atrioventricular block, including new criteria for the differential diagnosis between type I and type II block. Amer. J. Cardiol., *29*:111, 1972.
31. Langendorf, R., and Mehlman, J. S.: Blocked (nonconducted) A–V nodal premature systoles initiating first and second degree A–V block. Amer. Heart J., *34*:500, 1947.
32. Langendorf, R., Pick, A., and Katz, L. N.: Ventricular response in atrial fibrillation: Role of concealed conduction in the A–V junction. Circulation, *32*:69, 1965.
33. Lau, S. H., Bobb, G. A., and Damato, A. N.: Catheter recording and validation of left bundle-branch potentials in intact dogs. Circulation, *42*:375, 1970.
34. Lau, S. H., and Damato, A. N.: Mechanisms of A–V block. Cardiov. Clin., *2*:50, 1970.
35. Lau, S. H., et al.: A study of atrioventricular conduction in atrial fibrillation and flutter in man using His bundle recordings. Circulation, *40*:7, 1969.
36. Lewis, T., and Master, A. M.: Observations upon conduction in the mammalian heart: A–V conduction. Heart, *12*:209, 1925.
37. Ling, G., and Gerad, R. W.: The normal membrane potential of frog sorforius fibers. J. Cell Comp. Physiol., *34*:383, 1949.
38. Lister, J. W., et al.: Atrioventricular conduction in man: Effect of rate, exercise, isoproterenol and atropine on the P–R interval. Amer. J. Cardiol., *16*:516, 1965.
39. Matsuda, K., Hoshi, T., and Kameyama, S.: Action potential of the atrioventricular node (Tawara). Tohoku J. Exp. Med., *68*:8, 1958.
40. Moe, G. K., Abildskov, J. A., and Mendez, C.: An experimental study of concealed conduction. Amer. Heart J., *67*:338, 1964.
41. Moe, G., Mendez, C., and Han, J.: Aberrant A–V impulse propagation in the dog heart: A study of functional bundle branch block. Circ. Res., *16*:261, 1965.
42. Moore, E. N.: Observations on concealed conduction in atrial fibrillation. Circ. Res., *11*: 201, 1967.
43. Narula, O. S., et al.: Significance of His and left bundle recordings from left heart in man. Circulation, *42*:385, 1970.
44. Narula, O. S., and Samet, P.: Wenckebach and Mobitz II A–V block due to block within the His bundle and bundle branches. Circulation, *41*:947, 1970.
45. Narula, O. S., Scherlag, B. J., and Samet, P.: Pervenous pacing of the specialized conducting system in man. Circulation, *41*:77, 1970.
46. Narula, O. S., et al.: Atrioventricular block: Localization and classification by His bundle recordings. Amer. J. Med., *50*:146, 1971.
47. Narula, O. S., et al.: Localization of A–V conduction defects in man by recording of the His bundle electrogram. Amer. J. Cardiol., *25*:228, 1970.
48. Pick, A.: Aberrant ventricular conduction of escaped beats: Preferential and accessory pathways in the A–V junction. Circulation, *13*:702, 1956.
49. Pruitt, R., and Essex, H. E.: Potential changes attending the excitation process in the atrioventricular conduction system of bovine and canine hearts. Circ. Res., *8*:149, 1960.
50. Puech, P., et al.: L'enregistrement de l'activite electrique due faisceau de His dans les blocs A–V spontanes. Arch. Mal. Coeur, *63*:967, 1970.
51. Rosen, K., et al.: Site of heart block in acute myocardial infarction. Circulation, *42*:925, 1970.
52. Rosen, K. M., Rahimtoola, S. H., and Gunnar, R. M.: Pseudo A–V block secondary to premature non-propagated His bundle depolarizations. Documentation of His bundle electrocardiography. Circulation, *42*:367, 1970.
53. Rosen, K., et al.: Bundle branch and ventricular activation in man: A study utilizing catheter recordings of right and left bundle branch potentials. Circulation, *43*:193, 1971.
54. Sano, T., et al.: Resting and action potentials in the region of the atrioventricular node. Proc. Jap. Acad., *34*:558, 1958.
55. Sano, T., Tasaki, M., and Shimamoto, T.: Histologic examination of the origin of the action potential characteristically obtained from the region bordering the atrioventricular node. Circ. Res., *7*:700, 1959.
56. Scher, A. M., et al.: The mechanism of atrioventricular conduction. Circ. Res., *7*:54, 1959.

57. Scher, A. M.: Excitation of the heart. In: *Handbook of Physiology*. Washington, American Physiological Society, 1962.
58. Scherlag, B. J., Helfant, R. H., and Damato, A. N.: A catheterization technique for His bundle stimulation and recording in the intact dog. J. Appl. Physiol., *25*:425, 1968.
59. Scherlag, B. J., Kosowsky, B. D., and Damato, A. N.: Technique for ventricular pacing from the His bundle of the intact heart. J. Appl. Physiol., *22*:584, 1967.
60. Scherlag, B. J., et al.: Catheter technique for recording His bundle activity in man. Circulation, *39*:13, 1969.
61. Schuilenburg, R. M., and Durrer, D.: Conduction disturbances located within the His bundle. Circulation, *45*:612, 1972.
62. Sodi-Pallares, D., et al.: Electrograms of the conductive tissue in the normal dog's heart. Amer. J. Cardiol., *4*:459, 1959.
63. Steiner, C., et al.: Electrophysiologic documentation of trifascicular block as the common cause of complete heart block. Amer. J. Cardiol., *28*:436, 1971.
64. van der Kooi, M. W., et al.: Electrical activity in sinus node and atrioventricular node. Amer. Heart J., *51*:684, 1956.
65. Watanabe, Y., and Dreifus, L.: Second degree A–V block. In: *Mechanisms and Therapy of Cardiac Arrhythmias* (Dreifus, L., and Likoff, W., Eds.). New York, Grune and Stratton, 1966.
66. Watson, H., Emslie-Smith, D., and Lowe, K. G.: The intracardiac electrocardiogram of human atrioventricular conducting tissue. Amer. Heart J., *74*:66, 1967.
67. White, P. D., and Stevens, H.: Ventricular response to auricular premature beats and to auricular flutter. Arch. Intern. Med., *18*:712, 1916.

Chapter 7

PATHOPHYSIOLOGY OF SHOCK IN ACUTE MYOCARDIAL INFARCTION*

Jay N. Cohn, M.D., and Joseph A. Franciosa, M.D.

For more than 200 years, physicians have used the word "shock" to describe a complex pattern of signs appearing in patients suffering from a variety of physical disabilities.[110] Definition of this term has been impeded because of the multiplicity of causes of the syndrome and a lack of understanding of the mechanisms of the observed abnormalities.[202] In the years before the current era of quantitative physiology, shock was often viewed as a mysterious form of circulatory collapse originating in the central nervous system or the peripheral blood vessels. Although controversy still exists regarding many aspects of the problem, there is nearly unanimous agreement today that shock should be defined as a critical fall in capillary perfusion which reduces oxygen delivery to levels below the tissues' nutritional requirement for maintaining cellular integrity.[115,178,218] Furthermore, it is now generally accepted that this critical reduction in blood flow may result from inadequate venous return to the heart,

inability of one or more chambers of the heart to eject enough cardiac output, or some abnormality in the peripheral circulation which deprives certain capillary beds of their blood flow.[37,39,62,183] More than one of these factors often contribute to the perfusion deficiency.

The syndrome of shock accompanying acute myocardial infarction has been equally controversial. Although the typical clinical picture of the patient with severe shock and marked reduction in peripheral blood flow is well known, the absence of precise clinical criteria for diagnosis has led to marked variations in the severity of the circulatory abnormality labeled as shock. Even arterial pressure, often used as a guide to the presence of shock, provides little insight because it is now well known that pressures measured by sphygmomanometer may be grossly unreliable in shock.[39,130] If a cuff systolic pressure less than 90 mm Hg is used as a criterion for diagnosis, patients may be included with less severe circulatory abnormalities than if an intra-arterial systolic pressure less than 90 mm Hg is used. Since intra-arterial pressure

* Supported in part by U.S. Public Health Service Grant HE 09785 from the National Heart and Lung Institute.

207

now is being monitored directly in many coronary-care units, our contemporary understanding of the incidence and mortality rate of shock with myocardial infarction may be difficult to relate to historical experience.[151,197]

For the purposes of the present discussion we shall define shock in myocardial infarction as a syndrome of marked reduction in regional blood flow accompanied by progressive impairment of organ function occurring either immediately with or days after acute myocardial infarction and in the absence of any other severe medical illness which could account for the shock. The currently held view is that this complication of acute myocardial infarction is fatal in some 80 to 100 per cent of cases despite the use of a variety of medicinal agents.[88,191,224]

Data suggest that the mortality rate of myocardial infarction shock has not decreased in the past decade.[35,133] However, these statistics may be misleading. Shock may be less frequent today because more prompt recognition and treatment of correctable prodromal signs may improve the circulation of many patients who formerly drifted into a syndrome of shock. On the other hand, recognition and correction of arrhythmias have reduced the hospital incidence of sudden death in patients with massive infarction and provided a new reservoir of patients whose ultimate demise may be attributed to shock.[126] Thus, a changing pattern of hospital mortality from myocardial infarction related in part to improved treatment may not be detected by the usual data analysis.[144]

The terms "pump failure" and "power failure" have become popular in recent years to describe the functional cardiac abnormality in myocardial infarction shock. However, these phrases provide no real insight into mechanisms, and casual use of the terms could result in an easily treatable syndrome being assumed to represent irreversible end-stage cardiac impairment. If limited to situations where clinical and physiological data indicate that maximum attainable cardiac work is inadequate to provide suffi-

cient peripheral blood flow, then use of the term "power failure" is appropriate.

Although strict definition of the shock syndrome is mandatory for meaningful analysis of the results emanating from many clinics, it must be recognized at the outset that the circulatory complications of acute myocardial infarction represent a continuum from mild to severe. Thus, selection of rigid criteria for the diagnosis of shock may result in an arbitrary division into "shock" and "nonshock" which could obscure recognition of the spectrum of flow deficiencies and their rapid change with time. The pathophysiology of shock therefore cannot be considered independently from an analysis of the physiological abnormalities which accompany myocardial infarction in general. Indeed, it probably should be the goal of the physician to seek better means of detecting and treating the circulatory abnormalities occurring prior to the development of shock ("preshock") in hopes that early intervention will prevent its development or improve its prognosis.

This review will be concerned with an analysis of how the hemodynamic and metabolic events in myocardial infarction contribute to circulatory failure rather than with the semantic problem of the definition of shock. However, our understanding of the functional cardiac abnormalities in myocardial infarction is in transition. An awakened interest in the problem of acute myocardial infarction has led in the last few years to a profusion of new data which may eventually provide the basis for a better concept of the infarcted heart. This review should therefore be considered as a biased progress report in which the last chapter has not yet been written.

CLINICAL DIAGNOSIS

The reduction in regional blood flow which is the hallmark of cardiogenic shock results in a demonstrable impairment in tissue perfusion or organ function. Since early recognition of circulatory deficiency is probably the most important determinant of successful

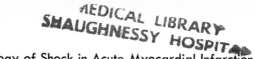

treatment, comprehensive evaluation of the adequacy of peripheral blood flow is a vital and continuing responsibility of the physician in the management of the patient with acute myocardial infarction. This evaluation should include the following measurements.

Skin Temperature

Warm skin indicates adequate cutaneous blood flow and usually, but not always, is associated with a fairly well-maintained cardiac output. Cool, clammy skin is a reflection of enhanced reflex sympatho-adrenal discharge leading to vasoconstriction of the cutaneous and often the visceral vascular beds, which may support arterial pressure in the face of a declining cardiac output.[121] Not all patients exhibit cutaneous vasoconstriction when cardiac output falls, and warm skin therefore can coexist with inadequate blood flow to other regional beds in acute myocardial infarction.[191]

Peripheral Pulses

Thready or absent radial or brachial pulses indicate either severe hypotension or reduction in extremity blood flow due to intense peripheral vasoconstriction, both of which demand prompt treatment.[44] When the skin is warm, weak pulses usually are indicative of arterial hypotension. The femoral pulses often are a better guide to the level of arterial pressure, since they are weak in hypotension and often bounding in the presence of peripheral vasoconstriction with adequate arterial pressure.

Auscultatory Blood Pressure

This is not a reliable measure of aortic pressure in shock. A low cuff pressure has the same significance as weak brachial or radial pulses. An absent auscultatory pressure is indicative of low blood flow which could result either from hypotension or forearm vasoconstriction.[39] In the early phase of shock, blood pressure may be only slightly reduced, normal, or even elevated while other signs of decreased perfusion are present.[40]

On the other hand, some patients with acute myocardial infarction manifest a low blood pressure without evidence of reduced perfusion. In the absence of signs of impaired regional flow this syndrome does not carry a grave prognosis and should not be classified as "shock."

Mentation

Agitation, restlessness, confusion, and somnolence are signs of inadequate cerebral blood flow and are usually associated with hypotension, although they occasionally occur at an arterial pressure only slightly below its usual range.

Urine Output

Urine flow less than 20 ml/hr with a low urine sodium concentration (less than 20 mEq/L) is evidence of inadequate renal blood flow which can contribute to the development of tubular necrosis.[217] Urine specific gravity and osmolality usually are high in the early phase of renal hypoperfusion unless there is preexisting renal disease.

Cardiac Signs

Persistent or recurrent chest pain or arrhythmias occurring in a patient with a low arterial pressure must be viewed as presumptive evidence of functional impairment of coronary blood flow to noninfarcted areas of the heart.

Acid-base Balance

Metabolic acidosis and elevated blood lactate levels are consistent with reduced tissue oxygenation. Hypocapnia may be the earliest finding in arterial blood before the arterial pH begins to fall. Therefore, arterial blood gases and pH are of great value in making the diagnosis of shock and in monitoring the response to therapy.[147,220]

If the above evaluation reveals one or more signs of inadequate tissue perfusion in a patient with an acute myocardial infarction, the diagnosis of shock should tentatively be made and intensive evaluation and monitoring should be undertaken to determine whether the flow deficiency is transient or progressive.

CLINICOPATHOLOGICAL CORRELATIONS

In an effort to shed light on the cause of myocardial infarction shock, pathologists have examined postmortem material from patients dying of acute myocardial infarction with shock and compared the cardiac findings to those in patients dying of acute myocardial infarction without shock. Divergent conclusions have been reached from these studies. Infarctions involving the anterior wall predominate in the shock group but also in the nonshock group.[88,146,150,151,164] A higher incidence of occluded coronary arteries in patients with shock has been noted in one series but not in others.[174,223] An unusually high incidence of occlusive lesions in secondary branches of the coronary arteries has been found in one series.[132] More recent studies indicate that the patient who dies with shock usually has an infarction involving more than 40 per cent of the total mass of the left ventricle.[96,174] Often the infarcted areas consist of old and new lesions.

These pathological studies have certain built-in deficiencies which reduce their value in elucidating the pathophysiology of shock in myocardial infarction. First of all, the clinical observation of the patients in these series often is deficient, and it therefore is not possible to be sure that patients whose hearts were examined indeed had shock as defined by the criteria given above. Secondly, the interval between the onset of shock and death is variable, and secondary myocardial changes consequent to shock may greatly alter the postmortem appearance of the heart.[23,154] Thirdly, postmortem material is obviously of limited help in arriving at an understanding of a disease process, since it is not possible to include in the study analysis of the hearts of patients who survive.

From the data available it probably can be concluded that the patient who dies from shock after acute myocardial infarction usually has a large infarct most commonly in the anterior wall, often accompanied by occlusion of one of the branches of the left coronary artery and frequently accompanied by evidence of old myocardial infarctions as well. It is not yet possible to conclude that the infarcts in shock are different either quantitatively or qualitatively from the infarcts in patients who do not develop shock.

CLINICAL SYNDROMES OF SHOCK

Signs of impaired regional perfusion may occur as transient or sustained episodes in a variety of settings in acute myocardial infarction. Although all of these syndromes may be referred to as shock, their management and prognosis vary widely.

Bradycardiac Shock

Shock occurs in association with a slow ventricular rate, usually less than 60 beats per minute. It may be observed at the onset of acute myocardial infarction when the patient is complaining of severe chest pain, or it may occur late in the course if heart block develops. The syndrome usually is reversible.[1,200,236]

Tachycardiac Shock

Shock is precipitated by a tachyarrhythmia of either supraventricular or ventricular origin, usually when the rate is over 140 beats per minute.[167,233] The shock may disappear when the rhythm is corrected but occasionally persists even after a sinus rhythm has been restored. It is important to separate a primary arrhythmia from the reflex sinus tachycardia which often accompanies a falling stroke volume in shock.

Cardiac Depression Shock

Shock is precipitated by the administration of negative inotropic drugs such as the antiarrhythmic compounds, especially propranolol, or anesthetics.[5,8,93,139,156,199] The duration of shock in such cases often is far longer than the pharmacological effect of the drug.

Hypovolemic Shock

Shock occurs some hours after acute myocardial infarction accompanied by a low or normal central venous pressure and left ventricular filling pressure, often in the setting of intense diaphoresis or after administration of sympathomimetic amines or diuretics.[6,41,43,143]

Power-failure Shock

The typical picture of progressive falling cardiac output is characteristic of severe myocardial infarction shock. Premonitory signs often appear minutes or hours before the full shock picture develops. The most common early signs are the increased perspiration of the forehead and neck associated with tachycardia, some weakening of the peripheral pulses and a fall in auscultatory pulse pressure. Urine output may still be adequate at this time, and some patients pass through this early phase without therapy and make an uneventful recovery.[104] In others, however, the signs of falling cardiac output and increasing peripheral vasoconstriction gradually become more prominent. A degree of stability may be attained during which the insufficiency of blood flow is only borderline and the shock progresses very slowly. When the arterial pressure begins to fall, however, the course may be telescoped into a few minutes of rapidly deteriorating circulatory function and death. Symptoms and signs of pulmonary congestion often but not always accompany this syndrome.

Cardiac Rupture Shock

The sudden onset of rapidly progressive heart failure or shock is precipitated by rupture of the left ventricular free wall, septum or a papillary muscle usually occurring two or more days after acute myocardial infarction.[58,138,198]

Nonvasoconstricted Shock

In this less common presentation falling blood pressure is not accompanied by signs of peripheral vasoconstriction or significant tachycardia. The earliest sign in such patients

may be changes in the sensorium as arterial pressure falls. The syndrome is seen most often in elderly patients or in individuals with severe underlying medical diseases which impair the reactivity of the sympathetic nervous system.[45] Hypertensive patients receiving treatment with sympathetic blocking agents also may exhibit this condition.

Impairment of the performance of the heart as a pump is an important, if not exclusive, basis for all of the syndromes of shock in acute myocardial infarction. An understanding of the mechanism of shock therefore requires knowledge of the mechanism and the nature of the functional cardiac disturbance which occurs in acute myocardial infarction.

MYOCARDIAL OXYGEN TENSION

Myocardial oxygen tension is determined by the balance between oxygen delivery to the heart and myocardial oxygen utilization.[92] Decreases in delivery or increases in consumption may result in a reduction in tissue oxygen tension. Oxygen for myocardial aerobic metabolism normally is supplied by relatively low coronary blood flow and high myocardial oxygen extraction. Since the venous drainage from the heart has the lowest oxygen content of any venous blood in the body, increases in myocardial oxygen demand must be met primarily by an increase in coronary blood flow.[4] Therefore, modest reductions in hemoglobin concentration or changes in oxygen-hemoglobin affinity may have profound effects on myocardial oxygen tension if increases in coronary blood flow are limited by coronary vascular disease.[89,91]

Myocardial Oxygen Consumption

The main determinants of myocardial oxygen consumption are ventricular-wall tension, heart rate and the state of contractility.[209] The wall tension, as described by the law of Laplace, is directly related to pressure within the chamber and its radius of curvature and inversely related to wall thickness.[186] Since both the radius and wall thickness vary in different areas of the left ventricle, oxygen consumption is not necessarily uniform throughout the myocardium.[36]

In the presence of acute infarction, marked regional metabolic changes occur. Oxygen consumption may be reduced in the infarcted area but increased in the region surrounding the infarct if localized distortion increases wall tension during systole.[149] Oxygen requirements also may rise in the distant normal myocardium if it exhibits a compensatory increase in contractility.[107] Thus, an unchanged total myocardial oxygen consumption might obscure regional alterations in the metabolic rate.[24]

Myocardial Oxygen Delivery

Oxygen delivery to the myocardium is affected by total coronary blood flow and the distribution of the blood flow. Coronary blood flow is a function of the effective perfusion pressure (aortic pressure minus intramyocardial or coronary venous pressure) and the coronary vascular resistance.[18] Because intramyocardial pressure fluctuates widely during the cardiac cycle, particularly at the endocardial surface,[7,128] the distribution of flow within the myocardium varies throughout the cycle. Thus, during left ventricular systole subendocardial pressure approximates aortic pressure and endocardial blood flow ceases, whereas subepicardial perfusion may continue. During diastole, however, the fall in intramyocardial pressure establishes a pressure gradient favoring coronary blood flow, which may be directed preferentially to the subendocardium because of localized reactive vasodilation induced by the transient systolic hypoxia.[161]

Coronary arteriolar resistance probably is altered by neural, humoral and metabolic influences.[18,69] The relative role of each in the control of coronary blood flow during physiological events is not entirely clear. Active changes in arteriolar resistance occurring when perfusion pressure is altered (autoregulation) may be due either to metabolic or local vascular phenomena[18,19,68,92,163]

which tend to maintain coronary blood flow constant in the face of moderate changes in arterial pressure. However, autoregulation of the coronary bed would appear to be teleologically less rational than that of other vascular beds, since in contrast to other organs the work of the heart is directly related to the arterial pressure. Some studies indicate that the most important factor in regulation of coronary vascular resistance may be local hypoxia, which induces prompt vasodilation by liberation of adenosine or adenine nucleotides.[17,195] Nonetheless, the integration of active changes in vascular resistance and passive effects of intramyocardial pressure normally serve to provide adequate myocardial blood flow and oxygen delivery to meet the continuously changing myocardial oxygen requirements.

In the presence of coronary-artery disease and myocardial infarction, considerable alteration in the normal pattern of coronary blood flow may occur.[108] Reduction of coronary perfusion pressure beyond a stenotic lesion may reduce total coronary blood flow or at least lead to redistribution of intramyocardial flow away from the subendocardium.[15,18,232] Furthermore, a rise in left ventricular end-diastolic pressure, which is a frequent accompaniment of transmural acute myocardial infarction,[95] might reduce subendocardial perfusion by reducing the effective diastolic perfusion pressure even in those myocardial areas remote from the acute infarction.[85,185] Since ischemia lasting over 20 to 30 minutes may produce necrosis of myocardial cells,[118] prompt restoration of perfusion is necessary to prevent infarction or to limit infarct size.

Although endocardial flow exceeds epicardial flow in the normal heart,[15,71,129] it is the subendocardial myocardium which is most vulnerable to tissue damage in the presence of coronary-artery disease.[119,185] This finding has been attributed to the higher intramyocardial tension and lower oxygen tension existing in the deep layers of the myocardium.[129] It has also been pointed out by Estes et al. that the branch vessels which penetrate to the deep layers come off the larger vessels at right angles and may therefore be more susceptible to decreases in perfusion pressure.[67] In the presence of cardiogenic shock, which usually is associated with low perfusion pressure and high left ventricular diastolic pressure, these factors may assume particular importance in reducing subendocardial flow.[33] The significance of an elevated left ventricular end-diastolic pressure has been shown by Salisbury's experiments; the most extensive ischemia was produced by the combination of low perfusion pressure and elevated end-diastolic pressure, while the area of ischemia was much smaller when similar hypotension was accompanied by a normal end-diastolic pressure.[185]

Collateral flow may play an important role in protection of the subendocardial myocardium.[116] Presumptive evidence for the functional significance of collaterals comes from the fact that the size of a myocardial infarction is always smaller than the total area supplied by the occluded vessel.[190] In experimental occlusion of the left anterior descending coronary artery, flow to the area adjacent to the infarct via branches of the anterior descending artery proximal to the occlusion was actually greater than flow through the nonobstructed circumflex artery.[181] Indeed, embolic occlusion of a major coronary branch may lead to an increase in flow in the other nonoccluded major branch.[103] Thus, collateral channels apparently open promptly in response to coronary occlusion. However, flow in these vessels is critically dependent on effective perfusion pressure, which may be markedly reduced in shock. It is not surprising, therefore, that shock may be associated with larger infarcts because of necrosis of the intermediate ischemic zone surrounding the central infarction.[52]

MYOCARDIAL METABOLISM

The myocardium normally utilizes a variety of substrates in oxidative metabolism. In the fed state glucose serves as the major fuel, whereas in the fasted state free fatty acids

(FFA) are the primary substrate.[20,171] Under anoxic conditions, however, FFA cannot be utilized for energy production and the myocardium depends totally on anaerobic glycolysis.[173,193] Since blood FFA concentration may be high in acute myocardial infarction,[131] FFA can accumulate in the myocardium even though they are not metabolized in the absence of oxygen.[173] Some studies indicate that the stored FFA have a deleterious effect on cardiac function.[170]

In the anoxic myocardium anaerobic glycolysis, which is an inefficient source of energy production, is incapable of maintaining adequate high-energy phosphate stores to support myocardial contractility.[12,26,168,173] Furthermore, the end-product of anaerobic glycolysis is lactate, the accumulation of which in the myocardium and systemic circulation[83,159] may lead to acidosis and direct depression of myocardial performance.[57,78,231] In the ischemic myocardium, where aerobic and anaerobic metabolism may coexist, the need for glucose to serve as substrate and insulin to accelerate its utilization is critical to the continued survival of the tissue.[25,228] Ordinarily, stores of glycogen, circulating glucose and endogenous insulin are probably adequate for optimal myocardial metabolism. However, the depression of insulin secretion demonstrated in some patients with acute myocardial infarction could limit glucose utilization by the myocardium.[215] Indeed, the glucose and insulin treatment popularized by Sodi-Pallares to prevent myocardial potassium loss[205] might have a quite different effect by providing substrate for an ischemic myocardium.

MYOCARDIAL FUNCTION

Systemic Hemodynamics

Cardiac output may range from normal to markedly depressed in patients with acute myocardial infarction.[30,73,75,80,95,166] Although a general relationship between the magnitude of reduction in output and the severity of the clinical syndrome can be demonstrated, the level of the cardiac index cannot itself serve as a guide to the presence of shock. The clinical picture of shock after acute myocardial infarction rarely coexists with a cardiac index (CI) over 2.5 L/min/M^2, and the CI is more commonly less than 2.0 L/min/M^2 in patients with the classical shock syndrome.[180] Yet cardiac outputs equally low are sometimes observed in patients with acute myocardial infarction without shock.[204,226] Apparently the regional distribution of this output and its effectiveness in providing tissue perfusion are of critical importance in preventing shock.

Certain derived hemodynamic data have been utilized to characterize cardiogenic shock (Fig. 1). Stroke volume, cardiac minute work and stroke work are usually markedly depressed in shock and the degree of their depression has been found to correlate

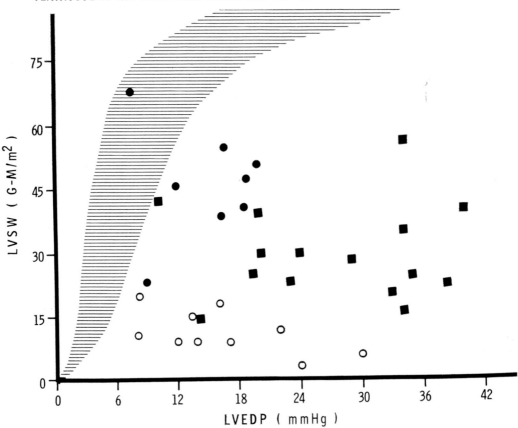

Fig. 1. Relationship between left ventricular end-diastolic pressure (LVEDP) and left ventricular stroke work (LVSW) in patients with acute myocardial infarction. Shaded area represents normal range of left ventricular performance. Patients with uncomplicated infarcts (dots) usually demonstrate moderate impairment of left ventricular function, whereas in patients with symptoms of heart failure (squares) stroke work is lower and LVEDP markedly elevated. Stroke work is profoundly depressed in shock (open circles) despite an elevated LVEDP. Unresolved question is whether patients with shock have an initial infarct quantitatively or qualitatively more severe than patients with heart failure, or whether the low stroke work in shock represents a shift in function from heart failure to shock because of the superimposition of positive feedback mechanisms.

with mortality.[180,201] As might be expected, the stroke work appears to provide the best single hemodynamic guide to severity of the clinical syndrome, since this measurement is reduced by a low cardiac output, fast heart rate and low arterial pressure, each of which independently probably has adverse prognostic significance in acute myocardial infarction.[176,192] Although these measurements, obtained from cardiac output data, imply considerable impairment of myocardial function after acute myocardial infarction, characterization of the ventricular functional deficit requires independent evaluation of each ventricle by more precise techniques.

Right Ventricle

Although myocardial infarction usually involves predominantly the left ventricle, the finding of some involvement of the right ventricle on postmortem examination is not uncommon.[136] In perhaps 2 per cent of hearts with myocardial infarction the lesion is predominant in the right ventricle.[225] Since the posterior surface of the right ventricle is most vulnerable, and the right coronary artery supplies the diaphragmatic and posterior walls of both the right and left ventricle, right ventricular infarction has been associated with right coronary-artery occlusion and electrocardiographic evidence of diaphragmatic infarction.[222] Little data are available on the hemodynamic significance of right ventricular infarction, but a disproportionately high central venous pressure has been noted in patients with diaphragmatic infarctions.[48] It is possible that this elevated right ventricular filling pressure is evidence for right ventricular dysfunction.

For many years, since the studies of Starr and his associates, it has been held that a functioning right ventricle is not necessary to maintain normal circulatory function.[212] Starr's work, confirmed by others, indicated that when the right ventricle was totally destroyed central venous pressure did not rise.[122] The conclusion was reached that pulmonary circulation could be maintained

in the absence of right ventricular function, perhaps in part by the passive pumping effect on the right ventricle of left ventricular contraction.[10] In recent studies in this laboratory, however, it was found that after infarction of the right ventricle of the dog plasma volume expansion produced a sharp rise in right ventricular end-diastolic pressure out of proportion to the rise in left ventricular end-diastolic pressure. The findings were in direct contrast to the response in hearts with left ventricular infarction, in which the rise in left ventricular end-diastolic pressure during volume expansion is far greater than the rise in right ventricular end-diastolic pressure.[87] It is therefore apparent that right ventricular infarction may have important and unique hemodynamic effects.

The role of right ventricular dysfunction in the genesis of pump failure in myocardial infarction is not known, but we have observed two patients with predominant right ventricular infarction who succumbed to shock with hemodynamic evidence of predominant right ventricular failure.[87] If the right ventricle was the cause of the circulatory failure in these patients, it must be assumed that refractory cardiogenic shock can exist in the absence of severe left ventricular disease.

Left Ventricle

The performance of the left ventricle is dependent on its preload, after-load and contractility. In the ischemic or infarcted ventricle, nonhomogeneity of involvement makes it necessary to consider the regional as well as the total performance of the left ventricle.

PRELOAD

Cardiac muscle demonstrates a direct relationship between its initial length and its contractile force. This property is translated into myocardial performance by the influence of acute changes in ventricular end-diastolic volume on ventricular stroke work.[177,211] This Frank-Starling relationship has been viewed as an important factor in alteration of left ventricular performance in response to changes in peripheral requirements for blood flow.[187] In view of this concept, dilatation of the left ventricle in diseased hearts has usually been assumed to represent a shift of ventricular performance to the right on a Frank-Starling curve, so that more work can be accomplished from a larger end-diastolic fiber length. However, the evidence that considerable dilation of the ventricular chamber may occur as a structural change in the absence of a change in fiber length requires that this traditional concept be reevaluated.[29,142]

In both experimental and clinical acute myocardial infarction, left ventricular filling pressure usually is considerably elevated.[95,107] Although an increase in left ventricular volume is sometimes observed, the rise in end-diastolic pressure appears to be considerably out of proportion to the rise in end-diastolic volume, suggesting a decrease in distensibility of the left ventricular chamber.[31,61,140,162,227] Thus the rise in end-diastolic pressure cannot necessarily be taken as evidence that the chamber has dilated and has utilized an increased end-diastolic fiber length to maintain contractile force. Manipulation of preload in acutely infarcted ventricles has provided data suggesting that the left ventricle usually is performing on a relatively flat function curve, so that large changes in end-diastolic pressure produce only small changes in stroke work.[27,31,184] Nonetheless, it can often be demonstrated that the infarcted ventricle has not fully utilized its Frank-Starling mechanism, for further increases in end-diastolic pressure may often augment stroke work and stroke volume even in the ventricles of patients in shock.[46] Once again, the relationship of these induced changes in end-diastolic pressure to changes in end-diastolic volume is not known.

The reduction in left ventricular compliance which has been described in experimental myocardial infarction,[162,227] angina pectoris[64] and clinical acute myocardial infarction[31,61] is not yet completely understood. Henderson, Parmley and Sonnenblick have demonstrated that the series elastic element of isolated papillary muscle becomes less compliant when placed in an hypoxic medium.[101] Teleologically, a decrease in compliance of hypoxic myocardium may be explained as an attempt to resist myocardial fiber elongation, which might increase force generation but at the same time would increase myocardial-wall tension and aggravate the underlying hypoxia. It must be recognized that an increase in ventricular volume not only increases wall tension at the onset of systole but, since the enlarged ventricle ejects stroke volume with a smaller than usual reduction in chamber radius, a smaller than usual reduction in wall tension will occur during systole and thus result in a considerable augmentation of myocardial oxygen consumption during the entire ejection phase.[36] Thus, the decrease in diastolic distensibility of the ventricle may be viewed as a device protecting the myocardium at the immediate expense of the circulation to the rest of the body.

Although it may be possible to increase myocardial fiber length by augmenting venous return in patients with cardiogenic shock, and this increase in myocardial fiber length may raise stroke volume or stroke work, this increase in fiber length in the noncompliant ventricle can be accomplished only with a considerable increase in filling pressure; this will further increase pulmonary capillary pressure, impair alveolar oxygen exchange and lead to symptomatic pulmonary congestion.[27]

AFTER-LOAD

The ventricular-wall tension during ejection is dependent on aortic pressure and left ventricular radius, and these factors constitute after-load. After-load is a simple concept in isolated muscle but not in the intact circulation, where the ventricle is partly responsible by virtue of its stroke volume for the level of aortic pressure, and this pressure as well as the ventricular volume is changing continuously during ejection. The normal ventricle, through mechanisms not totally understood, adjusts its performance to match the level of aortic pressure. Thus an increment in arterial pressure does not reduce the stroke volume from a normal ventricle; after a few beats the ventricle is able to accomplish a greater external work from the same end-diastolic pressure and perhaps from the same or only a slightly increased end-diastolic volume.[87,188] Similarly, a decrease in aortic pressure is not accompanied by a sustained increase in stroke volume and the ventricle performs less stroke work from a similar end-diastolic volume.[230] In contrast, the abnormal ventricle loses its ability to compensate for changes in after-load.[207] In patients with chronic heart disease increases in after-load induced by infusion of vasoconstrictor drugs or by performance of isometric handgrip induce a rise in left ventricular end-diastolic pressure with little change in stroke work.[100,141,182] Furthermore, reductions in after-load in such situations may induce a sustained increase in stroke volume from a reduced left ventricular filling pressure.[72,148] After-load therefore is a far more important determinant of left ventricular performance in the diseased than in the normal heart.

An increase in aortic pressure would be expected to reduce stroke volume of the infarcted left ventricle, whereas reduction of aortic pressure should augment stroke volume. Since ventricular wall tension is an important determinant of myocardial oxygen consumption, reduction of after-load also should improve the balance between myocardial oxygen consumption and supply in the ischemic ventricle. Furthermore, if a reduction in resistance to left ventricular outflow[112] (aortic impedance[230]) allows greater systolic emptying of the chamber and therefore provides a higher stroke volume, mean arterial pressure may be maintained by a higher flow and lower resistance while chamber size and after-load are reduced.

Despite these possible benefits of a low peripheral resistance, however, vasoconstrictor reflexes tend to maintain or even increase arterial pressure as output from the infarcted ventricle falls.[46] These neural adjustments may therefore support blood flow to certain vascular beds but at the expense of the myocardium, which must perform more pressure work. What may be lacking in this sometimes crude integrative system is a precise control mechanism which can "set" the arteriolar tone at a level consistent with optimal performance of the heart and optimal regional perfusion.

CONTRACTILITY

Contractility of the acutely infarcted ventricle in man is almost impossible to assess, because the measurements obtained probably reflect the net effect of a number of independent factors. The contractile element velocity measured in the whole heart will depend on the combined states of the normal, ischemic and infarcted myocardium and also on the degree of reflex neurohumoral stimulation which is present.[155,208] Furthermore, abnormalities in ventricular geometry during ejection may alter the significance of changes in contractile element velocity measured from pressure data.[169,176]

Most measurements made in experimental animals and in man with acute myocardial infarction indicate that myocardial contractility is diminished.[95,229] However, in view of the reservations alluded to, it probably is not valid to consider contractility of the infarcted left ventricle as a whole.

REGIONAL MYOCARDIAL CHANGES

The infarcted ventricle is characterized by a central area of muscle necrosis which shows permanent loss of contractile force,[172,216] a surrounding region of ischemia which demonstrates varying degrees of temporary depression of cardiac performance[52,124,153,189] and a distant area of presumably normal myocardium.[107] Because of this range of functional states of myocardium in different portions of the same ventricle, it is likely that compliance, systolic-wall tension (after-load) and contractility would differ if they could be measured independently in different areas of the heart. Thus if compliance were reduced only in the area of ischemia or infarction, the rise in end-diastolic pressure observed in acute myocardial infarction might actually be increasing myocardial fiber length considerably more in the normal areas of the ventricle than in the involved areas. Preload would then not be uniformly distributed through the ventricle. Similarly, if an area of ischemia or infarction bulges during contraction (dyskinesia)[99,102,216] its radius would actually be increasing during ejection and thus wall tension (after-load) would be higher in this area of the myocardium than in the neighboring areas which are contracting in a more normal fashion. Contractility may be normal, or because of neurohumoral influences actually increased in the noninfarcted areas of the myocardium, whereas it may be decreased in the areas of infarction and surrounding ischemic zones.[14] This nonhomogeneity of myocardial function in the infarcted left ventricle therefore makes meaningful analysis of myocardial performance by traditional concepts almost impossible.

The location of the infarction also may influence the hemodynamic response. Anterior-wall infarctions often produce serious circulatory effects[114] either because they tend to be larger or because they involve an area of the left ventricle which plays a dominant role in left ventricular ejection.[175,234] Anterior-wall akinesia and dyskinesia, therefore, often are associated with marked reduction in left ventricular stroke volume. Furthermore, if infarction or ischemia involves the papillary muscle, mitral regurgitation may complicate the left ventricular dysfunction.[34]

STRUCTURAL DISTORTION

Effective stroke volume may be further reduced after acute myocardial infarction if some of the contractile effort of the left ventricle is dissipated by ejecting blood which does not contribute to forward flow.[58] The most common example of this phenomenon is the dyskinetic or aneurysmal portion of infarcted ventricle which bulges with each systolic contraction.[216] Papillary muscle dysfunction and rupture produce acute mitral regurgitation which may significantly reduce forward flow. Rupture of the intraventricular septum or free wall of the left ventricle usually occurs several days after acute myocardial infarction, often as a dramatic event characterized by sudden onset or aggravation of left ventricular failure or shock.[58,138,198]

HYPERTROPHY

Hypertrophy is an invariable accompaniment of chronic coronary-artery disease associated with heart failure.[66] The stimulus for the development of myocardial hypertrophy in this setting is not known, but it is attractive to postulate that it is a response to a chronic increase in left ventricular-wall tension. Although hypertrophy is not usually viewed as an acute adaptive response of the heart to changes in work load, studies indicate that an increase in protein synthesis in response to acute overload can be noted within one hour, and considerable increase in left ventricular size can be noted within 24 to 48 hours.[194] In view of these more recent concepts of the dynamics of left ventricular hypertrophy, hypertrophy cannot be disregarded as a relatively acute response of the left ventricle to the stress of an acute myocardial infarction.

Although the development of hypertrophy probably does not play an important role in the immediate survival of a patient who develops shock after acute myocardial infarction, improvement in cardiac status as a result of hypertrophy might be expected within a relatively short period of time if life is sustained. This thesis of course depends on the concept that the hypertrophied ventricle can perform greater work loads than the normal ventricle and that hypertrophy is a useful protective device in ischemic heart disease.[99]

OTHER FACTORS AFFECTING CARDIAC OUTPUT

The output of the left ventricle in patients with shock may be affected by a number of factors not directly related to the myocardial damage. In managing the patient, the first priority is to recognize and correct any of these contributing factors.

Reduced Venous Return

A modest reduction in circulating plasma volume may not affect cardiac output in a normal individual, since stroke volume may be maintained even from a smaller end-diastolic volume by a reflex increase in ejection fraction. In the acutely infarcted ventricle the ejection fraction falls, and a larger than normal end-diastolic volume may be necessary to support stroke volume. Plasma volume often is reduced in acute myocardial infarction.[3] This hypovolemia may be related to increased external losses of extracellular fluid (sweating, vomiting), or internal shifts of intravascular fluid. Activation of the sympathetic nervous system is characteristic of acute myocardial infarction, as evidenced by high circulating levels of catecholamines,[77,94,145] high urinary excretion of catecholamines,[145,221] and increased circulating free fatty acids.[131] This adrenergic discharge may lead to sequestration of intravascular plasma in localized areas of low flow or extravasation of plasma out of the vascular space because of a rise in capillary hydrostatic pressure.[41] The net results of these changes are a reduction in plasma volume and a slight rise in hematocrit. Infusion of sympathomimetic drugs even for a short period of time may considerably reduce plasma volume and aggravate the relative hypovolemia when the drug infusion is stopped.[43]

Dysrhythmias

Alteration in the sequence of atrioventricular activation or profound alterations in heart rate may be critical factors in reducing cardiac output.[56] Bradycardia may reduce output if stroke volume is limited by intrinsic myocardial dysfunction or by inadequacy of venous return. Tachycardia may limit cardiac output if the diastolic filling period is markedly curtailed.[160] Furthermore, tachycardia increases oxygen consumption and may aggravate myocardial hypoxia in acute myocardial infarction.[209] When atrial contraction does not precede ventricular contraction, the loss of atrial "kick" to ventricular filling may contribute to a reduction in stroke volume.[28] It is important to attempt to separate those rhythm disturbances which result from the low output state and therefore should not receive primary attention from those which are contributing to the low cardiac output and should be treated promptly. Unfortunately, such a distinction is not always simple to make.

Cardiac Depressant Drugs

Administration of antiarrhythmic agents (lidocaine, quinidine, procainamide, propranolol) may result in direct myocardial depression, further reducing cardiac output. Propranolol even in the usual therapeutic doses may reduce myocardial contractility.[76] Lidocaine in doses over 2 mg/min may have a direct depressant effect on myocardial function, but even smaller doses may be deleterious in patients with acute myocardial damage.[8] Barbiturates and anesthetic agents also may have a profound negative inotropic effect.[93,156,199]

Acidosis and Hypoxemia

Hypoxia, an invariable finding in myocardial infarction shock, may aggravate myocardial ischemia and further impair cardiac function.[147] The development of lactic acidosis with shock also may be associated with deterioration of myocardial contractility because of a direct negative inotropic effect of the increased hydrogen-ion concentration.[57,78,231]

Circulating Toxic Substance

The role of humoral factors in the impairment of myocardial function is not known.

However, a myocardial depressant factor (MDF) has been characterized in experimental shock[137] and may also influence impairment of myocardial performance after experimental and clinical acute myocardial infarction.[53,82] It is likely that circulating humoral substances play a role in reduction of cardiac output only in the later stages of shock when tissue hypoxia has led to breakdown of lysosomal membranes.[117]

Fever

Temperature elevations often occur during the first week after acute myocardial infarction. If the temperature rises over 101 F a hemodynamic effect—including mild hypotension, tachycardia and a higher than usual cardiac output—would be expected. Malmcrona has reported higher cardiac output and lower peripheral vascular resistance in patients with fever than in those without fever in the first few days after acute myocardial infarction.[152] As previously implied, therefore, the infarcted left ventricle apparently is capable of increasing its output when the peripheral resistance is reduced by the vasodilating effect of an elevated body temperature. However, fever is likely to distribute much of the increased cardiac output to the skin and not to the more critical vascular beds which are underperfused in low-output states.

PERIPHERAL CIRCULATION

Active and passive changes in resistance and capacitance vessel function after acute myocardial infarction may result from the interplay of a variety of stimuli. Changes in total systemic vascular resistance result from the net effect of changes in length or caliber of all resistance vessels in the body combined with changes in viscosity of blood, as described by the formula of Poissieuille.[183] Changes in caliber of systemic capacitance vessels should be reflected in changes in total circulating blood volume or perhaps in the ratio of cardiopulmonary volume to total blood volume. Vessel caliber in myocardial infarc-

tion may be influenced by the following factors.

Reflex Vasoconstriction

A reduction in arterial pressure, pulse pressure, or rate of arterial pressure rise accompanying a fall in stroke volume would be expected to inhibit the carotid and aortic baroreceptors and result in a reflex increase in sympathetic discharge.[79] The effect should be an increase in vascular resistance in some if not all vascular beds, a rise in total systemic vascular resistance and an increase in venous tone.[105]

Several investigators have attempted to demonstrate the presence of receptors in the left ventricle which can inhibit reflex vasoconstriction.[32,51,125,214] Activation of these receptors in experimental and clinical acute myocardial infarction, perhaps by localized or generalized ventricular stretch or by myocardial ischemia, has been suggested to account for the lack of intense peripheral vasoconstriction and inappropriately small rise in systemic vascular resistance which sometimes accompany acute myocardial infarction.[2,74]

Alteration of Transmural Pressure

Reduction in intravascular pressure unaccompanied by a change in extravascular tissue pressure causes a passive reduction in vessel caliber. On the arterial side of the circulation a passive rise in vascular resistance would result. A reduction in venous pressure, due either to heightened prevenous resistance or to depletion of circulating blood volume, would reduce venous capacitance.

Autoregulation

Isolated from neurohumoral influences most vascular beds respond to a reduction in perfusion pressure by active arteriolar dilatation which tends to maintain flow constant. This autoregulation represents a response to metabolic or myogenic stimuli[120] which may play a role in regulating blood flow in hypotensive states even when vasoconstrictor influences appear to predominate.

Total Systemic Vascular Resistance

An increase in calculated total vascular resistance usually is observed when cardiac output falls after both experimental and clinical myocardial infarction. These changes in resistance probably are due at least in part to changes in arteriolar caliber, but changes in blood viscosity also could play a role. Since blood is a non-Newtonian fluid, reduction in flow velocity results in increased viscosity which could increase flow resistance in the microcirculation.[86]

Agress has stressed failure of peripheral resistance to rise as a factor contributing to the development of shock in coronary embolization in dogs.[2] Clinical studies have revealed a wide range in calculated resistance, from normal to very high. If hypotension is used as the criterion for the diagnosis of shock, either in animals or in man, then an attenuated rise in resistance may frequently be implicated. Total systemic vascular resistance more than three times normal has been observed in patients with hypovolemic or cardiogenic shock.[46] If these figures are used as an index of "maximal vasoconstriction," then arterial pressure should not fall until cardiac output is reduced to less than one-third of normal. Indeed, a mean arterial pressure reduced by more than one-third from normal levels could not exist in the presence of "maximal" vasoconstriction unless cardiac output were reduced to levels below those usually observed in patients with acute myocardial infarction and shock. From this standpoint, therefore, significant hypotension always implies "inadequate" vasoconstriction. However, it is the cardiac output which determines the maximal available flow for tissue perfusion. Vasoconstriction may support arterial pressure, but by increasing arterial impedance and left ventricular after-load the ultimate effects of vasoconstriction in myocardial infarction are

likely to be a further fall in cardiac output and a further aggravation of the flow deficiency. Thus, the failure of "maximal" vasoconstriction in myocardial infarction shock could be viewed as an "autoregulatory" device in which flow to at least some vascular beds may be partially preserved.

Total systemic resistance represents the sum of the resistances in the parallel vascular beds which make up the peripheral circulation. Since each of these beds may respond individually to vasoconstrictor and vasodilator influences, analysis of the responses of each bed is necessary to understand the integration of the cardiovascular system after myocardial infarction.

Regional Vascular Resistance

Cerebral Vascular Resistance

Cerebral blood flow normally constitutes approximately 15 per cent of the resting cardiac output and cerebral oxygen consumption about 20 per cent of total-body basal oxygen consumption.[135] Since cerebral vessels are relatively insensitive to neural stimuli and demonstrate efficient autoregulation over a wide range of arterial pressure, cerebral blood flow has been found to be quite constant at mean arterial pressures above 60 mm Hg in normal subjects.[206] Below this level, however, signs of cerebral ischemia may appear, and at perfusion pressures less than 35 mm Hg consciousness usually is lost.[70]

Clinical experience generally supports these physiological observations, since alterations in consciousness usually are not observed in shock when mean arterial pressures are above 60 mm Hg. However, patients occasionally exhibit confusion or coma out of proportion to the degree of hypotension. Such findings might be attributed to impaired vascular adjustments because of intrinsic vascular disease.[70] However, a reflex-induced rise in cerebral vascular resistance has been observed in patients with congestive heart failure,[65] and recent studies indicate that the cerebral circulation may be more sensitive than previously suspected to the vasoconstrictor effect of catecholamines.[158] Furthermore, catecholamines increase the cerebral metabolic rate and may aggravate cerebral hypoxia in shock.[127] Therefore, it may be an over-simplification to consider the cerebral vascular bed as entirely passive in acute myocardial infarction. Nonetheless, normal cerebral function in a patient with suspected shock indicates the presence of adequate arterial pressure.

RENAL VASCULAR RESISTANCE

Total renal vascular resistance is exquisitely sensitive to neural stimulation or to circulating catecholamines.[109,157] Furthermore, adrenergic stimuli may induce a redistribution of renal blood flow away from the superficial cortex and toward the juxtamedullary cortex.[38] Such changes in renal hemodynamics are important to the sodium retention and oliguria characteristic of shock.[196]

Several studies in experimental shock models have demonstrated no change in renal vascular resistance immediately after shock has developed.[11,63] However, patients with shock of diverse etiologies, including myocardial infarction, manifest a high renal vascular resistance and a reduced renal fraction of cardiac output some hours after shock develops.[219] Consequently the renal blood flow, which normally represents about 20 per cent of cardiac output, is made available to other vascular beds with greater immediate needs for perfusion.

Because of the sensitivity of the renal vascular bed to changes in systemic hemodynamics and the availability of urine flow measurement as an index of renal function, timed urine output serves as a crude but useful guide to the adequacy of renal blood flow in the diagnosis of shock and as a measure of response to therapy. Prolonged oliguria predisposes to the development of tubular necrosis,[217] which may be heralded by a spontaneous rise in urine sodium concentration to levels above 40 mEq/L.

CUTANEOUS VASCULAR RESISTANCE

The cutaneous bed constricts in response to activation of the sympathetic nervous system and dilates in response to raised body temperature.[84] The resistance at any moment is therefore dependent on the net effect of these vasoconstrictor and vasodilator influences. Because arteriolar and venous constriction of the skin vessels is easily observed at the bedside, and diaphoresis often is an early manifestation of reflex sympathetic discharge, observation of the skin serves as a useful guide to the diagnosis and course of shock. However, inhibition of cutaneous vasoconstriction because of fever or other neural or humoral mechanisms makes the skin a fallible guide to the intensity of systemic vasoconstriction.

SKELETAL VASCULAR RESISTANCE

The skeletal-muscle vascular bed is normally under considerable autonomic "tone," since its resting flow can be increased 15 to 20 times by inducing "maximal vasodilation."[235] Thus its capacity to enlarge is considerably greater than its capacity to contract, and in early shock skeletal-muscle resistance may actually fall.[13] In more severe shock, however, reflex vasoconstriction involves the muscle bed and the resultant anaerobic metabolism contributes to the accumulation of lactate in the peripheral blood.[210] The fall in skeletal-muscle flow in cardiogenic shock is largely responsible for the marked reduction in extremity blood flow which causes the disappearance of peripheral pulses and inaccuracy of auscultatory or palpatory blood-pressure measurements.[39]

SPLANCHNIC VASCULAR RESISTANCE

The splanchnic vascular bed consists of resistances in series separated by the portal vein. Changes in total splanchnic resistance are therefore dependent on the net effect of changes in preportal mesenteric or splenic resistance and intrahepatic vascular resistance. In the absence of significant prehepatic portasystemic shunting, the sum of these resistances determines total hepatic blood flow. The mesenteric resistance is markedly increased by adrenergic stimulation, and a reduction in hepatic blood flow is a constant finding in shock of diverse etiological factors.[49,50,106] Since hepatic blood flow normally represents about 30 per cent of the cardiac output, it can be appreciated that redistribution of blood flow away from the splanchnic bed could considerably augment the flow to other vascular beds.

Splanchnic vasoconstriction usually produces no clinically apparent signs, although mesenteric ischemia or infarction occasionally complicates the course of cardiogenic or other forms of shock. The reduction in hepatic blood flow impairs hepatocellular nutrition and markedly restricts the liver's ability to metabolize lactate. Therefore, hepatic lactate extraction is transformed into lactate production, contributing to the lactic acidosis of cardiogenic shock.[210]

LUNG

Hypoxemia is a common finding in acute myocardial infarction and its severity correlates well with the severity of the hemodynamic abnormality.[220] Only modest reductions in Po_2 are noted in uncomplicated infarcts; the Po_2 is lower in left ventricular failure and lowest in patients with shock.[95,147,179,213] During ventilation with 100 per cent oxygen, arterial Po_2 remains lower than the normally attained level, thus indicating that some form of veno-arterial shunting accounts for the hypoxemia.[9] Since the degree of hypoxemia correlates well in some studies with the left ventricular end-diastolic pressure,[95] interstitial or alveolar edema may be the most important factor in this functional shunt.[9]

Of perhaps greater importance is the syndrome of "shock lung," which occurs in patients with prolonged shock of any cause and is characterized by an infiltrative process and severe refractory hypoxemia.[21] Pathologically the lung is atelectatic, engorged and hemorrhagic, with fluid in the alveoli and interstitial spaces.[123] Although the cause of the syndrome remains obscure, microembolism, oxygen toxicity, loss of pulmonary surfactant and vascular or interstitial overload with noncolloid fluids have been implicated as possible factors.[16] Regardless of cause, this progressive pulmonary impairment with its accompanying mechanical and metabolic effects often is a preterminal event which prevents recovery of patients who might otherwise have survived an episode of shock.

Alterations in pulmonary vascular resistance in cardiogenic shock may result from a variety of causes. Sympathetic nervous system discharge may produce pulmonary arteriolar and venous constriction. Hypoxia also is associated with pulmonary vasoconstriction. Furthermore, pulmonary emboli are common after myocardial infarction and microthrombi could occur as a result of disseminated intravascular coagulation in the shock state.[97,134]

SHOCK VERSUS HEART FAILURE

Traditionally, left ventricular failure and shock have been considered as separate complications of acute myocardial infarction. Indeed, the clinical symptoms of these two disorders are quite different. The most prominent signs of left ventricular failure are pulmonary congestion and dyspnea associated with a ventricular diastolic gallop. Shock, on the other hand, presents predominant signs of reduced left ventricular output with or without coexistent signs of left ventricular failure. Physiologically, however, these two complications should represent somewhat different manifestations of the same basic problem: disturbed performance of the left ventricle.

From a conceptual standpoint it might be helpful to look upon left ventricular failure as predominant "backward failure" of the left heart and shock as predominant "forward failure."[111] The predominance of "backward" or "forward" manifestations of heart failure in this setting may change with time. Development of the high left ventricular filling pressure which characterizes "backward failure" may depend in part on gradual expansion of intravascular volume characteristic of chronic heart failure. In contrast, patients with acute myocardial infarction often exhibit a modest reduction in blood volume.[3,73] The increase in filling pressure characteristic of "backward failure" may help to maintain peripheral blood flow and protect against "forward failure."[46,184] However, when cardiac output falls blood pressure also falls and cardiac work is therefore reduced. This reduction in load on the left ventricle, combined with the reduction in venous return because of the fall in ventricular output, may actually relieve the backward failure as the forward failure is progressing. In support of this thesis are the data of Hamosh and Cohn, showing a left ventricular end-diastolic pressure significantly lower in patients in shock than in those with clinical heart failure after acute myocardial infarction.[95] Of course, such differences in end-diastolic pressure also could reflect differences in the diastolic compliance of the left ventricle in the two groups of patients.[29,140]

The much higher mortality rate in shock (80 to 100 per cent) than in heart failure (30 to 40 per cent)[22,203] indicates that either the damage to the heart is more severe in shock or that factors other than structural alterations of the left ventricle affect the circulatory deterioration of the patient in shock. Heart failure is basically a steady-state condition which with simple therapy or even no therapy at all may remain stable for hours or days unless some acute complication supervenes. Heart failure then is primarily a syndrome of negative feedbacks which tend to maintain circulatory stability. Shock, on the other hand, is an unstable process in which positive feedback mechanisms[90] supervene very early and contribute to progressive circulatory deterioration which may even be hastened by aggressive medical therapy. Therefore, when the patient with acute myocardial infarction develops shock the ventricular and peripheral circulatory func-

tions have usually already been affected by positive feedback mechanisms which did not originate from the initial myocardial damage. The fact that many patients with early left ventricular failure develop the syndrome of shock within minutes, hours or even days indicates that there may be no basic difference in the original myocardial insult in these two syndromes.

FEEDBACK MECHANISMS

The heart is in a unique position when compared to other organs, for its function is dependent, as are those of other organs, on its circulation, but its circulation is ultimately dependent on its own function. Such a self-regulatory system is designed to operate very efficiently when both the heart and its coronary arterial bed are normal, but it is obvious that the system invites disaster in the form of positive, destructive feedbacks in the presence of severe acute cardiac disease.

In diseases of the heart and its coronary bed it therefore is important to consider a number of regulatory events which may help to maintain integrity of the circulation or of the heart. These feedbacks tend to restore the entire system toward normal when they operate to the benefit of both cardiac function and circulation. The needs of these components of the cardiovascular system may not necessarily be in concert when disease has upset the fine regulatory balance. Therefore, a normally negative feedback mechanism may become a positive feedback mechanism when activated in a patient with coronary arterial disease and acute myocardial infarction.

Some of the possible protective and destructive adjustments which may occur in the patient with acute myocardial infarction are listed below and in Table 1.

Reflex Arteriolar Vasoconstriction

Baroreceptor inhibition induced by a fall in stroke volume, pulse pressure, rate of pressure rise or mean arterial pressure will induce reflex arteriolar vasoconstriction.[79]

Table 1.   Negative and Positive Feedback Mechanisms in Myocardial Infarction Shock

Physiological Event	Beneficial Effect	Deleterious Effect
Arteriolar constriction	Supports arterial pressure	Increases left ventricular work
Venoconstriction	Increases venous return	Pulmonary engorgement
Tachycardia	Increases cardiac output	Increases myocardial oxygen consumption
Inhibition of reflex vasoconstriction	Maintains flow to renal, splanchnic, skeletal and cutaneous beds	Fall in arterial pressure
Hypotension	Reduces left ventricular work	Reduces cerebral and coronary flow
Decreased LV compliance	Prevents chamber enlargement and reduces systolic-wall tension	High end-diastolic pressure
High end-diastolic pressure	Maintains stroke volume	Reduces subendocardial blood flow; increases pulmonary capillary pressure
Catecholamine release	Vasoconstriction, tachycardia	Arrhythmias, increased FFA levels
Slowed capillary flow	Improves oxygen extraction	Increases viscosity, intravascular clotting
Renal vasoconstriction	Expands intravascular volume	Pulmonary congestion; tubular necrosis
Splanchnic and skeletal vasoconstriction	Increases coronary and cerebral blood flow	Lactic acidosis

Support of arterial pressure normally helps to preserve coronary blood flow. However, when coronary arterial disease prevents the rise in aortic pressure from effecting an increase in coronary blood flow, the increase in cardiac work resulting from the rise in aortic pressure may aggravate an imbalance between myocardial oxygen demand and supply.

Venoconstriction Resulting from Baroreceptor Inhibition

Blood shifts centrally and, if the heart is able to respond appropriately to an increase in end-diastolic fiber length, an increase in stroke volume should result. However, if the heart is operating on a flat Frank-Starling curve, pulmonary congestion may develop without much change in stroke volume.

Reflex Stimulation of Cardiac Rate and Contractility

Cardiac output should be increased and the peripheral circulation improved. However, if myocardial oxygen consumption is increased to a greater extent than oxygen delivery, the protective effect of the reflex may give way to a destructive effect by aggravation of myocardial ischemia and further impairment of left ventricular performance.[54,113,165]

Decrease in Diastolic Compliance of the Left Ventricle

This response could prevent the ischemic left ventricle from increasing its radius of curvature, which would lead to an increase in wall tension and myocardial oxygen consumption. This feedback would therefore be immediately protective for the metabolic balance of heart muscle. However, inhibition of an increase in diastolic fiber length could limit the ventricle from reaching the peak of its Frank-Starling curve and thus contribute to an inadequate cardiac output. Furthermore, the resultant rise in intraventricular pressure during diastole may inhibit diastolic endocardial blood flow and aggravate endocardial ischemia.

Inhibition of Peripheral Vasoconstriction

A reflex response to stimulation of unknown afferent receptors[51,125,214] could be immediately beneficial for the heart, since it would allow aortic pressure to fall pari passu with cardiac output and therefore reduce the pressure work load on the left ventricle. A deleterious effect may result if aortic pressure falls below a critical level, since cerebral and coronary flow would then fall and immediate survival might be in jeopardy.

Reduction in Renal Perfusion

Urine output is reduced and sodium and water are retained. This feedback provides for a gradual expansion of extracellular volume and an increase in venous return to the heart. In hypovolemic states, or when the heart has not reached the peak of its Frank-Starling curve, this feedback should provide an increase in cardiac output. When output cannot rise correspondingly, however, the feedback becomes destructive by precipitating pulmonary congestion, hypoxemia, increased work of breathing, and even acute renal tubular necrosis.

Neurohumoral-induced Arteriolar Constriction

In skeletal muscle and the hepatic bed this is initially a protective reflex, since it redistributes the limited blood flow to more critical vascular areas such as the cerebral and coronary circulation. Persistence of the vasoconstriction is destructive, because lactic acidosis results from the reduced tissue perfusion and may directly impair function of the heart and other vascular tissue.

Slowed Capillary Flow

Increased oxygen extraction tends to maintain organ oxygen consumption constant. With slowing of flow, whole-blood viscosity rises, resistance to flow may increase and microthrombi or disseminated intravascular coagulation may occur.[97,134]

PATHOPHYSIOLOGY OF CLINICAL SYNDROMES

It may now be appropriate to reconsider the physiological basis of the clinical syndromes of shock which were previously outlined.

Bradycardiac Shock

This condition probably results from vagotonia which may represent a reflex response to coronary occlusion or a nonspecific response to apprehension and chest pain. Although the normal heart can maintain cardiac output despite bradycardia, the damaged left ventricle may have a limited stroke volume which allows cardiac output to fall with the heart rate. Furthermore, vagal stimulation may depress myocardial contractility and dilate the peripheral circulation, allowing arterial pressure to fall disproportionately.[55,59,98]

Tachycardiac Shock

The fall in cardiac output which occurs at rapid rates, the effect on ventricular contraction of an altered sequence of ventricular activation, or the more insidious metabolic effects of increased oxygen consumption on myocardial function may bring about tachycardiac shock. Correction of the arrhythmia may not necessarily lead to prompt restoration of the circulation, because positive feedbacks initiated during the tachycardia may have further depressed circulatory function.

When tachycardia occurs as a reflex response to a primary impairment in stroke volume, attempts at slowing of the heart rate usually are unsuccessful. Treatment in this situation must be directed at improving the stroke volume by other means.

Cardiac Depression Shock

This should be suspected when administration of a negative inotropic agent appears to be temporally related to further decompensation of the circulation in a patient who already manifests signs of severe left ventricular dysfunction. Anesthetics and antiarrhythmic drugs are the most frequent causes. Since positive feedbacks again may influence the course, it is important to recognize that the shock may persist longer than the expected duration of action of the drug. Therefore, shock in a patient who has received such a medication should always be considered potentially reversible if temporary circulatory support can be provided.

Hypovolemic Shock

Diagnosis can be made only after volume loading has resulted in enough improvement in cardiac output to correct the inadequate regional blood flow. It must be recognized that hypovolemia in this setting is superimposed on severe left ventricular dysfunction and that volume expansion with dextran or albumin may correct the shock but precipitate some degree of pulmonary congestion.

Power-failure Shock

This syndrome is responsible for severe left ventricular low-output failure when other iatrogenic or mechanistic precipitating events cannot be found. It is here that the appropriateness of various therapeutic measures is highly controversial, since each drug recommended has both potential beneficial and deleterious effects. Mechanical cardiac assistance may be the only entirely rational means of treatment, but even this form of therapy usually fails when it is administered after the shock state has developed. It is apparent that the greatest need may be for means of detecting and effectively treating at an early stage of acute myocardial infarction those patients with a high risk of developing power failure.

Cardiac Rupture Shock

This surgical emergency, if recognized and treated in time, may have a better prognosis than the above power-failure syndrome.

Nonvasoconstricted Shock

Again, the prognosis may be better, since the cardiac output usually is higher than in the typically vasoconstricted patient with shock. Of course, the higher output in this group could result from the lower peripheral vascular resistance. The syndrome may result from constitutional, drug-induced or vagal reflex-induced inactivity of the sympathetic nervous system. Temporary pharmacological support of the arterial pressure, if needed, may carry the patient through the shock episode, especially if attention is paid to maintenance of plasma volume; this may be reduced if sympathomimetic agents are administered.

SUMMARY

The common denominator of all circulatory complications after acute myocardial infarction is impairment of myocardial performance. However, it is apparent from the foregoing review that loss of contractility in the infarcted muscle is not the sole cause of the progressive reduction in peripheral blood flow which characterizes shock. The challenge to the physician is to sort out and treat those correctable hemodynamic and metabolic factors which may be at work. The need for urgency in this task is obvious, for with every passing moment new pathophysiological mechanisms supervene and established ones become more difficult to reverse.

Indeed, experience to date with the rational management of shock in myocardial infarction suggests that success will continue to be limited until therapy is instituted at a stage of the disease considerably earlier than that at which shock is currently being recognized —perhaps at the moment of onset of acute myocardial infarction. Until improved means of recognition or treatment become available, however, the physician finds himself in the classical dilemma: to treat effectively those disorders which can be improved, not to treat those disorders which cannot be improved, and to possess the wisdom to distinguish between them.

REFERENCES

1. Adgey, A. A., et al.: Incidence, significance and management of early bradyarrhythmias complicating acute myocardial infarction. Lancet, 2:1097, 1968.

2. Agress, C. M., and Binder, M. J.: Cardiogenic shock. Amer. Heart J., 54:458, 1957.

3. Agress, C. M., et al.: Blood volume changes in protracted shock resulting from experimental myocardial infarction. Amer. J. Physiol., 166:603, 1951.

4. Alella, A., et al.: Interrelation between cardiac oxygen consumption and coronary blood flow. Amer. J. Physiol., 183:570, 1955.

5. Allard, J. R., Ware, W. H., and Bennett, L. L.: Negative chronotropism and inotropism of procaine amide in the heart. J. Lab. Clin. Med., 55:120, 1960.

6. Allen, H. N., Danzig, R., and Swan, H. J. C.: Incidence and significance of relative hypovolemia as a cause of shock associated with acute myocardial infarction. Circulation, 36 (Suppl. 2):50, 1967.

7. Armour, J. A., and Randall, W. C.: Canine left ventricular intramyocardial pressures. Amer. J. Physiol., 220:1833, 1971.

8. Austen, W. G., and Moran, J. M.: Cardiac and peripheral vascular effects of lidocaine and procainamide. Amer. J. Cardiol., 16:701, 1965.

9. Ayres, S. M., et al.: The lung in shock. Alveolar-capillary gas exchange in the shock syndrome. Amer. J. Cardiol., 26:588, 1970.

10. Bakos, A. C. P.: The question of the function of the right ventricle. Proc. Soc. Exp. Biol. Med., 71:69, 1949.

11. Balint, P., Kiss, E., and Sturez, J.: Influence of nonshocking hemorrhage on cardiac output and renal blood flow. Acta Physiol. Acad. Sci. Hung., 15:249, 1959.

12. Ballinger, W. F., and Vollenweider, H.: Anaerobic metabolism of the heart. Circ. Res., 11:681, 1962.

13. Barcroft, H., et al.: Post-hemorrhagic fainting. Lancet, 1:489, 1944.

14. Baxley, W. A., and Reeves, T. J.: Abnormal regional myocardial performance in coronary artery disease. Progr. Cardiov. Dis., 13:405, 1971.

15. Becker, L. C., Fortuin, N. J., and Pitt, B.: Effect of ischemia and antianginal drugs on the distribution of radioactive microspheres in the canine left ventricle. Circ. Res., 28:263, 1971.

16. Bergofsky, E. H.: The adult acute respiratory insufficiency syndrome following nonthoracic trauma: The lung in shock. Amer. J. Cardiol., 26:619, 1970.

17. Berne, R. M.: Cardiac nucleotides in hypoxia: Possible role in regulation of coronary blood flow. Amer. J. Physiol., 204:317, 1963.

18. Berne, R. M.: Regulation of coronary blood flow. Physiol. Rev., 44:1, 1964.

19. Berne, R. M., De Geest, H., and Levy, M. N.: Influence of the cardiac nerves on coronary resistance. Amer. J. Physiol., 208:763, 1965.

20. Bing, R. J.: Cardiac metabolism. Physiol. Rev., 45:171, 1965.

21. Blaisdell, F. W., Lim, R. C., Jr., and Stallone, R. J.: The mechanism of pulmonary damage following traumatic shock. Surg. Gynec. Obstet., 130:15, 1970.

22. Bloomfield, D. K., et al: Survival in acute myocardial infarction before and after the establishment of a coronary care unit. Chest, 57: 224, 1970.

23. Blumgart, H., Schlesinger, M., and Zoll, P.: Multiple fresh coronary occlusions in patients with antecedent shock. Arch. Intern. Med., 68:181, 1941.

24. Braasch, W., et al.: Early changes in energy metabolism in the myocardium following acute coronary artery occlusion in anesthetized dogs. Circ. Res., 23:429, 1968.

25. Brachfeld, N., and Scheuer, J.: Metabolism of glucose by the ischemic dog heart. Amer. J. Physiol., 212:603, 1967.

26. Brachfeld, N.: Maintenance of cell viability. Circulation, 40 (Suppl. 4):202, 1969.

27. Bradley, R. D., Jenkins, B. S., and Brathwaite, M. A.: The influence of atrial pressure on cardiac performance following myocardial infarction complicated by shock. Circulation, 42:827, 1970.

28. Braunwald, E., and Frahm, C. J.: Studies on Starling's law of the heart. IV. Observations on the hemodynamic functions of the left atrium in man. Circulation, 24:633, 1961.

29. Braunwald, E., and Ross, J., Jr.: Ventricular end-diastolic pressure. Amer. J. Med., 34:147, 1963.

30. Broch, O. J., et al.: Hemodynamic studies in acute myocardial infarction. Amer. Heart J., 57:522, 1959.

31. Broder, M. I., and Cohn, J. N.: Evolution of abnormalities in left ventricular function after acute myocardial infarction. Circulation, in press.

32. Brown, A. M.: Excitation of afferent cardiac sympathetic nerve fibers during myocardial ischemia. J. Physiol., 190:35, 1967.

33. Buckberg, G. D., et al.: Experimental subendocardial ischemia in dogs with normal coronary arteries. Circ. Res., 30:67, 1972.

34. Burch, G. E., De Pasquale, N. P., and Phillips, J. H.: Clinical manifestations of papillary muscle dysfunction. Arch. Intern. Med., 112:112, 1963.

35. Burch, G. E., and Giles, T. D.: A study of the effectiveness of the coronary care unit. Southern Med. J., *64*:435, 1971.

36. Burton, A. C.: The importance of the shape and size of the heart. Amer. Heart J., *54*:801, 1957.

37. Byrne, J. J.: Shock. New Eng. J. Med., *275*: 543, 1966.

38. Carriere, S., et al.: Intrarenal distribution of blood flow in dogs during hemorrhagic hypotension. Circ. Res., *19*:167, 1966.

39. Cohn, J. N.: Blood pressure measurement in shock. Mechanisms of inaccuracy in auscultatory and palpatory methods. JAMA, *199*: 972, 1967.

40. Cohn, J. N.: Paroxysmal hypertension and hypovolemia. New Eng. J. Med., *275*:643, 1966.

41. Cohn, J. N.: Relationship of plasma volume changes to resistance and capacitance vessel effects of vasopressor drugs and dextran. Clin. Sci., *30*:267, 1966.

42. Cohn, J. N.: Treatment of shock following myocardial infarction. Mich. Med., *68*:803, 1969.

43. Cohn, J. N.: Venous hypotension as related to cardiac output in shock. In: *Shock and Hypotension* (Mills, L. C., and Moyer, J. H., Eds.). New York, Grune and Stratton, 1965.

44. Cohn, J. N., and Luria, M.: Studies in clinical shock and hypotension: The value of bedside hemodynamic observations. JAMA, *190*:891, 1964.

45. Cohn, J. N., and Luria, M.: Studies in clinical shock and hypotension. IV. Variations in reflex vasoconstriction and cardiac stimulation. Circulation, *34*:823, 1966.

46. Cohn, J. N., et al.: Studies in clinical shock and hypotension. V. Hemodynamic effects of dextran. Circulation, *35*:316, 1967.

47. Cohn, J. N., and Tristani, F. E.: Studies in clinical shock and hypotension. VI. Relationship between left and right ventricular function. J. Clin. Invest., *48*:2008, 1969.

48. Collins, J. V., et al.: Central venous pressure in acute myocardial infarction. Lancet, *1*: 373, 1971.

49. Corday, E., and Williams, J. H., Jr.: Effect of shock and of vasopressor drugs on the regional circulation of the brain, heart, kidney, and liver. Amer. J. Med., *29*:228, 1960.

50. Corday, E., et al.: Effect of systemic blood pressure and vasopressor drugs on coronary blood flow and the electrocardiogram. Amer. J. Cardiol., *3*:626, 1959.

51. Constantin, L.: Extracardiac factors contributing to hypotension during coronary occlusion. Amer. J. Cardiol., *11*:205, 1963.

52. Cox, J. L., et al.: The ischemic zone surrounding acute myocardial infarction. Its morphology as detected by dehydrogenase staining. Amer. Heart J., *76*:650, 1968.

53. Crampton, R. S., et al.: Production of a myocardial depressant factor in shock following

acute myocardial infarction: Preliminary evaluation of treatment with methylprednisone. Amer. J. Cardiol., *29*:257, 1972.

54. Cronin, R. F.: Effect of isoproterenol and norepinephrine on myocardial function in experimental cardiogenic shock. Amer. Heart J., *74*:387, 1967.

55. Daggett, W. M., et al.: Influence of vagal stimulation on ventricular contractility, O_2 consumption, and coronary flow. Amer. J. Physiol., *212*:8, 1967.

56. Dalle, S., Meltzer, E., and Kravitz, B.: A new look at ventricular tachycardia. Acta Cardiol., *22*:519, 1967.

57. Darby, T. D., et al.: Effects of metabolic acidosis on ventricular isometric systolic tension and the response to epinephrine and levarterenol. Circ. Res., *8*:1242, 1960.

58. De Busk, R. F., and Harrison, D. C.: The clinical spectrum of papillary muscle disease. New Eng. J. Med., *281*:1458, 1969.

59. De Geest, H., et al.: Depression of ventricular contractility by stimulation of the vagus nerves. Circ. Res., *17*:222, 1965.

60. De Haan, R. L., and Field, J.: Mechanism of cardiac damage in anoxia. Amer. J. Physiol., *197*:449, 1959.

61. Diamond, G., and Forrester, J. S.: Effect of coronary artery disease and acute myocardial infarction on left ventricular compliance in man. Circulation, *40*:11, 1972.

62. Dietzman, R. H., et al.: Mechanisms in the production of shock. Surgery, *62*:645, 1967.

63. Dow, R. W., and Fry, W. J.: Hemorrhagic shock: Changes in renal blood flow and vascular resistance. Arch. Surg., *94*:190, 1967.

64. Dwyer, E. N.: Left ventricular pressure-volume alterations and regional disorders of contraction during myocardial ischemia induced by atrial pacing. Circulation, *42*:1111, 1970.

65. Eisenberg, S., Madison, L., and Sensenbach, W.: Cerebral hemodynamics and metabolic studies in patients with congestive heart failure. II. Observations in confused subjects. Circulation, *21*:704, 1960.

66. Ellis, L. B., et al.: Relation of the degree of coronary-artery disease and of myocardial infarction to cardiac hypertrophy and chronic congestive heart failure. New Eng. J. Med., *266*:525, 1962.

67. Estes, E. H., et al.: The vascular supply of the left ventricular wall. Amer. Heart J., *71*:58, 1966.

68. Fam, W. M., and Mc Gregor, M.: Pressure-flow relationships in the coronary circulation. Circ. Res., *25*:293, 1969.

69. Feigl, E. O.: Parasympathetic control of coronary blood flow in dogs. Circ. Res., *25*:509, 1969.

70. Finnerty, F. A., Witkin, L., and Fazekas, J. F.: Cerebral hemodynamics during cerebral ischemia induced by acute hypotension. J. Clin. Invest., *33*:1227, 1954.

71. Fortuin, N. J., et al.: Regional myocardial blood flow in the dog studied with radioactive microspheres. Cardiov. Res., 5:331, 1971.

72. Franciosa, J. A., et al.: Improved left ventricular function during nitroprusside infusion in acute myocardial infarction. Lancet, 1:650, 1972.

73. Freis, E. D., et al.: Hemodynamic alterations in acute myocardial infarction. I. Cardiac output, mean arterial pressure, total peripheral resistance, "central" and total blood volumes, venous pressure and average circulation time. J. Clin. Invest., 31:131, 1952.

74. Friedberg, C. K.: Cardiogenic shock in acute myocardial infarction. Circulation, 23:325, 1961.

75. Gammill, J. F., et al.: Hemodynamic changes following acute myocardial infarction using the dye injection method for cardiac output determination. Ann. Intern. Med., 43:100, 1955.

76. Gander, M., et al.: Cardiac hemodynamics under β-receptor blockade in dogs. Cardiologia, 49:1726, 1966.

77. Gazes, P. C., Richardson, J. A., and Woods, E. F.: Plasma catecholamine concentrations in myocardial infarction and angina pectoris. Circulation, 19:657, 1959.

78. Gelet, T. R., Altschuld, R. A., and Weissler, A. M.: Effects of acidosis on the performance and metabolism of the anoxic heart. Circulation, 40 (Suppl. 4):60, 1969.

79. Gero, J., and Gerova, M.: The role of parameters of pulsating pressure in the stimulation of intracarotid receptors. Arch. Int. Pharmacodyn., 140:35, 1962.

80. Gilbert, R. P., Goldberg, M., and Griffin, J.: Circulatory changes in acute myocardial infarction. Circulation, 9:847, 1954.

81. Gilmore, J. P., et al.: Physical factors and cardiac adaptation. Amer. J. Physiol., 211:1219, 1966.

82. Glenn, T. M., et al.: Production of a myocardial depressant factor in cardiogenic shock. Amer. Heart J., 82:78, 1971.

83. Gorlin, R.: Evaluation of myocardial metabolism in ischemic heart disease. Circulation, 40 (Suppl. 4):155, 1969.

84. Greenfield, A. D. M.: The circulation through the skin. In: Handbook of Physiology, Vol. 2. Washington, American Physiological Society, 1963.

85. Gregg, D. E.: Physiology of the coronary circulation. Ann. N.Y. Acad. Sci., 90:145, 1960.

86. Guest, M. M.: Circulatory effects of blood clotting, fibrinolysis, and related hemostatic processes. In: Handbook of Physiology, Vol. 3. Washington, American Physiological Society, 1965.

87. Guiha, N. H., et al.: Predominant right ventricular failure in clinical and experimental right ventricular infarction. Clin. Res., 20:375, 1972.

88. Gunnar, R. M., et al.: Myocardial infarction with shock. Hemodynamic studies and results of therapy. Circulation, 33:753, 1966.

89. Guy, C., Salhany, J., and Eliot, R.: Disorders of hemoglobin-oxygen release in ischemic heart disease. Amer. Heart J., 82:824, 1971.

90. Guyton, A. C., and Crowell, J. W.: Cardiac deterioration in shock. I. Its progressive nature. Int. Anesth. Clin., 2:159, 1964.

91. Guz, A., Kurland, G. S., and Freedberg, A. S.: Relation of coronary flow to oxygen supply. Amer. J. Physiol., 199:179, 1960.

92. Haddy, F. J.: Physiology and pharmacology of the coronary circulation and myocardium, particularly in relation to coronary artery disease. Amer. J. Med., 47:274, 1969.

93. Hamilton, W. K., et al.: Effect of cyclopropane and halothane on ventricular mechanics. J. Pharmacol. Exp. Ther., 154:566, 1966.

94. Hamosh, P., et al.: Systolic time intervals and left ventricular function in acute myocardial infarction. Circulation, 45:375, 1972.

95. Hamosh, P., and Cohn, J. N.: Left ventricular function in acute myocardial infarction. J. Clin. Invest., 50:523, 1971.

96. Hanarayan, C., et al.: Study of infarcted myocardium in cardiogenic shock. Brit. Heart J., 32:728, 1970.

97. Hardaway, R. M.: Syndromes of Disseminated Intravascular Coagulation with Special Reference to Shock and Hemorrhage. Springfield, Charles C Thomas, 1966.

98. Harman, M. A., and Reeves, T. J.: Effects of efferent vagal stimulation on atrial and ventricular function. Amer. J. Physiol., 215:1210, 1968.

99. Harrison, T. R.: Some unanswered questions concerning enlargement and failure of the heart. Amer. Heart J., 69:100, 1965.

100. Helfant, R. H., deVilla, M. A., and Meister, S. G.: Effect of sustained isometric handgrip exercise on left ventricular performance. Circulation, 44:982, 1971.

101. Henderson, A. H., Parmley, W. W., and Sonnenblick, E. H.: The series elasticity of heart muscle during hypoxia. Cardiov. Res., 5:10, 1971.

102. Herman, M. V., and Gorlin, R.: Implications of left ventricular asynergy. Amer. J. Cardiol., 23:538, 1969.

103. Herzberg, R. M., Rubio, R., and Berne, R. M.: Coronary occlusion and embolization: Effect on blood flow in adjacent arteries. Amer. J. Physiol., 210:169, 1966.

104. Heyer, H. E.: A clinical study of shock occurring during acute myocardial infarction. An analysis of 58 cases. Amer. Heart J., 62:436, 1961.

105. Heymans, C., and Neil, E.: Reflexogenic Areas of the Cardiovascular System. Boston, Little, Brown and Co., 1958.

106. Hinshaw, D. B., et al.: Regional blood flow in hemorrhagic shock. Amer. J. Surg., 102:224, 1961.

107. Hood, W. B., Jr.: Experimental myocardial infarction. III. Recovery of left ventricular function in the healing phase: Contribution of increased fiber shortening in noninfarcted myocardium. Amer. Heart J., 79:531, 1970.
108. Hood, W. B., Jr.: Pathophysiology of ischemic heart disease. Progr. Cardiov. Dis., 14:297, 1971.
109. Houck, C. R.: Alterations in renal hemodynamics and function in separate kidneys during stimulation of renal artery nerves in dogs. Amer. J. Physiol., 167:523, 1951.
110. Hunter, A. R.: Old unhappy far-off things: Some reflections on the significance of the early work in shock. Ann. Roy. Coll. Surg. Eng., 40:289, 1967.
111. Hurst, J. W., and Logue, R. B.: The Heart, 2nd ed. New York, McGraw-Hill, 1970.
112. Imperial, E. S., Levy, M. N., and Zieske, H.: Outflow resistance as an independent determinant of cardiac performance. Circ. Res., 9:1148, 1961.
113. Irving, M. H.: Sympatho-adrenal hyperactivity —the key to irreversible shock. Postgrad. Med. J., 45:523, 1969.
114. Isomakie, H., Takala, J., and Rasanen, O.: Influence on the site of myocardial infarction on mortality rate. Acta Med. Scand., 185:227, 1969.
115. Jacobson, E. D.: A physiologic approach to shock. New Eng. J. Med., 278:834, 1968.
116. James, T. N.: The velocity and distribution of coronary collateral circulation. Chest, 58:183, 1970.
117. Janoff, A., et al.: Pathogenesis of experimental shock. IV. Studies on lysosomes in normal and tolerant animals subjected to lethal trauma and endotoxemia. J. Exp. Med., 116:451, 1962.
118. Jennings, R. B.: Early phase of myocardial ischemic injury and infarction. Amer. J. Cardiol., 24:753, 1969.
119. Jennings, R. B., et al.: Myocardial necrosis induced by temporary occlusion of a coronary artery in the dog. Arch. Path., 70:68, 1960.
120. Johnson, P. C.: Review of previous studies and current theories of autoregulation. Circ. Res., 15 (Suppl. 2):9, 1964.
121. Joly, H. R., and Weil, M. H.: Temperature of the great toe as an indication of the severity of shock. Circulation, 39:131, 1969.
122. Kagan, A. M.: Dynamic responses of the right ventricle following extensive damage by cauterization. Circulation, 5:816, 1952.
123. Kamada, R. M., and Smith, J. R.: The phenomenon of respiratory failure in shock: The genesis of "shock lung." Amer. Heart J., 83:1, 1972.
124. Katz, A. M.: Effects of interrupted coronary flow upon myocardial metabolism and contractility. Progr. Cardiov. Dis., 10:450, 1968.
125. Kezdi, P., et al.: The role of vagal afferents in acute myocardial infarction. Amer. J. Cardiol., 26:642, 1970.
126. Killip, T., and Kimball, J. T.: Treatment of myocardial infarction in a coronary care unit. Amer. J. Cardiol., 20:457, 1967.
127. King, B. D., Sokoloff, L., and Wechsler, R. L.: The effects of l-epinephrine and l-norepinephrine upon cerebral circulation and metabolism in man. J. Clin. Invest., 31:273, 1951.
128. Kirk, E. S., and Honig, C. R.: An experimental and theoretical analysis of myocardial tissue pressure. Amer. J. Physiol., 207:361, 1964.
129. Kirk, E. S., and Honig, C. R.: Nonuniform distribution of blood flow and gradients of oxygen tension within the heart. Amer. J. Physiol., 207:661, 1964.
130. Kroetz, F. W., Leon, D. F., and Leonard, J. J.: The diagnosis of acute circulatory failure. Progr. Cardiov. Dis., 10:262, 1967.
131. Kurien, V. A., and Oliver, M. F.: Serum free fatty acids after acute myocardial infarction and cerebral vascular occlusion. Lancet, 2:122, 1966.
132. Kurland, G. S., Weingarten, C., and Pitt, B.: The relation between the location of coronary occlusions and the occurrence of shock in acute myocardial infarction. Circulation, 31:646, 1965.
133. Langhorne, W. H.: The coronary care unit revisited. Chest, 57:550, 1970.
134. Lasch, H. G.: Coagulation disturbances in shock. Postgrad. Med. J., 45:539, 1969.
135. Lassen, N. A.: Cerebral blood flow and oxygen consumption in man. Physiol. Rev., 39:183, 1959.
136. Laurie, W., and Woods, J. D.: Infarction (ischemic fibrosis) in the right ventricle of the heart. Acta Cardiol., 18:399, 1963.
137. Lefer, A. M.: Role of a myocardial depressant factor in the pathogenesis of hemorrhagic shock. Fed. Proc., 29:1836, 1970.
138. Lewis, A. J., Burchell, H. B., and Titus, J. L.: Clinical and pathologic features of postinfarction cardiac rupture. Amer. J. Cardiol., 23:43, 1969.
139. Lieberman, N. A., et al.: The effects of lidocaine on the electrical and mechanical activity of the heart. Amer. J. Cardiol., 22:375, 1968.
140. Linhart, J. W., et al.: Left heart hemodynamics during angina pectoris induced by atrial pacing. Circulation, 40:483, 1969.
141. Linhart, J. W., et al.: Myocardial function in patients with coronary artery disease. Amer. J. Cardiol., 23:379, 1969.
142. Linzbach, A. J.: Heart failure from the point of view of quantitative anatomy. Amer. J. Cardiol., 5:370, 1960.
143. Loeb, H. S., et al.: Hypovolemia in shock due to acute myocardial infarction. Circulation, 40:653, 1969.
144. Lown, B., et al.: Unresolved problems in coronary care. Amer. J. Cardiol., 20:494, 1967.
145. Lukomsky, P. E., and Organov, R. G.: Blood plasma catecholamines and their urinary excretion in patients with acute myocardial infarction. Amer. Heart J., 83:182, 1972.

146. MacDonald, J., and Bentley, W.: Acute myocardial infarction: A ten year study. New Eng. J. Med., 244:743, 1951.

147. MacKenzie, G. J., et al.: Circulatory and respiratory studies in myocardial infarction and cardiogenic shock. Lancet, 2:825, 1964.

148. Majid, P. A., Sharma, B., and Taylor, S. H.: Phentolamine for vasodilator treatment of severe heart failure. Lancet, 2:719, 1971.

149. Majno, G., and Bauchardy, B.: Early stage of myocardial infarction. New methods for microscopic and macroscopic study. Schweiz. Med. Wschr., 102:271, 1972.

150. Malach, M., and Rosenberg, B. A.: Acute myocardial infarction in a city hospital. I. Clinical review of 264 cases. Amer. J. Cardiol., 1:682, 1958.

151. Malach, M., and Rosenberg, B. A.: Acute myocardial infarction in a city hospital. III. Experience with shock. Amer. J. Cardiol., 5: 487, 1960.

152. Malmcrona, R.: Haemodynamics in myocardial infarction. Acta Med. Scand., 176: 417, 1964.

153. Maroko, P. R., et al.: Factors influencing infarct size following experimental coronary artery occlusion. Circulation, 43:67, 1971.

154. Martin, A. M., et al.: Human myocardial zonal lesions. Arch. Path., 87:339, 1969.

155. Mason, D. T.: Usefulness and limitations of the rate of rise of intraventricular pressure (dp/dt) in the evaluation of myocardial contractility in man. Amer. J. Cardiol., 23:516, 1969.

156. McDowall, D. G.: Cardiac output under anaesthesia. Ann. Roy. Coll. Surg. Eng., 46: 128, 1970.

157. Mehrizi, A., and Hamilton, W. F.: Effect of levarterenol on renal blood flow and vascular volume in dog. Amer. J. Physiol., 197:1115, 1959.

158. Meyer, J. S., Yoshida, K., and Sakamoto, K.: Autonomic control of cerebral blood flow measured by electromagnetic flowmeters. Neurology, 17:638, 1967.

159. Michal, G., et al.: Metabolic changes in heart muscle during anoxia. Amer. J. Physiol., 197:1147, 1959.

160. Miller, D. E., et al.: Effect of ventricular rate on the cardiac output in the dog with heart block. Circ. Res., 10:658, 1962.

161. Moir, T. W., and De Bra, D. W.: Effect of left ventricular hypertension, ischemia, and vasoactive drugs on the myocardial distribution of coronary blood flow. Circ. Res., 21:65, 1967.

162. Monroe, R. G., et al.: Left ventricular performance and coronary flow after coronary embolization with plastic microspheres. J. Clin. Invest., 50:1656, 1971.

163. Mosher, P., et al.: Control of coronary blood flow by an autoregulatory mechanism. Circ. Res., 14:250, 1964.

164. Motterham, P., and Buchanan, M.: Cardio-

165. Mueller, H., et al.: Effect of isoproterenol, l-norepinephrine, and intraaortic counterpulsation on hemodynamics and myocardial metabolism in shock following acute myocardial infarction. Circulation, 45:335, 1972.

166. Murphy, G. W., et al.: Cardiac output in acute myocardial infarction. Amer. J. Cardiol., 11: 587, 1963.

167. Nakano, J., and McCloy, R. B.: Effects of atrial and ventricular tachycardia on systemic and coronary circulation and myocardial oxygen consumption in control dogs and in dogs with adrenergic blockade. Cardiov. Res., 4:180, 1970.

168. Neill, W. A., et al.: Myocardial anaerobic metabolism in intact dogs. Amer. J. Physiol., 204:427, 1963.

169. Noble, M. I. M.: Problems concerning the application of concepts of muscle mechanics to the determination of the contractile state of the heart. Circulation, 45:252, 1972.

170. Opie, L. H.: Metabolic response during impending myocardial infarction. I. Relevance of studies of glucose and fatty acid metabolism in animals. Circulation, 45:483, 1972.

171. Opie, L. H.: Metabolism of the heart in health and disease. Amer. Heart J., 77:100, 1969.

172. Orias, O.: Dynamic changes in ventricles following ligation of ramus descendens anterior. Amer. J. Physiol., 100:629, 1932.

173. Owen, P., et al.: Comparison between metabolic changes in local venous and coronary sinus blood after acute experimental coronary arterial occlusion. Amer. J. Cardiol., 25:562, 1970.

174. Page, D. L., et al.: Myocardial changes associated with cardiogenic shock. New Eng. J. Med., 285:133, 1971.

175. Pairolero, P. C., et al.: Experimental production and hemodynamic effects of left ventricular akinesis. Amer. J. Cardiol., 25:120, 1970.

176. Parmley, W. W., et al.: Clinical evaluation of left ventricular pressures in myocardial infarction. Circulation, 45:358, 1972.

177. Patterson, S. W., Piper, H., and Starling, E. H.: Regulation of the heart beat. J. Physiol., 48: 465, 1914.

178. Pierce, C. H.: The enigma of shock. Canad. Med. Assoc. J., 103:621, 1970.

179. Ramo, B. W., et al.: Hemodynamic findings in 123 patients with acute myocardial infarction on admission. Circulation, 42:567, 1970.

180. Ratshin, R. A., Rackley, C. E., and Russell, R. O.: Hemodynamic evaluation of left ventricular function in shock complicating myocardial infarction. Circulation, 45:127, 1972.

181. Redding, V. J., and Rees, J. R.: Experimental myocardial infarction: A comparison of myocardial flow rates in the vicinity of the infarct with that in more distant muscle. Brit. Heart J., 31:392, 1969.

genic shock in acute myocardial infarction. Med. J. Aust., 2:347, 1967.

182. Ross, J., Jr., and Braunwald, E.: The study of left ventricular function in man by increasing resistance to ventricular ejection with angiotensin. Circulation, 29:739, 1964.

183. Rushmer, R. F.: *Cardiovascular Dynamics.* Philadelphia, W. B. Saunders, 1970.

184. Russell, R. O., Jr., et al.: Effects of increasing left ventricular filling pressure in patients with acute myocardial infarction. J. Clin. Invest., 49:1539, 1970.

185. Salisbury, P. F., Cross, C. E., and Rieben, P. A.: Acute ischemia of inner layers of ventricular wall. Amer. Heart J., 66:650, 1963.

186. Sandler, H., and Dodge, H. J.: Left ventricular tension and stress in man. Circ. Res., 13:91, 1963.

187. Sarnoff, S. J., and Berglund, E.: Ventricular function. I. Starling's law of the heart studied by means of simultaneous right and left ventricular function curves in the dog. Circulation, 9:706, 1954.

188. Sarnoff, S. J., et al.: Homeometric autoregulation in the heart. Circ. Res., 8:1077, 1960,

189. Savranoglu, N., Boucek, R. J., and Casten, G. G.: The extent of reversibility of myocardial ischemia in dogs. Amer. Heart J., 58:726, 1959.

190. Schaper, W.: Pathophysiology of the coronary circulation. Progr. Cardiov. Dis., 14:275, 1971.

191. Scheidt, S., Ascheim, R., and Killip, T.: Shock after acute myocardial infarction. Amer. J. Cardiol., 26:556, 1970.

192. Scheidt, S., et al.: Objective assessment of prognosis after acute myocardial infarction. Circulation, 42 (Suppl. 3):196, 1970.

193. Scheuer, J.: Myocardial metabolism in cardiac hypoxia. Amer. J. Cardiol., 19:385, 1967.

194. Schreiber, S. S., et al.: Effect of acute overload on cardiac muscle mRNA. Amer. J. Physiol., 215:1250, 1968.

195. Scott, J. B., et al.: Role of chemical factors in regulation of flow through kidney, hindlimb, and heart. Amer. J. Physiol., 208:813, 1965.

196. Selkurt, E. E., and Elpers, M. J.: Influence of hemorrhagic shock on renal hemodynamics and osmolar clearance in the dog. Amer. J. Physiol., 205:147, 1963.

197. Selzer, A.: The hypotensive state following acute myocardial infarction. I. Clinical observations. Amer. Heart J., 44:1, 1952.

198. Selzer, A., Gerbode, F., and Kerth, W.: Clinical, hemodynamic, and surgical considerations of rupture of the ventricular septum after myocardial infarction. Amer. Heart J., 78:598, 1969.

199. Servinghaus, J. W., and Cullen, S. C.: Depression of myocardium and body oxygen consumption with fluothane. Anesthesiology, 19:165, 1958.

200. Shillingford, J. P., and Thomas, M.: Treatment of bradycardia and hypotension syndrome in patients with acute myocardial infarction. Amer. Heart J., 75:843, 1968.

201. Shubin, H., et al.: Objective index of hemodynamic status for quantitation of severity and prognosis of shock complicating myocardial infarction. Cardiov. Res., 2:329, 1968.

202. Simone, F. A.: Some issues in the problem of shock. Fed. Proc. 20 (Suppl. 9):3, 1961.

203. Sloman, G., and Brown, R.: Hospital registration in patients with acute myocardial infarction. Amer. Heart J., 79:761, 1970.

204. Smith, H. J., et al.: Hemodynamic studies in cardiogenic shock. Circulation, 35:1084, 1967.

205. Sodi-Pallares, D. N., et al.: Potassium, glucose and insulin treatment for acute myocardial infarction. Lancet, 1:1315, 1969.

206. Sokoloff, L.: The cerebral circulation. In: *Shock and Hypotension* (Mills, L. C., and Moyer, J. H., Eds.). New York, Grune and Stratton, 1965.

207. Sonnenblick, E. H., and Downing, S. E.: Afterload as a primary determinant of ventricular performance. Amer. J. Physiol., 204:604, 1963.

208. Sonnenblick, E. H., Parmley, W. W., and Urschel, C. W.: The contractile state of the heart as expressed by force-velocity relations. Amer. J. Cardiol., 23:488, 1969.

209. Sonnenblick, E. H., and Skelton, C. L.: Myocardial energetics: Basic principles and clinical implications. New Eng. J. Med., 285:668, 1971.

210. Sriussadaporn, S., and Cohn, J. N.: Lactate metabolism in clinical and experimental shock. Clin. Res., 16:519, 1968.

211. Starling, E. H.: *Principles of Human Physiology,* 3rd ed. Philadelphia, Lea and Febiger, 1920.

212. Starr, I., Jeffers, W. A., and Meade, R. H.: The absence of conspicuous increments of venous pressure after severe damage to the right ventricle of the dog, with a discussion of the relation between clinical congestive failure and heart disease. Amer. Heart J., 26:291, 1943.

213. Sukumalchantra, Y., et al.: The mechanism of arterial hypoxemia in acute myocardial infarction. Circulation, 41:641, 1970.

214. Toubes, D. B., and Brody, M. J.: Inhibition of reflex vasoconstriction after experimental coronary embolization in the dog. Circ. Res., 26:211, 1970.

215. Taylor, S. H., et al.: Insulin secretion following myocardial infarction with particular reference to the pathogenesis of cardiogenic shock. Lancet, 2:1373, 1969.

216. Tennant, R., and Wiggers, C. J.: Effect of coronary occlusion on myocardial contraction. Amer. J. Physiol., 112:351, 1935.

217. Teschan, P. E., and Lawson, N. L.: Studies in acute renal failure: Prevention by osmotic diuresis and observations on the effect of plasma and extracellular volume expansion. Nephron, 3:1, 1966.

218. Thal, A. P., and Kinney, J. M.: On the definition and classification of shock. Progr. Cardiov. Dis., 9:527, 1967.

219. Tristani, F. E., and Cohn, J. N.: Studies in clinical shock and hypotension. VII. Renal hemodynamics before and during treatment. Circulation, 42:839, 1970.

220. Valentine, P. A., et al.: Blood-gas changes after acute myocardial infarction. Lancet, 2:837, 1966.

221. Valori, C., Thomas, M., and Shillingford, J.: Free noradrenaline and adrenaline excretion in relation to clinical syndromes following myocardial infarction. Amer. J. Cardiol., 20: 605, 1967.

222. Wade, W. G.: The pathogenesis of infarction of the right ventricle. Brit. Heart J., 21:545, 1959.

223. Walston, A., Hackel, D. B., and Estes, E. H.: Acute coronary occlusion and the "power failure" syndrome. Amer. Heart J., 79:613, 1970.

224. Wan, S., et al.: Cardiogenic shock. A review of one year's experience. Med. J. Aust., 1: 1000, 1971.

225. Wartman, W. B., and Hellerstein, H. K.: Incidence of heart disease in 2,000 consecutive autopsies. Ann. Intern. Med., 28:41, 1948.

226. Weil, M. H., and Shubin, H.: Shock following myocardial infarction. Current understanding of hemodynamic mechanisms. Progr. Cardiov. Dis., 11:1, 1968.

227. Weisse, A. B., et al.: Left ventricular function during the early and late stages of scar formation following experimental myocardial infarction. Amer. Heart J., 79:370, 1970.

228. Weissler, A. M., et al.: Role of anaerobic metabolism in the preservation of functional capacity and structure of anoxic myocardium. J. Clin. Invest., 47:403, 1968.

229. Wiggers, C. J.: Dynamics of ventricular contraction under abnormal conditions. Circulation, 5:321, 1952.

230. Wilcken, D. E. L., et al.: Effects of alterations in aortic impedance on the performance of the ventricles. Circ. Res., 14:283, 1964.

231. Wildenthal, K., et al.: Effects of acute lactic acidosis on left ventricular performance. Amer. J. Physiol., 214:1352, 1968.

232. Winbury, M., Howe, B., and Weiss, R.: Effect of nitroglycerine and dipyridamole on epicardial and endocardial oxygen tension. Further evidence for redistribution of myocardial blood flow. J. Pharmacol. Exp. Ther., 176:184, 1971.

233. Wolff, L.: Clinical aspects of paroxysmal rapid heart action. New Eng. J. Med., 226:640, 1942.

234. Zaret, B. L., Pitt, B., and Ross, R. S.: Determination of the site, extent, and significance of regional ventricular dysfunction during acute myocardial infarction. Circulation, 45:441, 1972.

235. Zierler, K. L.: The skeletal muscle circulation. In: Shock and Hypotension (Mills, L. C., and Moyer, J. H., Eds.). New York, Grune and Stratton, 1965.

236. Zipes, D. P.: The clinical significance of bradycardic rhythms in acute myocardial infarction. Amer. J. Cardiol., 24:814, 1969.

Chapter 8

MEDICAL THERAPY FOR SHOCK IN ACUTE MYOCARDIAL INFARCTION*

Mark G. Perlroth, M.D., and Donald C. Harrison, M.D.

Death ensuing after acute myocardial infarction usually occurs in either of two distinct ways: the abrupt onset of a lethal arrhythmia or the rapid, progressive hemodynamic deterioration of cardiogenic shock. In this second decade of utilizing coronary-care units for the treatment of patients with infarction, the first problem, that of primary lethal arrhythmias, has been effectively dealt with, if not completely abolished.[81] The second problem, that of "pump failure" including cardiogenic shock, is now much better understood, but treatment remains largely ineffective.[117]

DEFINITION

Shock is defined as a circulatory state of sustained inadequate tissue perfusion, acute in onset, and incompatible with life for more than a short time. When due to pump failure, a fall in cardiac output and associated hypotension typically occur. Tachycardia, vasoconstriction and other signs of sympathetic autonomic discharge are usually

* This work was supported in part by NIH Grants HE-5709 and HE-5866.

present. There is decreased function of the brain, kidneys, and other vital organs, with systemic accumulation of lactic acid.

Thus, in addition to hypotension, the clinical findings include pallor, sweating, obtundation, oliguria, and acidosis. In the case of cardiogenic shock, a primary injury to the myocardium, such as myocardial infarction, will also be present. It is important to note that the shock syndrome may occur without hypotension if the fall in cardiac output is sufficiently compensated for by a rise in total peripheral resistance.

Since the circulatory system depends on the heart for the contractile energy required to maintain organ perfusion, diminished flow to the heart, regardless of etiology, will further impair hemodynamic status. Where shock is due to myocardial infarction, diminution in blood supply to an already ischemic heart exacerbates the original injury and accelerates the development of severe circulatory failure.

The prognosis for a patient with cardiogenic shock is dismal[117] and to a large extent depends on the definitions used by authors of various published series.[10,11,91] The stricter the criteria for inclusion, the more likely that the mortality will approach 100 per cent.[91] Factors influencing survival, in addition to definition, are duration of shock,[72,117] time of onset after myocardial infarction,[117] age, and associated clinical conditions. Despite a prolonged experience with cardiogenic shock and a failure to increase survival with any present method of treatment, there are no clear data concerning the course of untreated cardiogenic shock, nor is there any prospective controlled, randomized study of the effect of any one therapy on survival.

ALTERNATIVE ETIOLOGIES

The diagnosis of cardiogenic shock often is understood to mean the shock syndrome associated with the occurrence of recent myocardial infarction. It is worth stressing that an admitting diagnosis of myocardial infarction followed by shock is not uniformly due to pump failure secondary to extensive myocardial necrosis. The clinician should keep in mind a number of alternatives (Table 1), all of which can usually be diagnosed if considered. In addition, despite their infrequency, they may be readily repaired.

PATHOLOGY

SIZE OF INFARCT

This discussion will be limited to cardiogenic shock resulting from myocardial infarction secondary to atherosclerotic heart disease.

Quantitation of myocardial injury in hearts of patients with cardiogenic shock has been limited to autopsy specimens. Recent studies[53,96] showed 40 to 70 per cent myocardial loss in hearts of patients with cardiogenic shock, with 40 per cent or less in deaths not associated with cardiogenic shock. The entire extent of destruction was not necessarily acute, since previous old infarction accounted for up to 30 per cent of the loss. There was no predilection for any particular anatomical site.[96]

The data strongly suggest that shock secondary to myocardial infarction is primarily a reflection of pump failure reducing cardiac function to a level which cannot be compensated for by endogenous or exogenous attempts to restore homeostasis.

Table 1.   Shock Associated with Myocardial Infarction: Alternative Etiologies

1. Arrhythmias, especially marked tachy- and bradycardias

2. Iatrogenic causes
   A. Narcotics
   B. Tranquilizers
   C. Diuretics and Na⁺ restriction
   D. Antihypertensives
   E. Phlebotomy
   F. Intermittent positive-pressure respiration

3. Other cardiopulmonary causes
   A. Cardiac tamponade, especially in presence of central-venous[1] or pacemaker catheters
   B. Pulmonary embolism
   C. Dissecting aneurysm of the aorta
   D. Pneumothorax or hydrothorax (especially with subclavian central-venous pressure catheter)

4. Misdiagnosis, e.g. pancreatitis, perforated viscus

5. Myocardial infarction with additional diagnosis, e.g. septicemia, gastrointestinal hemorrhage

6. Specific complications of myocardial infarction
   A. Ventricular septal defect
   B. Ruptured papillary muscle or severe papillary-muscle dysfunction
   C. Ventricular aneurysm

PROGRESSION OF MYOCARDIAL LESION

Histological examination revealed small foci of scattered cell necrosis in hearts from patients in shock, but not in hearts from patients who died suddenly.[96] It may be that these lesions were related to therapy as much as to the shock syndrome per se.[106] All of the patients with cardiogenic shock in the study cited[96] had received isoproterenol.

The presence of a variable number of damaged cells outside the zone of infarction, the extent of which increased with the duration of shock, suggested that injury was progressive with the passage of time.[96]

The pathological picture in cardiogenic shock followed by recovery, although occurring only in a minority of cases, remains uncertain, yet it is precisely this group which needs definition. Techniques for accomplishing this will be discussed.

PATHOPHYSIOLOGY

STROKE VOLUME—STARLING CURVE

Myocardial infarction typically involves the left ventricle and is marked by an area of necrosis surrounded by an ischemic viable zone, which has impaired contraction.[16,28] The diminution in contractile mass leads to a decreased ejection fraction and a larger diastolic volume.[105] Thus, there is simultaneously a decrease in stroke volume and an elevation in left ventricular end-diastolic and left atrial mean pressures.[50,105] A consequence of this is that the normal (Starling) curve is depressed, flattened, and shifted to the right. In progressive cardiogenic shock, a descending limb may also be described.[13,103,104] This has been shown after coronary-artery ligation in animals.[114] With large infarctions (such as those leading to cardiogenic shock) the depressed stroke volume may be relatively fixed.[13]

PAPILLARY MUSCLE

If the papillary muscle becomes ischemic or necrotic, mitral regurgitation may occur due to either impaired contractility or rupture.

These complications will additionally decrease the stroke volume and elevate the left atrial pressure, accentuating the displacement of the Starling curve. The appearance of murmurs of mitral regurgitation in a setting of acute myocardial infarction is approximately 50 per cent.[57] The incidence of papillary-muscle rupture is much smaller, but more than 120 cases have been reported to date.[55]

CORONARY VERSUS SYSTEMIC CIRCULATION

The coronary and systemic circulations form two parallel circuits. Therefore, with a fixed, lowered cardiac output, efforts to increase flow to the systemic circulation by peripheral vasodilation are done at the expense of myocardial perfusion. Conversely, elevation of the peripheral resistance will divert blood toward the heart. Attempts to increase cardiac output sufficiently to meet both systemic and myocardial needs elevate myocardial oxygen requirements in an already ischemic heart. This is evidenced by increases in coronary sinus lactate concentrations.[91] The survival of the ischemic myocardium is then jeopardized.[16] This is, in fact, one of the central issues limiting the success of customary pharmacological intervention.

LEFT VENTRICLE

Perfusion of the left ventricle takes place primarily during diastole[48] and is therefore limited during tachycardia. Aortic diastolic hypotension and left ventricular diastolic hypertension, both common in experimental and clinical shock,[13,50,104,105] act together to diminish the pressure gradient across the left ventricle. Because of coronary-artery atherosclerosis, intraluminal pressure in coronary arterioles is even less than that measured in the central aorta during diastole.

If acute cardiac failure causes left ventricular dilatation, myocardial energy requirements will rise as a consequence of increased systolic wall tension.[113,123] Conversely, if ventricular dimensions diminish, external cardiac work may increase at no cost in terms of myocardial oxygen requirement. When more than 20 to 25 per cent of the ventricle is noncontractile, increased fiber shortening of the remaining viable myocardium is required to maintain stroke volume, usually in concert with an increase in ventricular end-diastolic pressures.[59]

ATRIAL KICK

Loss of atrial "kick" requires higher mean left ventricular diastolic and left atrial pressures for the same left ventricular end-diastolic pressure as was available with normal sinus rhythm. Therefore, atrial infarction, fibrillation, or atrioventricular dissocation each may contribute to hemodynamic deterioration.

NERVOUS CONTROL

The discharge from the sympathetic nervous system precipitated by the effects of myocardial injury has been alluded to earlier, and from it emerge the clinical signs of the cardiogenic-shock syndrome. However, departures from the expected effects are common. Thus, sinus bradycardia is frequently seen in myocardial infarction.[2] If associated with extensive myocardial injury and small stroke volume, this may severely limit cardiac output and lead to shock. Although sympathetic discharge produces an increase in total peripheral resistance, some vascular beds may be vasodilated, since mean total peripheral resistance has been found normal or low in as many as half of the patients in cardiogenic shock.[50,91,119] The mechanism is uncertain. It may be due to a reflex response to myocardial injury[27] or to reflexes from the left ventricle which produce a fall in total peripheral resistance in the presence of left ventricular systolic and diastolic hypertension.[109] Some patients are agonal, and local autoregulation of vascular resistance, from accumulation of metabolites, may override sympathetic vasoconstrictor activity. It is tempting to hypothesize that there may be an occasional patient with a reflex decrease in total peripheral resistance as a homeostatic mechanism lowering left ventricular end-diastolic pressure and left atrial mean pressures, and thus decreasing pulmonary congestion. In this regard, it is of interest that left ventricular end-diastolic pressure in cardiogenic shock after myocardial infarction is slightly lower than is such pressure in congestive heart failure after myocardial infarction. This is true in animals[105] as well as in man.[50]

CENTRAL VENOUS PRESSURE

The constrictor activity of sympathetic discharge increases venous tone and raises the central venous pressure and mean right atrial pressure. In the presence of arterial hypotension, this diminishes the pressure gradient across the systemic circulation. The acute central venous pressure elevation effectively increases right-sided filling pressures, but does not reflect any real increase in total blood volume. When the central venous pressure is low, effective hypovolemia may be presumed, but when it is elevated hypervolemia is not necessarily present.[43]

In the absence of pulmonary vascular obstruction, the central venous pressure is also useful, in that it is less than or equal to pulmonary-artery wedge pressure.[13,41,50] Thus, although a low central venous pressure does not exclude elevation of pulmonary-artery wedge pressure, a high central venous pressure, representing the lower limit of the pulmonary-artery wedge pressure, assures an equal or still higher wedge pressure and increases the likelihood of pulmonary congestion. Shubin and Weil[121] have suggested that central venous pressure response to fluid challenge may be a useful physiological test of vascular volume. This may be helpful with low central venous pressure, or when direct pulmonary-artery wedge pressure measurement is unavailable, but it seems an unnecessary maneuver when the central venous pressure is elevated (>15 cm H_2O), or direct pulmonary-artery wedge pressure determination is at hand.

HYPOXEMIA

In addition to the hemodynamic consequences noted above, arterial hypoxemia is frequent and often severe[7,83] in cardiogenic shock. This finding is not duplicated in experimental cardiogenic shock in dogs.[33] In animal models, abnormalities existed in the distribution of pulmonary blood flow with redistribution favoring blood flow to the highest (antigravity) pulmonary segments, as a consequence of elevated left atrial mean and pulmonary venous pressures. Perivascular edema was described, a finding not present in lungs of animals suffering hemorrhagic shock. Hyperventilation was also documented. Decreased pulmonary blood flow in cardiogenic shock may predispose to atelectasis by diminishing pneumocyte function and surfactant production.

Depression of respiratory reflexes due to cerebral ischemia and/or depressant drugs may also play a role in the development of atelectasis by causing shallow respiration and less frequent sighing respiration.[87] Low systemic arterial saturation and low cardiac output with increased tissue extraction of oxygen accentuate the hypoxemic effect of veno-arterial shunting through atelectatic segments of the lung.[7] Concomitant pleural effusions, intra-alveolar edema, pulmonary embolism and/or intrinsic pulmonary disease are frequent additional factors worsening hypoxemia.

IRREVERSIBILITY

The concept of "irreversibility" is vague, due to often erratic correlation between hemodynamic, clinical and mortality data. It is frequently attributed to the progress of a "vicious cycle"[96,99] or to the extent of myocardial necrosis per se.[96] Evidence of a humoral cardiodepressant substance has also been described.[75] However, as shock progresses, underperfused tissues show an increase in anaerobic metabolism marked by lactate production.[18,98] Systemic acidosis is increased by the failure of renal excretion of hydrogen ions and occasionally by carbon dioxide retention with severe pulmonary failure.[4]

As cellular hypoxia and acidosis worsen, lysosomal membranes become more permeable and release lytic enzymes into the cytoplasm.[60,130] With destruction of mitochondrial and nuclear integrity, the cell is unable to resume aerobic metabolism, even if circulation is restored. Both functional and microscopic injuries to mitochondria have been documented in shock.[60,61,86,125] Nuclear injury may prevent repair of partially destroyed organelles. It is probably at this time and at this tissue level that irreversibility and anaerobic metabolism become fixed and ultimate mortality is determined. This is supported by studies showing that mortality in shock of all causes is a direct function of the elevation of serum lactate concentration.[18]

METHODS

CLINICAL CONSIDERATIONS

The definition of shock correctly identifies a group of patients at high risk who require immediate and aggressive therapy. It does not accurately distinguish within that group those patients who have irreparable and extensive damage from those who are salvageable. In the latter group, techniques are needed to separate those who would benefit from early mechanical assistance from those who are likely to improve with drug therapy alone. Even the choice of drug therapy is likely to be more efficacious if the hemodynamics of cardiogenic shock in any given patient are defined before and during treatment.

Clinical observation of the patient in the coronary-care unit now includes routine monitoring of vital signs, electrocardiogram, central venous pressure and central venous oxygen saturation.

Measurement of urinary output in cardiogenic shock is mandatory, both as a clinical guide and in order to calculate fluid balance. Although voluntary voiding at regular intervals may be sufficient, catheterization of the bladder, with hourly urine measurements, is preferred. Urine output in cardiogenic shock is usually below 20 ml/hr. Occasionally, even transient hypotension (4 to 6 hours) is sufficient to produce acute tubular necrosis with persistent oliguria, despite return of adequate renal blood flow.

COMPUTER ECG MONITORING

Continuous electrocardiographic observation is now routine in coronary-care units. Tape recording and computer monitoring of electrocardiograph records permit quantitation of abnormal rhythms and immediate electronic identification of arrhythmias associated with hemodynamic instability.[49]

CATHETERS AND HEMODYNAMICS

Although cuff measurements of arterial pressure are usually correct, peripheral arterial constriction may lead to erroneously low readings when compared with intra-arterial catheter measurements.[23] The presence of an arterial line also permits sampling of arterial blood gases as a guide to oxygen administration and ventilatory assistance.

In addition to these relatively conventional techniques, several other procedures have been introduced which provide more direct information about left atrial pressures and cardiac output. Indwelling pulmonary-artery catheters, utilizing pulmonary-artery diastolic pressures as a close approximation of left ventricular end-diastolic pressure,[13,69,104] usually but not always[12] provide accurate reflections of left ventricular end-diastolic pressures. An inflatable balloon-tipped catheter[41,44] has facilitated pulmonary-arterial wedge pressure monitoring. The advantages of a right-sided catheter distal to the right atrium include the opportunity to sample mixed venous blood for Fick cardiac outputs, the ability to detect left-to-right shunting at the level of the right ventricle in cases of suspected ventricular septal defect secondary to myocardial infarction, and the means to note accurately phasic measurements of the pulmonary-artery wedge pressure, permitting

diagnosis and quantitation of mitral regurgitation when present.

With a thermistor-tipped catheter as a sensor, the thermodilution technique permits repeated cardiac-output measurements without the disadvantages of collection of expired gases or the necessity of steady-state conditions required by the Fick method.[14] In comparison with the dye-dilution method, repeated output measurements may be made without accumulation of dye indicators in the circulation, and without repeated withdrawal of blood. Relative proximity of injection and sampling sites also avoids the errors inherent in early recirculation.[95]

The simultaneous measurement of cardiac output and central venous pressures allows calculation of the total peripheral resistance and will also allow immediate identification of the entire range of hemodynamic effects of therapeutic intervention.

Placement of pulmonary catheters has been aided greatly by the fluoroscopic equipment and radiolucent beds which are now available in coronary-care units.

New techniques for continuous monitoring of stroke volume in man, such as echocardiography[100] and central arterial pulse-curve analyses,[3] are also being studied.

ANGIOGRAPHY

Emergency angiography of the coronary circulation and left ventricle has been gaining wider acceptance in conjunction with emergency surgery for coronary-artery bypass grafts,[92] for ventricular aneurysm,[37] for mitral regurgitation,[6] and for acute ventricular septal defect associated with myocardial infarction and cardiogenic shock.[11,16,63]

RADIONUCLIDE SCANNING

Left ventricular dysfunction and dyskinesis can also be examined in a less invasive manner by scintigrams requiring only intravenous injection of radionuclides.[134] This technique is not widespread and lacks the resolution of conventional radiographic methods.

Scanning techniques showing the extent

of myocardial uptake[56] of radionuclides or reflecting distribution of capillary flow by macro-aggregated albumin[102,127] after selective injection into the coronary circulation are being developed in a few centers. These permit *premortem* estimation of viable myocardium and could play an invaluable role in determining the choice of appropriate therapy early in the patient's course.

Drawbacks

The hazards of an aggressive approach to patient monitoring in cardiogenic shock include the obvious one involving the use of radiopaque agents with myocardial depressant properties[45] and the difficulties of working with isotopes. Numerous catheters require constant slow infusions, and frequent flushes may provide a substantial fluid load for the oliguric patient; the catheters also provide a percutaneous portal of entry for systemic infection. Hematoma formation and/or thrombosis of vessels may occur. The passage of catheters into the ventricles and coronary arteries may trigger ventricular arrhythmias, ventricular fibrillation, and/or myocardial infarction.

MEDICAL THERAPY

Volume

It is axiomatic that hypovolemia, manifested by low ventricular filling pressures, will reduce cardiac output. The limitations regarding use of the central venous pressure have been mentioned earlier. If direct or indirect (pulmonary-artery diastolic or pulmonary-artery wedge) measurements of left ventricular end-diastolic pressures are available, then well-informed decisions regarding volume replacement (with low-molecular-weight dextran or plasma) can be made.[24,94,103,104] Changes in cardiac output, in response to challenges with dextran, have been used as a measure of cardiac reserve, and increases have suggested a favorable prognosis.[104,121] Generally, the injured myocardium in cardiogenic shock responds subnormally to fluid

challenge.[13] Conversely, marked elevation of left ventricular end-diastolic pressure has justified phlebotomy, with occasional rise in cardiac output.[104] A level of 20 to 24 mm Hg has been suggested as optimal for left ventricular end-diastolic pressure with acute myocardial infarction.[103]

Ventilation and pH

In addition to manipulating volume to optimize pressure measurements in the heart and lungs, pH and blood gases must be restored toward normal. Sodium bicarbonate is an effective base for the treatment of metabolic acidosis. However, attempts to restore pH entirely to normal may lead to overshoot as the circulation is restored and lactate production ceases.

Hypoxemia and hypercarbia should be treated with oxygen and assisted ventilation, respectively. With severe pulmonary congestion accompanying cardiogenic shock, endotracheal intubation and positive-pressure ventilation may be useful, both as an antagonist to alveolar edema and as a source of very high concentrations of inspired oxygen.[90]

A diligent search should be made for any additional etiological factors contributing to the hypotension (Table 1).

Drugs

Drugs are available which can selectively increase or decrease heart rate, inotropism, total peripheral resistance, and specific organ vascular resistance (in some cases). No discussion of standard antiarrhythmic drugs is included here. It is the basic paradox of drug therapy for cardiogenic shock that myocardial minute-oxygen consumption is correlated with the velocity of contraction[124] and the time-tension index[115] and that, as a rule, drugs which bolster the failing circulation do so by augmenting the same factors which stimulate myocardial oxygen demand. In cardiac tissue already damaged by ischemia, the magnitude of the lesion is likely to increase under the influence of pharmacological therapy with positive inotropic influence.[16]

Before outlining the effects of individual drugs, it is worth repeating that carefully controlled prospective studies in comparable patient groups are totally lacking. Evidence supporting the actions of given drugs is typically drawn from small series of patients or from experimental studies in animals, usually dogs.

Despite attempts to provide unifying theories for the common pathogenesis of all forms of shock,[79] there are important differences in response among different species and conclusions from nonprimate animal studies should be regarded as only tentative when generalized to human clinical experience.[93]

Ideally a drug utilized to treat cardiogenic shock should: increase cardiac output; raise blood pressure; increase cardiac and peripheral tissue perfusion; have a quick onset of action; be rapidly metabolized even during depressed renal and hepatic function; keep left ventricular end-diastolic pressure and myocardial minute-oxygen consumption at a minimum while achieving these effects; and

be free of undesired side effects (i.e. arrhythmias). No drug presently used achieves all these benefits. However, different drugs are capable of some of these effects (Table 2).

CATECHOLAMINES

Because of the ability of catecholamine derivatives to stimulate predominantly alpha-sympathetic (vasoconstrictor) or beta-sympathetic (chronotropic, inotropic, vasodilator) receptors, a variety of responses can be elicited with this group of drugs. A brief review of these agents and their mode of action has appeared recently.[88] The commonly used drugs in this class are norepinephrine, isoproterenol and, increasingly, dopamine.

Norepinephrine

Norepinephrine (levarterenol) causes both alpha- and beta-receptor stimulation, with the former predominating. It is the naturally occurring sympathetic neurotransmitter substance[36] and has been in use for the treatment of cardiogenic shock for many years. Careful metabolic and hemo-

Table 2. Effects of Drugs in Cardiogenic Shock

Drug	α/β	HR	CO	LVEDP	TPR	RBF	ΔMVO_2
Isoproterenol	β	↑↑↑	↑↑↑	↓	↓	±↑	↑
Norepinephrine	α,β	↑,0	0,↑	↑,0	↑	↓	±
Dopamine	β,α	↑	↑↑	?↓	±	↑	↑
Digitalis	—	↓	0,↑	±,↓	±,↑	±	↑?
Glucagon	—	↑	↑	?↓	↓?	0?	0,↑

Key:
α = alpha-receptor sympathetic stimulation
β = beta-receptor sympathetic stimulation
HR = heart rate
CO = cardiac output
LVEDP = left ventricular end-diastolic pressure
TPR = total peripheral resistance
RBF = renal blood flow
ΔMVO_2 = change in rate of myocardial oxygen requirement (assuming no change in heart size)
↑ = increase
↓ = decrease
0 = no change
± = variable
? = uncertain

dynamic studies[91] have shown levarterenol to increase arterial pressure with little change in cardiac index. A decrease in myocardial lactate production or a change-over to lactate extraction was measured by simultaneous arterial and coronary-sinus samples. There was no improvement in survival.

Measurements of left ventricular end-diastolic pressure in animals[38] and man[29] show an increase after norepinephrine administration. Because its local vasoconstrictor properties are so intense, it must be delivered intravenously, and necrosis may result if extravasation occurs. This can be treated by local infiltration with phentolamine (Regitine), an alpha blocker.

The onset and offset of action are rapid. Ventricular arrhythmias may occur with rapid infusion. The rise in systolic pressure will exacerbate any preexisting mitral or aortic regurgitation. The dose should be delivered in a concentration sufficient to titrate arterial blood pressure within a desired range without excessive fluid load.

Metaraminol

Metaraminol (Aramine), a synthetic catecholamine, is a false neurotransmitter with similar but weaker properties than norepinephrine. It also acts indirectly, releasing norepinephrine from adrenergic-nerve terminals. The duration of action of metaraminol is somewhat longer because its metabolism is slower. Its action is decreased by prolonged use or prior depletion of body stores of norepinephrine.[54] Because it is a less potent vasoconstrictor, it may be injected intramuscularly without fear of local tissue sloughing. It has no other advantages, and it is used infrequently.

Isoproterenol

Isoproterenol (Isuprel) is a synthetic catecholamine with almost pure beta-receptor stimulating properties. Its positive inotropic effect is striking. Even in the presence of cardiogenic shock, increases in cardiac index

have averaged 61 per cent.[80,91] Although its vasodilatory effect offers increased blood flow to the systemic circulation, mean blood pressure usually remains constant, with a fall in diastolic pressure and diastolic time per minute. These latter effects decrease myocardial oxygen supply relative to increased needs. Thus, in one study[91] coronary-sinus lactate reflected either increased production or decreased extraction of lactate in all patients in cardiogenic shock while on isoproterenol. Experimental studies have shown this compound to increase the size and extent of topical S-T elevation over the ventricle after coronary-artery occlusion.[16]

The chronotropic effect of the drug may produce marked sinus tachycardia and/or ventricular arrhythmias. The occurrence of either of these contingencies calls for diminution or cessation of infusion.

Isoproterenol should be given intravenously, and administration should be titrated by appropriate clinical responses. It may, in contrast with norepinephrine, be expected to increase urine output and cause improvement in skin circulation. Patients with mitral regurgitation and cardiogenic shock may be benefited.[99] Increased pulmonary arteriovenous shunting due to increased cardiac output through underventilated lung has caused hypoxemia.[39]

Dopamine

This drug has been gaining recognition for the treatment of cardiogenic shock since favorable reports of its clinical use were published by MacCannell and associates.[82] It is the biochemical precursor of norepinephrine,[49] and shares the strong inotropic effects of other catecholamines.[80] The increased cardiac output and arterial blood pressure are accompanied by a fall in left ventricular end-diastolic pressure,[80,104,133] by selective dilation of the renal vasculature[84,85] and by increased urine output. Moreover, since there is less chronotropic effect than with isoproterenol, there is less increase in myocardial oxygen demand. Increased oxygen delivery

9

to the myocardium may occur, secondary to its effects on aortic and left ventricular end-diastolic pressures.

This drug is presently under investigation, but its use is becoming more widespread. Given intravenously, it acts rapidly. Metabolism of dopamine is brisk. Infusion at a rate of 1 to 17 μg/kg/min may attain the desired clinical effects.

Angiotensin II

This extremely potent pressor is not in general use for the treatment of shock. It lacks inotropic effect.[101,108] It is mentioned here for those rare cases where conventional drugs have failed to reverse severe hypotension. It should also be considered in the event of a marked fall in blood pressure after administration of alpha blockers (phenoxybenzamine or phentolamine) when levarterenol is likely to be ineffective.

Alpha-receptor Blockade and Vasodilation

Phentolamine (Regitine) and phenoxybenzamine (Dibenzyline) have been advocated for the treatment of shock[57,132] to decrease peripheral vasoconstriction. If cardiac output remains fixed, a fall in total peripheral resistance will simply result in further hypotension and cardiac deterioration, despite signs of peripheral vasodilation. Discussions of the merits and hazards of these agents in cardiogenic shock are presented elsewhere,[99] and we agree with published recommendations that they be avoided.[89]

Perhaps the only situation in which these agents may be helpful is as an adjunct to mechanical circulatory assistance, when cardiac output can be augmented by an external power source. Chlorpromazine in small doses has been used for this purpose.[72]

Beta-receptor Blockade

Beta blockade with propranolol has been investigated in the treatment of shock.[34,38] Although its negative inotropic effect[35] may diminish oxygen demand by the heart, further depression of cardiac output and/or elevation of left ventricular end-diastolic pressure would probably not be tolerated by the patient in cardiogenic shock. Beta-blocking agents have been demonstrated by electrophysiological and biochemical techniques to decrease the area of peripheral necrosis surrounding myocardial infarction in animals.[16] These drugs may also impair atrioventricular conduction. They cannot be recommended alone, but a potential role in combination with mechanical assistance has not been described.

Digitalis

The inotropic effect of digitalis has led to its reevaluation for the treatment of cardiogenic shock.[25,80,104] Optimally, digitalis produces an increase in cardiac output with a decrease in left ventricular end-diastolic pressure. In congestive heart failure, its direct effect of increasing total peripheral resistance is usually gradual and is compensated for by a reflex diminution in sympathetic tone, so that total peripheral resistance remains the same or diminishes.[15] When more than 25 per cent of myocardial muscle mass is destroyed, digitalis has had little effect on cardiac output.[62] Perhaps because of this inadequate myocardial response, studies in man[25] have shown biphasic responses to intravenously administered digitalis with early (<5- to 10-min) rises in total peripheral resistance, arterial pressure, and left ventricular end-diastolic pressure. One patient developed acute pulmonary edema immediately after digitalization. Inotropic responses occurred 15 to 20 minutes after injection.[25] If the increased contractility of noninfarcted muscle segments requires increased oxygen supply, the net effect may be deleterious.

In contrast with the catecholamines, digitalis slows the sinus rate, and it has a longer time for onset of action. Depending on the preparation used, digitalis can be given orally, intramuscularly, or intravenously. In cardiogenic shock, the intravenous route is indicated. Clearance of commonly used preparations may be impaired.

In the setting of renal insufficiency, assisted ventilation and electrolyte disturbances, marked variation in serum potassium may occur, thus altering the threshold of digitalis toxicity.[131] Ventricular arrhythmias are frequent in cardiogenic shock, and their presence in the digitalized patient may be confused with digitalis toxicity. For these reasons, digitalis is probably best avoided in cardiogenic shock. Its use in myocardial infarction should probably be reserved for patients with stable renal function and congestive heart failure and/or supraventricular tachycardias such as atrial fibrillation.

GLUCAGON

Interest in glucagon derives from identification of its positive inotropic effect in man.[97] This action was not associated with a rise in total peripheral resistance, although blood pressure rose. Heart rate, cardiac output, and left ventricular dp/dt increased also. Left ventricular end-diastolic pressure was unchanged. These studies were not performed during cardiogenic shock. More recent studies of glucagon in experimental myocardial infarction in conscious dogs suggest that the beneficial hemodynamic effects of this drug are coupled with no significant change in myocardial minute-oxygen consumption (perhaps due to a decrease in left ventricular volume) and no increase in ventricular arrhythmias.[73]

Glucagon has a brief (1-hour) effect and must be given parenterally. Continuous infusion may produce nausea and vomiting, a major clinical limitation. Its stimulation of the heart is minimized in the presence of chronic congestive heart failure.[5] It may be of use when prior administration of a beta blocker antagonizes the effect of catecholamines. It is a peptide and is potentially antigenic. Finally, the rise in blood glucose may lower serum potassium, a possible hazard in the previously digitalized patient.[131] The

role of glucagon in cardiogenic shock is still uncertain.

CORTICOSTEROIDS

These agents in pharmacological doses (i.e. 1 to 3 gm of hydrocortisone q.d.) have been used in the therapy of shock from a variety of causes, including cardiogenic shock.[32] The mechanism, if any, is uncertain. Hemodynamic actions described include alpha blockade[32] and potentiation of the vasoconstriction of norepinephrine[74] and angiotensin.[76] Other studies have indicated that no significant cardiovascular response ensued.[19,76,120] Side effects of chronic large doses of steroids are not seen when it is used for less than one week. The drug may be discontinued or rapidly tapered off over a few days.

It is possible that the membrane-stabilizing effects of these agents may be the basis for whatever value they have in shock, regardless of etiology. If membranes at capillary, cell-membrane, and especially lysosomal surfaces are maintained during stress by high concentrations of corticosteroid,[67,130] then mitochondria and other cell organelles might be spared, permitting resumption of normal cellular metabolic activity after restoration of adequate blood flow. If pump failure persists despite therapeutic efforts, the potential value of this treatment will not be recognized. Although case reports of the beneficial effects of steroids in cardiogenic shock after heart surgery have appeared,[74,78,79] clinical studies have not yet suggested a systematic role for corticosteroids in cardiogenic shock as they have for shock of other etiologies.[20,129] Short-term toxicity has not been a problem.

ATROPINE

This drug has long been used for the treatment of sinus bradycardia and first- and second-degree atrioventricular block occurring in the wake of an acute myocardial infarction. The role of heart rate in maintaining cardiac output in situations of small, fixed stroke volumes has been stated earlier.

Intravenous atropine has been shown to increase cardiac output, lower venous pressure and raise heart rate in man.[9] However, this effect is very short-lived (<15 min), and there is controversy regarding inotropic action.[116]

Experimental evidence for vagal afferent impulses from the heart producing sympathetic inhibition has been proposed as a mechanism for hypotension after myocardial infarction. This afferent loop can be interrupted by vagotomy, but not by atropine.[71]

Atropine should be given intravenously in doses of 1.0 mg at 4- to 8-hour intervals. Its action is rapid. Deleterious effects include rapid sinus tachycardia. Occasionally, atropine toxicity is seen when high doses are used. The warm, dry, red skin and mental confusion may suggest fever and sepsis.

OXYGEN

Oxygen has been almost universally administered to patients with cardiogenic shock for decades. This practice is based on the hypothesis that hypoxia is frequently observed in patients with cardiogenic shock[83] and results in increases in heart rate and left ventricular filling pressures, with decreases in cardiac contractility. While the circulatory system has a number of compensatory mechanisms for reacting to hypoxia, studies have shown that these compensatory mechanisms are inadequate in the heart damaged by infarction.[118]

The argument against administering oxygen to all patients with cardiogenic shock is based on the finding that hypoxia results in increases in total peripheral resistance, decreases in cardiac output, and slowing of the heart rate.[42] Those changes in circulatory dynamics observed were small and, if arterial oxygen saturations are reduced significantly, oxygen administration will enhance cardiac function and improve the circulatory state of the patient with cardiogenic shock. Thus, for the present time, it seems appropriate to offer oxygen to all patients in cardiogenic shock. Monitoring of blood gases is mandatory if the patient is being artificially ventilated through a nasotracheal tube.

SURGERY

Conventional Surgery

The presence of a noncontractile, marginally perfused, yet viable segment of myocardium at the border of an infarct[28] suggests that aortocoronary bypass surgery as an emergency procedure in cardiogenic shock may be justified. Case reports documenting successful recovery after such surgery have appeared.[11,16,92]

Infarctectomy has been proposed[11,58] as a surgical remedy for cardiogenic shock because of data indicating that infarction of more than 25 per cent of the ventricle dilutes the effectiveness of the remaining contractile tissue[59] and renders inotropic drugs impotent.[62] Results of this approach have not as yet altered long-term survival. Resection of myocardium is more likely to be effective if a classical ventricular aneurysm is present at the same time that a fresh myocardial infarction supervenes, producing cardiogenic shock. Then resection of the true aneurysm may be lifesaving.[37]

The occurrence of rupture of a papillary muscle or of the interventricular septum as a sequel to acute myocardial infarction is now a well-known syndrome. It is marked by rapid hemodynamic deterioration and the onset of a loud systolic murmur, often with a thrill, over the lower precordium.[55,63] Repair of the ruptured septum[11,16,63] and replacement of the mitral valve[6] have each been successful in reversing cardiogenic shock. Such events are usually symptomatic of large infarctions and extensive coronary-artery disease. Prognosis is therefore often grim,[112] even with technically expert surgery. Silent mitral insufficiency due to valve prolapse has been diagnosed with the use of a balloon-tipped pulmonary-artery catheter to monitor pulmonary-artery wedge phasic pressures after acute myocardial infarction. One patient with this syndrome was hypotensive and was surgically helped.[40]

Cardiac Transplantation

The concept of surgical replacement[8] of the diseased heart has achieved much publicity in the last few years, despite the uncertain availability of donor hearts. Early results so far indicate that the prognosis is guarded, with 33 per cent survival at one year.[21] Recent experience at Stanford shows that 40 to 45 per cent one-year survival can be expected in young patients. The quality of the life prolonged is limited by the necessity for geographical proximity to the mother institution, by the susceptibility to rejection and infection, and by many of the side effects of chronic corticosteroid administration. Psychological stresses with this procedure are unique. Cardiac transplantation will probably never completely solve the problem of cardiogenic shock, and must be considered at present as an important experimental procedure which speaks directly to the need for a new pump in the case of pump failure.

ASSISTED CIRCULATION

Principles (Table 3)

Assisted circulation has been succinctly reviewed elsewhere.[26,111] Basically, it is capable of enhancing perfusion of all tissues, without increasing myocardial oxygen demand, by utilizing an external energy source. This is a goal which cannot be realized by pharmacological intervention alone.

The effects of cardiogenic shock and hypotension are reversed, with return of function to vital organs and minimization of ischemia at border zones. If the heart heals sufficiently, assistance may be discontinued without recurrence of shock. If the heart continues to beat during assistance, synchronization of the assist device with cardiac contractions is desirable. This allows the pumping device to raise aortic pressure during diastole and to lower it at the onset of systole, decreasing the time of isometric contraction, decreasing myocardial oxygen demand, and increasing the ejection fraction, thus lowering the left ventricular end-diastolic pressure. Such synchronization requires recognition of QRS complexes even when bizarre, as well as during arrhythmias.

Circulatory-assist devices may also provide support during a critical period between the onset of shock and subsequent emergency surgery.[92] If cardiac activity is replaced completely, as in total cardiopulmonary assist[68,110] or in mechanical ventricular assistance,[122] circulatory function will be maintained even with cardiac arrest.

The various modes of external circulatory assistance range from manual compression of the sternum to complete cardiopulmonary bypass, as utilized during cardiac surgery (Table 3).

Balloon Pumping

Of the various interventions in use, only one has received extensive clinical trial in cardiogenic shock secondary to myocardial infarction, and that is intra-aortic balloon pumping.[17,70,72,77,89,126] This procedure utilizes the principle of counterpulsation, in that aortic diastolic pressures are augmented and aortic systolic pressures remain the same or lower, while aortic mean pressures rise.

Balloon pumping has been used for periods ranging from only a few hours to more than three days.[90] Most studies of hemodynamic effects have shown increased systemic pressures and perfusion, with a diminution of ventricular end-diastolic pressures.[90,126]

Effects on myocardial metabolism and blood flow have shown both erratic[77] and uniformly beneficial[90] results. The latter study showed an increase in coronary blood flow of approximately 25 per cent, without change in myocardial oxygen consumption, and with a return of myocardial lactate extraction.

Hemolysis is minimal compared to mechanical counterpulsation.[17,70] Only a femoral

Table 3. Circulatory Assistance*

	Heparin	Effective with Arrest	Hemolysis	Mechanism	References
A. Noninvasive					
1. External counterpulsation	—	—	—	Modified counter-pulsation	22, 31
B. Catheterization of peripheral arteries/veins					
1. Veno-arterial pulsatile circulatory assistance	+	+	+	Cardiopulmonary bypass	110
2. Counterpulsation	++	—	+	Counterpulsation	64, 107
					17, 70, 72
3. Intra-aortic balloon pump	++	—	+|—	Modified counter-pulsation	77, 89, 126
C. Thoracotomy without cardiac incision					
1. Mechanical ventricular assistance	—	+	—	Ventricular compression	122
D. Thoracotomy with cardiac incision					
1. Left ventricular bypass	±	—	±	Parallel pump	30, 128

*This is not an exhaustive list. It is designed to give examples of current techniques and is arranged in increasing order of required surgical effort.

arteriotomy is required. Heparin is used for anticoagulation.

A modification of the "omnidirectional" balloon has been introduced[17] with a double balloon-tipped catheter. A proximal balloon first occludes the aorta and a distal balloon then expands so that the blood is preferentially distributed to the heart, brain and upper extremities. Measurements of proximal aortic pressure indicate that coronary perfusion is possibly superior with this system. It has been combined with vacuum withdrawal of gas from the aorta to cope with the problem of severe aortic systolic hypotension and insufficient balloon collapse. This added feature prevents obstruction (by an incompletely deflated balloon) to distal aortic runoff during cardiac systole. It also has been designed to include a second balloon in series with the first, outside the body, which prevents overdistension of the intra-aortic balloon. Carbon dioxide is used to limit the consequences of balloon rupture.

The limitations of the intra-aortic balloon pump are that diastolic stroke volume is limited to balloon size (approximately 30 cc[17]) and that severe aorto-iliac atherosclerosis may make retrograde passage of the balloon impossible. An electrical control system to time the balloon phase with the cardiac cycle must recognize the R wave, even when QRS and rhythm are bizarre. A competent aortic valve is also required for maximum effectiveness. Because of its principle of action and small stroke volume, this form of intervention cannot maintain circulation in the event of cardiac arrest. Circulation to the distal aorta is minimized. Rupture of the balloon has been reported.[91] Although carbon dioxide, because of its solubility in blood, was originally used,[89] the relative inertia and viscosity of this gas have led to its replacement with helium.[90,126] Trauma to the aorta with mural hemorrhage has been reported,[70] but this has not appeared to be a major drawback. Femoral-artery circulation distal to catheter insertion is severely compromised and may require bypass to prevent serious ischemia.[70,90] Wound infection has also been a hazard.[70]

Survival during balloon pumping has largely been confined to the period of actual assistance. Although there have been some suggestions of occasional increased long-term survival in patients who have received circulatory assistance,[72,90] it is likely that without correction of the underlying defect (extensive noncontractile myocardium) mortality will change little. Nevertheless, the small proportion of patients in cardiogenic shock after myocardial infarction who presently do recover suggests that perfusion of ischemic, potentially viable areas, and the possible expansion of dormant collateral channels[64,65] may be lifesaving, especially if performed soon after the onset of shock.

A second major area of application of intra-aortic balloon pumping may be the support of a fragile patient in cardiogenic shock, or one with a rapidly failing circulation, whose candidacy for surgical procedures such as aortocoronary bypass graft and aneurysmectomy requires additional studies. Since the passage of time and the administration of contrast agents for coronary arteriography and left ventricular angiography are both hazardous, circulatory assistance will prevent or offset hemodynamic deterioration during the hours in which definitive evaluation may be completed and the patient brought to the operating room.

COMMENT

Present practice for the treatment of cardiogenic shock secondary to myocardial infarction begins with its recognition by traditional clinical signs. Cardiac rhythm, venous and arterial pressures, and arterial gases and pH are monitored and treated as necessary with oxygen, ventilatory assistance, antiarrhythmic drugs, volume replacement, pressors and inotropic agents. If, after prolonged treatment, the patient is still refractory to therapy, he undergoes more sophisticated study to measure left-sided hemodynamics, cardiac output and myocardial metabolism. At this point, circulatory assistance may be initiated. If the patient cannot tolerate withdrawal of mechanical assistance, he may undergo special angiographic studies and possibly emergency surgery.

Such a strategy offers little likelihood of exploiting whatever benefits may be available from surgery or from newer techniques for defining physiological and anatomical abnormalities. The immediate aim of management should be to restore adequate circulation in *as short a time as possible*, to minimize damage to the heart. Circulatory assistance provides a physiological umbrella for the gathering of radiological and hemodynamic data. Such an approach may well offer more support, more information, and more therapeutic alternatives early in the patient's course than is presently the case.

SUMMARY

Cardiogenic shock following myocardial infarction is a syndrome of inadequate tissue perfusion, usually due to acute depression of cardiac output following loss of more than 40 per cent of the total contractile ventricle. The decrease in stroke volume is usually coupled with a rise in left ventricular end-diastolic pressure, which causes pulmonary congestion and further depresses left ventricular perfusion. There is probably progressive extension of infarction throughout the period of hypotension.

Since return of contractility will not occur in the infarct, medical therapy is limited to prevention of extension of the infarct and maintenance of myocardial perfusion. The effects of isoproterenol, norepinephrine, dopamine, digitalis and glucagon in the management of patients with cardiogenic shock are presented, and the role of emergency surgery is considered.

Various forms of circulatory assistance are in use, but the most extensive experience to date has been with the intra-aortic balloon pump, which offers circulatory support with a minimum of surgery and utilizes the principle of counterpulsation. During mechanical assistance, radiological and hemodynamic studies demonstrating coronary-artery and left ventricular anatomy, as well as patterns of myocardial perfusion, can be safely completed, allowing better-informed decisions regarding possible surgical therapy.

REFERENCES

1. Adar, R., and Mozes, M.: Fatal complications of central venous catheters. Brit. Med. J., 3:746, 1971.
2. Adgey, A. A. J., et al.: Incidence, significance and management of early bradyarrhythmia complicating acute myocardial infarction. Lancet, 2:1097, 1968.
3. Alderman, E. L., et al.: Evaluation of the pulse contour method of determining stroke volume in man. Circulation, 46:546, 1972.
4. Anthonisen, N. R., and Smith, H. J.: Respiratory acidosis as a consequence of pulmonary edema. Ann. Intern. Med., 62:991, 1965.
5. Armstrong, P. W., et al.: Hemodynamic evaluation of glucagon in symptomatic heart disease. Circulation, 44:67, 1971.
6. Austen, W. G., Sokol, D. M., DeSanctis, R. W., and Sanders, C. A.: Surgical treatment of papillary-muscle rupture complicating myocardial infarction. New Eng. J. Med., 278: 1137, 1968.
7. Ayres, S. M., et al.: The lung in shock. Alveolar-capillary gas exchange in the shock syndrome. Amer. J. Cardiol., 26:588, 1970.
8. Barnard, C. N.: A human cardiac transplant: An interim report of a successful operation performed at Groote Schuur Hospital, Cape Town, S. Afr. Med. J., 41:1271, 1967.
9. Berry, J. N., Thompson, H. K., Jr., Miller, D. E., and McIntosh, H. D.: Changes in cardiac output, stroke volume and central venous pressure induced by atropine in man. Amer. Heart J., 58:204, 1959.
10. Binder, M., et al.: Therapy of shock following acute myocardial infarction. Amer. J. Med., 18:622, 1955.
11. Bolooki, H., et al.: Clinical, surgical and pathologic correlation in patients with acute myocardial infarction and pump failure. Circulation, 44:1034, 1971.
12. Bouchard, R. J., Gault, J. H., and Ross, J., Jr.: Evaluation of pulmonary arterial end-diastolic pressure in patients with normal and abnormal left ventricular performance. Circulation, 44:1072, 1971.
13. Bradley, R. D., Jenkins, B. S., and Branthwaite, M. A.: The influence of atrial pressure on cardiac performance following myocardial infarction complicated by shock. Circulation, 42:827, 1970.

14. Branthwaite, M. A., and Bradley, R. D.: Measurement of cardiac output by thermal dilution in man. J. Appl. Physiol., 24:434, 1968.

15. Braunwald, E., Bloodwell, R. D., Goldberg, L. I., and Morrow, A. G.: Studies on digitalis. IV. Observations in man on the effects of digitalis preparations on the contractility of the non-failing heart and on total vascular resistance. J. Clin. Invest., 40:52, 1961.

16. Braunwald, E., et al.: Research on the diagnosis and treatment of myocardial infarction. Calif. Med., 114:44, 1971.

17. Bregman, D., et al.: Clinical experience with the unidirectional dual-chambered intra-aortic balloon assist. Circulation, 43(Suppl. I):82, 1971.

18. Broder, G., and Weil, M. H.: Excess lactate: Index of reversibility of shock in human patients. Science, 143:1457, 1964.

19. Chou, C. C., Rudko, M., and Haddy, F. J.: Effects of hydrocortisone on forelimb resistance responses to vasoactive agents in intact and adrenalectomized dogs. Clin. Res., 16:433, 1968.

20. Christy, J. H.: Treatment of gram-negative shock. Amer. J. Med., 50:77, 1971.

21. Clark, D. A., et al.: Cardiac transplantation in man. VI. Prognosis of patients selected for cardiac transplantation. Ann. Intern. Med., 75:15, 1971.

22. Cohen, L. S., Mullins, C. B., and Mitchell, J. H.: Sequenced external counterpulsation and intra-aortic balloon pumping in cardiogenic shock. Circulation, 42 (Suppl. III):81, 1970.

23. Cohn, J. N.: Blood pressure measurement in shock. Mechanism of inaccuracy in auscultatory and palpatory methods. JAMA, 199:972, 1967.

24. Cohn, J. N., Luria, M. H., Daddario, R. C., and Tristani, F. E.: Studies in clinical shock and hypotension. V. Hemodynamic effects of dextran. Circulation, 35:316, 1967.

25. Cohn, J. N., Tristani, F. E., and Khatri, I. M.: Studies in clinical shock and hypotension. VI. Relationship between left and right ventricular function. J. Clin. Invest., 48:2008, 1969.

26. Cooper, T., and Dempsey, P. J.: Assisted circulation. I, II. Mod. Conc. Cardiov. Dis., 37:95, 1968.

27. Costantin, L.: Extracardiac factors contributing to hypotension during coronary occlusion. Amer. J. Cardiol., 11:205, 1963.

28. Cox, J. L., McLaughlin, V. W., Flowers, N. C., and Horan, L. G.: The ischemic zone surrounding acute myocardial infarction. Its morphology as detected by dehydrogenase staining. Amer. Heart J., 76:650, 1968.

29. Cudkowicz, L.: Effect of l-norepinephrine on left ventricular diastolic pressures in man. Thorax, 23:63, 1968.

30. DeBakey, M. E.: Left ventricular bypass pump for cardiac assistance. Amer. J. Cardiol., 27:3, 1971.

31. Dennis, C.: External counterpulsation as a means to reduce the work of the left ventricle. In: Mechanical Devices to Assist the Failing Heart. Washington, National Academy of Sciences—National Research Council, 1966.

32. Dietzman, R. H., and Lillehei, R. C.: The treatment of cardiogenic shock. V. The use of corticosteroids in the treatment of cardiogenic shock. Amer. Heart J., 75:274, 1968.

33. Edelman, N. H., et al.: Experimental cardiogenic shock: Pulmonary performance after acute myocardial infarction. Amer. J. Physiol., 219:1723, 1970.

34. Entman, M. L., et al.: Phasic myocardial blood flow in hemorrhagic hypotension. Amer. J. Cardiol., 21:881, 1968.

35. Epstein, S. E., Robinson, B. F., Kahler, R. L., and Braunwald, E.: Effects of beta-adrenergic blockade on the cardiac response to maximal and submaximal exercise in man. J. Clin. Invest., 44:1745, 1965.

36. Euler, U. S. von: Noradrenaline: Chemistry, Physiology, Pharmacology and Clinical Aspects. Springfield, Charles C Thomas, 1956.

37. Favaloro, R. G., et al.: Ventricular aneurysm —clinical experience. Ann. Thorac. Surg., 6:227, 1968.

38. Fearon, R. E.: Comparison of norepinephrine and isoproterenol in experimental coronary shock. Amer. Heart J., 75:634, 1968.

39. Fordham, R. M. M., and Resnekov, L.: Arterial hypoxemia, a side effect of intravenous isoprenaline used after cardiac surgery. Thorax, 23:19, 1968.

40. Forrester, J. S., et al.: Silent mitral insufficiency in acute myocardial infarction. Circulation, 44:877, 1971.

41. Forrester, J. S., Diamond, G., McHugh, T. J., and Swan, H. J. C.: Filling pressures in the right and left sides of the heart in acute myocardial infarction. New Eng. J. Med., 285:190, 1971.

42. Foster, G. L., Casten, G. G., and Reeves, T. J.: The effects of oxygen breathing in patients with acute myocardial infarction. Cardiov. Res., 3:179, 1969.

43. Friedman, E., Grable, E., and Fine, J.: Central venous pressure and direct serial measurements as guides in blood-volume replacement. Lancet, 2:609, 1966.

44. Ganz, W. W., et al.: A new flow-directed catheter technique for measurement of pulmonary artery and capillary wedge pressures without fluoroscopy. Amer. J. Cardiol., 25:96, 1970.

45. Gensini, G. G., Dubiel, J., Huntington, P. P., and Kelly, M. S.: Left ventricular end-diastolic pressure before and after coronary arteriography. Amer. J. Cardiol., 27:453, 1971.

46. Gianelly, R., von der Groeben, J. O., Spivack, A. P., and Harrison, D. C.: Effect of lidocaine on ventricular arrhythmias in patients with coronary heart disease. New Eng. J. Med., 277:1215, 1967.
47. Goldman, R. H., et al.: Measurement of central venous oxygen saturation in patients with myocardial infarction. Circulation, 38:941, 1968.
48. Gregg, D. E., and Fisher, L. C.: Blood supply to the heart. In: Handbook of Physiology, Vol. II, Section 2. Baltimore, American Physiological Society, 1962.
49. Gurin, S., and Delluva, A.: The biologic synthesis of radioactive adrenalin from phenylalanine. J. Biol. Chem., 170:545, 1947.
50. Hamosh, P., and Cohn, J. N.: Left ventricular function in acute myocardial infarction. J. Clin. Invest., 50:523, 1971.
51. Hardaway, R. M., et al.: Influence of vasoconstrictors and vasodilators on disseminated intravascular coagulation in irreversible hemorrhagic shock. Surgery, 119:1053, 1964.
52. Hardaway, R. M., et al.: Intensive study and treatment of shock in man. JAMA, 199:779, 1967.
53. Harnarayan, C., Bennett, M. A., Pentecost, B. L., and Brewer, D. B.: Quantitative study of infarcted myocardium in cardiogenic shock. Brit. Heart J., 32:728, 1970.
54. Harrison, D. C., Chidsey, C. A., and Braunwald, E.: Studies on the mechanism of action of metaraminol (Aramine). Ann. Intern. Med., 59:297, 1965.
55. Harrison, D. C., Isaeff, D., and DeBusk, R. F.: Papillary muscle syndromes. In: Disease-a-month. Chicago, Yearbook Medical Publishers, 1972.
56. Hayden, W., and Kriss, J.: Radionuclide coronary arteriography in man using 99mTc-pertechnetate and 43K-chloride. In preparation.
57. Heikkila, J.: Mitral incompetence as a complication of acute myocardial infarction. Acta Med. Scand., Suppl. 475, 1967.
58. Heimbecker, R. O., and Chen, C.: Surgery for acute myocardial infarction: An experimental study of emergency infarctectomy, with a preliminary report on the clinical application. Circulation, 36 (Suppl. II):138, 1967.
59. Herman, M. V., and Gorlin, R.: Implications of left ventricular asynergy. Amer. J. Cardiol., 23:538, 1969.
60. Hift, H., and Strawitz, J. G.: Structure and function of mitochondria in reversible hemorrhagic shock. II. Proc. Soc. Exp. Biol. Med., 98:235, 1958.
61. Holden, W. D., DePalma, R. G., Drucker, W. R., and McKalen, A.: Ultrastructural changes in hemorrhagic shock: Electron microscopic study of liver, kidney and striated muscle cells in rats. Ann. Surg., 162:517, 1965.
62. Hood, W. B., Jr., McCarthy, B., and Lown, B.: Myocardial infarction following coronary ligation in dogs: Hemodynamic effects of isoproterenol and acetylstrophanthidin. Circ. Res., 21:191, 1967.
63. Iben, A. B., Pupello, D. F., Stinson, E. B., and Shumway, N. E.: Surgical treatment of postinfarction ventricular septal defects. Ann. Thorac. Surg., 8:252, 1969.
64. Jacobey, J. A.: Results of counterpulsation in patients with coronary artery disease. Amer. J. Cardiol., 27:137, 1971.
65. Jacobey, J. A., Taylor, W. J., and Smith, G. T.: A new therapeutic approach to acute coronary occlusion. II. Opening dormant coronary collateral channels by counter pulsation. Amer. J. Cardiol., 11:218, 1963.
66. Janoff, A., Weissman, G., Zweifach, B. W., and Thomas L.: Pathogenesis of experimental shock. IV. Studies on lysosomes in normal and tolerant animals subjected to lethal trauma and endotoxemia. J. Exp. Med., 116:451, 1962.
67. Janoff, A., and Zeligs, J. D.: Vascular injury and lysis of basement membrane in vitro by neutral protease of human leukocytes. Science, 161:702, 1968.
68. Joseph, W. L., and Maloney, J. V., Jr.: Extracorporeal circulation as an adjunct to resuscitation of the heart. JAMA, 193:683, 1965.
69. Kaltman, A. J., Herbert, W. H., Conroy, R. J., and Kossman, C. E.: Gradient in pressure across the pulmonary vascular bed during diastole. Circulation, 34:377, 1966.
70. Kantrowitz, A., et al.: Phase-shift balloon pumping in medically refractory cardiogenic shock. Arch. Surg., 99:739, 1969.
71. Kezdi, P., et al.: The role of vagal afferents in acute myocardial infarction. Amer. J. Cardiol., 26:642, 1970.
72. Krakauer, J. S., et al.: Clinical management ancillary to phase-shift balloon pumping in cardiogenic shock. Amer. J. Cardiol., 27:123, 1971.
73. Kumar, R., et al.: Experimental myocardial infarction: X. Efficacy of glucagon on acute and healing phase in intact conscious dogs: effects on hemodynamics and myocardial oxygen consumption. Circulation, 45:55, 1972.
74. Kurland, G. S., and Freedberg, A. S.: Potentiating effect of ACTH and of cortisone on pressor response to intravenous infusions of l-norepinephrine. Proc. Soc. Exp. Biol. Med., 78:28, 1951.
75. Lefer, A. M.: Role of a myocardial depressant factor in the pathogenesis of circulatory shock. Fed. Proc., 29:1836, 1970.
76. Lefer, A. M., Manwaring, J. L., and Verrier, R. L.: Effect of corticosteroids on the cardiovascular responses to angiotensin and norepinephrine. J. Pharmacol. Exp. Ther., 154:83, 1961.

77. Leinbach, R. C., et al.: Effects of intra-aortic balloon pumping on coronary flow and metabolism in man. Circulation, *43* (Suppl. I):77, 1971.

78. Lillehei, R. C., Dietzman, R. H., and Movsas, S.: Treatment of septic shock. Mod. Treatm., *4*:321, 1967.

79. Lillehei, R. C., Longerbeam, J. K., Bloch, J., and Manax, W. G.: The nature of irreversible shock: Experimental and clinical observations. Ann. Surg., *160*:682, 1964.

80. Loeb, H. S., et al.: Acute hemodynamic effects of dopamine in patients with shock. Circulation, *44*:163, 1971.

81. Lown, B., Fakhro, A. M., Hood, W. B., Jr., and Thorn, G. W.: The coronary care unit. JAMA, *199*:188, 1967.

82. MacCannell, K. L., McNay, J. L., Meyer, M. B., and Goldberg, L. I.: Dopamine in the treatment of hypotension and shock. New Eng. J. Med., *275*:1389, 1966.

83. MacKenzie, G. J., et al.: Circulatory and respiratory studies in myocardial infarction and cardiogenic shock. Lancet, *2*:825, 1964.

84. McDonald, R. H., Jr., Goldberg, L. D., McNay, J. L., and Tuttle, G. P., Jr.: Effects of dopamine in man: Augmentation of sodium excretion, glomerular filtration rate, and renal plasma flow. J. Clin. Invest., *43*:1116, 1964.

85. McNay, J. L., McDonald, R. H., Jr., and Goldberg, L. I.: Direct renal vasodilation produced by dopamine in the dog. Circ. Res., *16*:510, 1965.

86. Martin, A. M., and Hackel, D. B.: An electron microscopic study of the progression of myocardial lesions in the dog after hemorrhagic shock. Lab. Invest., *15*:243, 1966.

87. Mead, J., and Collier, C.: Relation of volume history of lungs to respiratory mechanics in anesthetized dogs. J. Appl. Physiol., *14*:669, 1959.

88. Moran, N. C.: Evaluation of the pharmacologic basis for the therapy of circulatory shock. Amer. J. Cardiol., *26*:570, 1970.

89. Moulopoulos, S. D., Topaz, S., and Kolff, W. J.: Diastolic balloon pumping (with carbon dioxide) in the aorta: Mechanical assistance to the failing circulation. Amer. Heart J., *63*:669, 1962.

90. Mueller, H., et al.: The effects of intra-aortic counterpulsation on cardiac performance and metabolism in shock associated with acute myocardial infarction. J. Clin. Invest., *50*:1885, 1971.

91. Mueller, H., et al.: Hemodynamics, coronary blood flow and myocardial metabolism in coronary shock; response to *l*-norepinephrine and isoproterenol. J. Clin. Invest., *49*:1885, 1970.

92. Mundth, E. D., et al.: Myocardial revascularization for the treatment of cardiogenic shock complicating acute myocardial infarction. Surgery, *70*:78, 1971.

93. Nies, A. S., Forsyth, R. P., Williams, H. E., and Melmon, K. L.: Contribution of kinins to endotoxin shock in unanesthetized rhesus monkeys. Circ. Res., *22*:155, 1968.

94. Nixon, P. G. F., Taylor, D. J. E., and Morton, S. D.: Left ventricular diastolic pressure in cardiogenic shock treated by dextrose infusion and adrenaline. Lancet, *1*:1230, 1968.

95. Oriol, A., and McGregor, M.: Indicator-dilution methods in estimation of cardiac output in clinical shock. Amer. J. Cardiol., *20*:826, 1967.

96. Page, D. L., et al.: Myocardial changes associated with cardiogenic shock. New Eng. J. Med., *285*:133, 1971.

97. Parmley, W. W., Glick, G., and Sonnenblick, E.: Cardiovascular effects of glucagon in man. New Eng. J. Med., *279*:12, 1968.

98. Peretz, D. I., et al.: The significance of lacticacidemia in the shock syndrome. Ann. N.Y. Acad. Sci., *119*:1133, 1965.

99. Perlroth, M. G., and Harrison, D. C.: Cardiogenic shock: A review. Clin. Pharmacol. Ther., *10*:449, 1969.

100. Popp, R. L., and Harrison, D. C.: Ultrasonic cardiac echography for determining stroke volume and valvular regurgitation. Circulation, *41*:493, 1970.

101. Puri, P. S., and Bing, R. J.: Effects of drugs on myocardial contractility in the intact dog and in experimental myocardial infarction: Basis for their use in cardiogenic shock. Amer. J. Cardiol., *21*:886, 1968.

102. Quinn, J. L., III, Serratto, M., and Kardi, T.: Coronary artery bed photoscanning using radioiodine albumin macroaggregates (RAMA). J. Nucl. Med., *7*:107, 1966.

103. Rackley, C. E., and Russell, R. O., Jr.: Left ventricular function in acute myocardial infarction and its clinical significance. Circulation, *45*:231, 1972.

104. Ratshin, R. A., Rackley, C. E., and Russell, R. O., Jr.: Hemodynamic evaluation of left ventricular function in shock complicating myocardial infarction. Circulation, *45*:127, 1972.

105. Regan, T. J., et al.: Influence of scar on left ventricular performance at the onset of myocardial ischemia: Shock versus heart failure. J. Clin. Invest., *50*:534, 1971.

106. Reichenbach, D. D., and Benditt, E. P.: Catecholamines and cardiomyopathy: The pathogenesis and potential importance of myofibrillar degeneration. Hum. Path., *1*:125, 1970.

107. Rosensweig, J., Chatterjee, S., and Merino, F.: Treatment of acute myocardial infarction by counterpulsation. J. Thorac. Cardiov. Surg., *59*:243, 1970.

108. Ross, J., Jr.: Left ventricular contraction and the therapy of cardiogenic shock. Circulation, *35*:611, 1967.

109. Ross, J., Jr., Frahm, C. J., and Braunwald, E.: The influence of intra-cardiac baroreceptors on venous return, systemic vascular volume and peripheral resistance. J. Clin. Invest., *40*:563, 1961.

110. Rosselot, E., et al.: Venoarterial pulsatile circulatory assist in the treatment of resistant ventricular fibrillation. Amer. J. Cardiol., 27:46, 1971.

111. Sanders, C. A., Buckley, M. J., and Austen, W. G.: Mechanical circulatory assistance: Current status. New Eng. J. Med., 285:348, 1971.

112. Sanders, R. J., Neubuerger, K. T., and Ravin, A.: Rupture of papillary muscles: Occurrence of rupture of posterior muscle in posterior myocardial infarction. Dis. Chest, 37: 316, 1957.

113. Sandler, H., and Dodge, H. T.: Left ventricular tension and stress in man. Circ. Res., 13: 91, 1963.

114. Sarnoff, S. J., and Berglund, E.: Ventricular function. I. Starling's law of the heart studied by means of simultaneous right and left ventricular function curves in the dog. Circulation, 9:706, 1954.

115. Sarnoff, S. J., et al.: Hemodynamic determinants of oxygen consumption of the heart with special reference to the tension-time index. Amer. J. Physiol., 192:148, 1958.

116. Sarnoff, S. J., and Mitchell, J. H.: The control of the function of the heart. In: Handbook of Physiology, Vol. I, Section 2. Baltimore, American Physiological Society, 1962.

117. Scheidt, S., Ascheim, R., and Killip, T.: Shock after acute myocardial infarction. Amer. J. Cardiol., 26:556, 1970.

118. Schroll, M., Robison, S. C., and Harrison, D. C.: Circulatory responses to hypoxia in experimental myocardial infarction. Cardiov. Res., 5:498, 1971.

119. Shillingford, J. P., and Thomas, M.: Acute myocardial infarction, hypotension and shock: Their pathological physiology and therapy. Mod. Conc. Cardiov. Dis., 36:13, 1967.

120. Shubin, H., and Weil, M. H.: Failure of corticosteroid to potentiate sympathomimetic pressor response during shock. JAMA, 197: 808, 1966.

121. Shubin, H., and Weil, M. H.: Practical considerations in the management of shock complicating acute myocardial infarction. Amer. J. Cardiol., 26:603, 1970.

122. Skinner, D. B.: Experimental and clinical evaluations of mechanical ventricular assistance. Amer. J. Cardiol., 27:146, 1971.

123. Sonnenblick, E. H., Ross, J., and Braunwald, E.: Oxygen consumption of the heart, newer concepts of its multifactorial determination. Amer. J. Cardiol., 23:328, 1968.

124. Sonnenblick, E. H., Jr., et al.: Velocity of contraction as a determinant of myocardial oxygen consumption. Amer. J. Physiol., 209:919, 1965.

125. Strawitz, J. G., and Hift, H.: Structure and function of mitochondria in reversible hemorrhagic shock. I. Proc. Soc. Exp. Biol. Med., 91:641, 1956.

126. Summers, D. N., et al.: Intra-aortic balloon pumping. Arch. Surg., 99:733, 1969.

127. Tanaka, T., and Sakakibara, S.: The direct diagnosis of human myocardial ischemia using ^{131}I-MAA via the selective coronary catheter. Amer. Heart J., 80:498, 1970.

128. Trinkle, J. K., and Bryant, L. R.: Mechanical support of the circulation: A new approach. Arch. Surg., 101:740, 1970.

129. Weil, M. H., Shubin, J., and Biddle, M.: Shock caused by gram-negative micro-organisms. Analysis of 169 cases. Ann. Intern. Med., 60: 384, 1964.

130. Weissmann, G., and Thomas, L.: Studies on lysosomes. I. The effects of endotoxin, endotoxin tolerance, and cortisone on release of acid hydrolases from a granular fraction of rabbit liver. J. Exp. Med., 116:433, 1962.

131. Williams, J. R., Klocke, F. J., and Braunwald, E.: Studies on digitalis. XIII. Comparison of the effects of potassium on the inotropic and arrhythmia producing actions of ouabain. J. Clin. Invest., 45:346, 1968.

132. Wilson, R. F., Jablonski, D. V., and Thal, A. P.: The usage of dibenzyline in clinical shock. Surgery, 56:172, 1964.

133. Wintroub, B., et al.: Hemodynamic response to dopamine in experimental myocardial infarction. Amer. J. Physiol., 217:1716, 1969.

134. Zaret, B. L., et al. A noninvasive scintiphotographic method for detecting regional ventricular dysfunction in man. New Eng. J. Med., 284:1165, 1971.

Chapter 9

SUBSTRATE UTILIZATION BY EXERCISING MUSCLE IN MAN*

John Wahren, M.D.

Muscle tissue accounts for some 40 per cent of the body weight of the average man. Even in the resting state, as much as 40 per cent of the body's oxygen consumption occurs in skeletal muscle; during physical exercise the percentage is considerably higher. The requirements of muscle, particularly during exercise, are thus a major determinant of the body's total energy metabolism. Thus the nature and sources of the fuel used by muscle are highly relevant for an understanding of physical performance and its limitations under different conditions.

The basic concepts of substrate utilization by skeletal muscle have been revised drastically in recent decades. Not long ago carbohydrate substrates were considered the predominant, if not the only, fuel used for the generation of energy required for muscular work. This view, however, has been modified by a growing awareness of the physiological importance of plasma free fatty acids (FFA). Direct measurements with the use of biopsy techniques and isotopic tracers, determina-

tions of organ or tissue blood flows and arteriovenous (A–V) concentration differences of substrates have facilitated a more detailed understanding of the changing patterns of substrate utilization in a variety of physiological conditions.

This review, which does not claim to be comprehensive, is concerned with the description and evaluation of recent studies on fuel utilization by exercising muscle, with the emphasis on quantitative human data. Unless otherwise stated, the studies discussed below have been performed in the post-absorptive state after 12 to 14 hours of fasting. However, it should be recognized that as man proceeds from the fed to the adapted fasting state, important biochemical and hormonal changes occur by which a continuous supply of fuel is maintained to meet metabolic expenditures. Since the adaptation to fasting proceeds for several days, exercise studies after only 12 to 14 hours of fasting involve two superimposed states—the transition from the fed to the fasting state and the metabolic response to exercise—which may be of consequence for the interpretation of results

* Supported by Grants 19X-722 and 19X-3108 from the Swedish Medical Research Council.

from studies including prolonged periods of exercise.

CARBOHYDRATE METABOLISM

Carbohydrate Stores

Table 1 summarizes the estimated substrate depots in normal man. The amount of free glucose in the body is small (about 20 gm) and unevenly distributed, being limited to extracellular water and the intracellular compartment of the liver cells. In the resting basal state, the dominant glucose-consuming tissue is the brain, while the liver is the sole organ producing quantitatively important amounts of glucose.[17] The hepatic glucose output derives from glycogenolysis (75 to 80 per cent) and de novo synthesis from glucose precursors such as lactate, pyruvate, glycerol and amino acids, taken up from the blood.

The hepatic glycogen concentration in subjects ingesting a mixed diet is reported to be approximately 50 gm/kg wet tissue.[75] Assuming a liver weight of 1500 to 1800 gm, the total glycogen store in the liver is 75 to 90 gm. This substrate depot has an important function in the body's adjustment to energy requirements. After 10 to 12 hours of fasting, mobilization of liver glycogen— to maintain the blood glucose level—proceeds at a rate of approximately 50 mg/min per kg

liver.[75] As discussed below, this rate accelerates substantially during physical exertion. Although we do not know just how large a part of the liver glycogen is available for mobilization during exercise, the fact that the liver is almost entirely depleted after a week on a carbohydrate-free diet[75] suggests the possibility that the major part can be utilized during exercise, too. The liver depot of glycogen refills relatively slowly, 12 to 36 hours (depending on diet and physical activity) being required for full restitution after a period of severe exercise. When a carbohydrate-rich diet is ingested after an exercise period, the liver glycogen content recovers to levels which exceed the control value.[75]

The introduction of a needle-biopsy technique by Bergström,[12] by which repeated samples can be obtained from the lateral portion of the quadriceps femoris muscle in man, has opened up a particularly fruitful research area in that sequential changes in muscle composition can be followed. This technique has been used in numerous studies of local energy metabolism during exercise in man, showing that the content of glycogen in muscle is approximately 9 to 16 gm/kg wet muscle; the values are lowest in arm and shoulder muscles and highest in samples from the lower extremities.[71] The muscle glycogen concentration does not seem to vary with

Table 1. Estimated Substrate Depots in Normal Man

Fuel	Weight (kg)	Energy (kcal)
Tissues		
Fat (adipose triglycerides)	15	141,000
Protein (mostly muscle)	6	24,000
Glycogen (muscle)	0.350	1,400
Glycogen (liver)	0.085	340
		166,740
Circulating fuels		
Glucose (extracellular water)	0.020	80
Free fatty acids (plasma)	0.0004	4
Triglycerides (plasma)	0.003	30
		114

either age or sex. Assuming that the total muscle mass accounts for approximately 40 per cent of body weight, the glycogen depot in skeletal muscle can be estimated to be 300 to 400 gm, making this the largest carbohydrate store of the body. This estimate agrees quite well with indirect evaluations based on determination of respiratory quotient (RQ) and prolonged exhaustive exercise.[25]

The muscle glycogen content does not vary under resting basal conditions and decreases only slowly during prolonged fasting.[72] Physical exercise is the major physiological means by which muscle glycogen is utilized, as discussed below. Muscle tissue lacks glucose-6-phosphatase[89] and, since there is no hydrolysis of phosphorylated glycolytic intermediary metabolites, quantitatively significant amounts of glucose do not leave muscle either at rest or during exercise. Consequently, only the local glycogen store of the exercising muscle can be utilized as fuel; the glycogen content of a resting muscle does not change even when other muscle groups are exercised to exhaustion.[15]

Recent studies have emphasized the profound differences in muscle glycogen restitution after exercise in subjects ingesting different diets. A diet rich in carbohydrate greatly enhances glycogen resynthesis after exercise; the glycogen content recovers to a peak higher than the preexercise level, an overshoot that is confined to the glycogen-depleted muscle.[73] With a diet consisting mainly of protein and fat, on the other hand, the resynthesis of glycogen after rigorous exercise is greatly delayed.[2,13]

The key enzyme in the regulation of glycogen synthesis is glycogen synthetase, of which there are two forms, one (D form) being dependent and the other (I form) independent of glucose-6-phosphate for its activity.[30,124] It is widely accepted that most physiological alterations involving accelerated glycogen synthesis can be explained by increased activity of the I-form synthetase. However, this does not seem to apply either to the increase in glycogen synthesis following a

period of exercise or to the overshoot in muscle glycogen content observed on a carbohydrate-rich diet.[14,15,71] Although glycogen resynthesis clearly depends on substrate availability as well as on the I-form synthetase, a more detailed understanding of the mechanisms behind the above phenomena will have to await further investigation.

The blood glucose pool, the glycogen stored in the liver and the glycogen in muscle are thus the quantitatively important depots of carbohydrate. Their relative importance for providing fuel during exercise depends on the type and duration of the exercise performed. Although muscle glycogen is the largest depot, its use is limited to its site, whereas the smaller store of liver glycogen is mobilized to the blood and can thus be delivered to the muscle actually engaged in exercise.

Muscle Glycogen Utilization

Although it has long been known that muscle glycogen is utilized during exercise, it was thought until recently that this was mainly for anaerobic metabolism and the production of lactate. While it is true that the lactate produced at the onset of exercise, as well as that formed during very strenuous exertion, is likely to be derived from glycogen, the metabolic fate of the glucosyl units of muscle glycogen is mainly terminal oxidation. The important role of glycogen in aerobic muscle metabolism was identified by Bergström and Hultman,[14] and much work has subsequently been devoted to characterizing the utilization of muscle glycogen under different physiological conditions.

There appear to be two main determinants of glycogen consumption during exercise: the duration and the intensity of the work performed. Concerning duration, it has been found that the glycogen content of muscle decreases in a curvilinear fashion during prolonged submaximal exercise[65,72] (Fig. 1). At the onset of work there is a rapid initial decline in concentration, accompanied by a sharp increase in blood lactate levels.

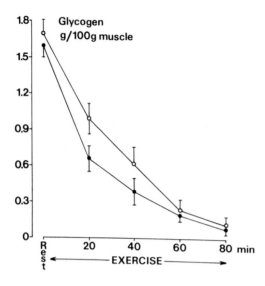

Fig. 1. Glycogen content of the lateral portion of the quadriceps muscle at rest and during exercise in groups of trained (○—○) and untrained (●—●) individuals (mean ±SE). (Data kindly furnished by Dr. B. Saltin.)

After 5 to 10 minutes of exercise, the rate of glycogen utilization slows down, possibly because circulatory adaptation to exercise makes other substrates available to the muscle. As exercise proceeds beyond 60 to 90 minutes the rate of glycogen utilization drops still further; there is now a relative lack of muscle glycogen and the consumption of substrates taken up from the blood gradually increases.

The effect of work intensity on the rate of glycogenolysis in exercising muscle has been demonstrated indirectly[27] as well as by direct measurements of muscle glycogen consumption. The rate of muscle glycogen consumption displays a curvilinear relationship to work load both for dynamic work[65] and for isometric contractions.[5] The rise in the rate of utilization is more pronounced at heavier work loads. The most rapid rate of muscle glycogenolysis is seen during short-term heavy isometric contractions, when the rates may be ten times those recorded during heavy dynamic work.[5]

Subjects exercising at heavy work loads generally have to desist at about the time the glycogen content of muscle approaches zero. Studies in subjects with differing muscle glycogen contents (as a result of ingesting carbohydrate-rich or protein- and fat-rich diets) have illustrated how the size of the carbohydrate stores affects the capacity to perform heavy work.[2,13,80] The initial glycogen content of muscle correlates closely with the subject's capacity to tolerate prolonged, heavy, bicycle exercise, and it has been suggested that the size of the glycogen depot in muscle is a limiting factor here. It is still not clear, however, why glycogen depletion should coincide with fatigue, when large amounts of substrate in the form of fatty acids are still available. The associations among glycogen depletion, fatigue and reduced physical working capacity have been debated recently: in a study of glycogen utilization rates in selected leg muscles[29] it was found that prolonged treadmill runs elicited fatigue even though the level of glycogen in the quadriceps, gastrocnemius and soleus muscles was still substantial.

These studies were performed in the post-absorptive, basal state. As some form of nutrition, usually rich in carbohydrate, is often taken in connection with heavy daily exercise or athletics, it would be of interest to know whether less glycogen is used during exercise if extra glucose is supplied. The data available suggest that this is not the case with heavy exercise lasting 30 to 60 minutes. At a lower work load, however, the infusion of glucose significantly reduces glycogen consumption.[3,4] Similarly, the administration of nicotinic acid to inhibit the mobilization of FFA from adipose tissue[19] is associated with an augmented utilization of muscle glycogen during work, particularly during the latter part of a 90-minute exercise period.[16] Thus it can be concluded that, although glycogen utilization plays an important and at times a dominant role in aerobic muscle metabolism, its rate of consumption is modified to a certain extent by alterations in the supply of blood-borne fuels.

Blood Glucose Turnover

GLUCOSE UPTAKE BY MUSCLE

It is generally recognized that blood glucose is taken up to some extent by exercising muscle in man, but its quantitative importance in total substrate utilization by muscle and the relationships between blood glucose utilization and the duration or intensity of work have long been controversial. Recent studies have shed some light on these matters and will be discussed below.

The forearm is a useful experimental model for quantitative metabolic studies inasmuch as it permits the accurate measurement of both brachial artery blood flow[119] and A-V differences in the metabolites utilized or produced by forearm muscle tissue, thus allowing quantitative determinations of the net uptake or production of the metabolites in question. This experimental model has accordingly been used in several studies of the glucose metabolism of skeletal muscle, both at rest and during exercise.

At rest, glucose shows a small positive A-V difference across the forearm.[8,120] At the onset of exercise this difference is reduced and after 1 to 2 minutes it is reversed, indicating a net release of glucose from the forearm.[79,120] Similar observations have been reported for stimulated dog skeletal muscle during tetanus.[28] Since the enzyme glucose-6-phosphatase is absent in muscle tissue[89] the mechanism behind this finding probably does not involve hydrolysis of glucose-6-phosphate. Some clues may be provided by the breakdown pattern of glycogen, in which most of the glycosyl units are converted to glucose phosphate by the action of myophosphorylase, but where debranching of the glycogen molecules (catalyzed by amylo-1,6-glucosidase and oligo-1,4-1,4-glucantransferase) involves the formation of free glucose corresponding to 8 to 10 per cent of the glycogen.[39] During conditions of low to moderate rates of glycogenolysis this glucose is probably phosphorylated rapidly in the hexokinase reaction, whereas during heavy exercise with very rapid glycogen degradation increased amounts of glucose will be formed at a time when the hexokinase reaction may be operating slowly or not at all; this is due in part to inhibition by accumulating glucose-6-phosphate[28,110] and in part to substrate deficiency as a consequence of lowered levels of adenosine triphosphate (ATP). Under such circumstances it is conceivable that glucose transport across the cell membrane into the cell is slowed down and actually reversed. This transient release of glucose to the blood is quantitatively insignificant, but the observation may help explain the divergent results reported for glucose uptake by muscle during exercise in man; it emphasizes the importance of relating such measurements both to the duration and to the intensity of the exercise performed.

After the initial phase of exercise there is a net uptake of glucose to the forearm muscles.[79] The A-V difference for glucose then increases gradually during a 60-minute exercise period. At the same time there is a small rise in blood flow to the forearm. Quantitative calculations show that net glucose uptake by the forearm has increased 15 times above the resting value after 10 minutes of exercise and as much as 35 times after 60 minutes.

Glucose participation in the carbohydrate and total oxidative metabolism of forearm muscles can be estimated on the basis of the local RQ and the A-V differences for oxygen, glucose and lactate.[49] Such calculations show that under resting conditions carbohydrate oxidation plays a minor role, free fatty acids being the dominant fuel. After 10 minutes of exercise this situation has altered: the major part of the oxygen uptake is now being used for carbohydrate oxidation, about half of which can be accounted for by the glucose uptake. Glycogen breakdown is probably quite rapid at this time and could contribute the remaining carbohydrate substrate. At the end of a 60-minute exercise period the situation has changed again: the RQ value indicates that about half of the oxidative metabolism is now carbohydrate combustion, and the entire carbohydrate oxidation can be accounted for by the uptake of glucose from the blood.[79] Thus, glycogen utilization does not constitute a significant energy supply to the exercising muscle at this time.

Because of the small muscle volume involved, glucose utilization during prolonged forearm exercise does not substantially challenge the blood glucose homeostasis. During exercise with large muscle groups, however, total glucose turnover increases markedly[107] and an augmented hepatic production[113] is needed to maintain the arterial blood glucose concentration. In a study of healthy individuals exercising on a bicycle ergometer at work loads of 400, 800 and 1200 kpm/min, the arterial levels of glucose were unchanged or moderately increased during a 40-minute exercise period[121] (Fig. 2). At all levels of work intensity the A-V difference for glucose and the leg blood flow both increased, indicating that exercise markedly augmented net glucose uptake by the leg. The magnitude of this augmentation may be estimated from the product of leg blood flow and the A-V difference for glucose, according to which net glucose uptake by the leg increases 7-fold above the resting value

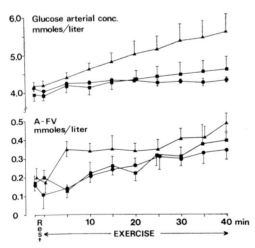

Fig. 2. Arterial glucose concentrations and arterio-femoral venous (A-FV) glucose differences at rest and during exercise at work loads of 400 (●), 800 (■) and 1200 (▲) kpm/min (mean ± SE).

after 40 minutes of light exercise (400 kpm/min) and 10- and 20-fold at work intensities of 800 and 1200 kpm/min, respectively (Fig. 2). Leg muscle uptake showed a gradual increase during the course of exercise, in keeping with the observations from forearm exercise. For leg exercise, blood glucose oxidation accounts for a growing fraction of both total and carbohydrate oxidation of the leg during progressive exercise at all levels of work intensity, thereby substituting in part for the gradually diminishing endogenous muscle stores of carbohydrate. Muscle glycogen is likely to be the dominant carbohydrate substrate during the initial phase of exercise, but the utilization of blood glucose thus rises steadily with time. After 40 minutes of exercise, blood glucose can (assuming that the glucose taken up by the leg muscles is completely oxidized) sustain as much as 75 to 90 per cent of the carbohydrate metabolism and 28 to 37 per cent of the total oxidative metabolism of the leg.[121] It can thus be concluded that during exercise with the large muscle groups of the leg, as in the case of rhythmic work with the forearm flexors, blood glucose is a quantitatively important substrate for muscle oxidation.

It seems clear that the above rates of hepatic glucose production can be maintained for only a limited period of time. From the findings for exercise at 1200 kpm/min[121] it can be estimated that after an hour's exercise about 30 gm glycogen of the 75 to 90 gm available in the liver have been mobilized. The remaining hepatic glycogen store may thus suffice for 1 to 1½ hours of continued exercise at this work load, after which the subject will either become more dependent on utilization of fat-derived substrates or face hypoglycemia.

Glucose turnover is also augmented during very prolonged forms of exercise. Twice the basal turnover was found in healthy subjects who walked on a treadmill for 13 hours at a rate which caused their oxygen uptake to rise to a third of the maximal value.[125] Since the hepatic glycogen stores are insufficient to maintain this rate of glucose turnover for as long as 13 hours, an increased rate of hepatic gluconeogenesis must be postulated for this type of work. In keeping with this hypothesis, the study showed an accelerated incorporation of labeled lactate into blood glucose.[125]

It has been claimed on the basis of indirect evidence that part of the increased uptake of blood glucose to the exercising muscles is provided for by a reduced uptake to inactive muscle and brain, and even by an actual liberation from nonexercising muscle.[58,115] Subsequent studies have failed to confirm these findings. The cerebral glucose uptake remains unchanged during an hour's exercise at a work load sufficient substantially to augment the glucose uptake by exercising muscle.[7] Moreover, during one-leg exercise the net glucose uptake to the inactive leg is slightly increased or unchanged, and in no instance was release of glucose to the blood detectable.[6]

With respect to the mechanism of the rise in glucose uptake to muscle during exercise, it is noteworthy that the plasma insulin concentration falls significantly in conjunction with exercise.[76,121] The opposite responses of circulating glucose and insulin, particularly with strenuous exercise, suggest that insulin secretion is in fact inhibited during physical work, perhaps as a consequence of increased liberation of catecholamines.[77] It has been postulated that exercise-induced hypoinsulinemia serves to limit blood glucose uptake by muscle, thereby increasing its availability to the brain,[104] but this is not supported by more recent data which demonstrate that increased muscle glucose uptake during exercise does not depend on ability to secrete increased quantities of insulin.[121]

HEPATIC GLUCOSE PRODUCTION DURING EXERCISE

From the data presented above it is apparent that the turnover of the glucose pool accelerates to a varying but significant extent during exercise with large muscle groups.

This suggests that, since the arterial glucose concentration is maintained or even increased during strenuous exertion, the pool is replenished continuously during exercise. The kidney can synthesize significant amounts of glucose, particularly in the prolonged fasted state,[96] but no renal glucose production can be detected from direct measurements during exercise.[121] Since the liver is the only other organ capable of significant gluconeogenesis and since muscle glycogenolysis, in the absence of glucose-6-phosphatase in muscle, is unlikely to contribute significantly to the blood glucose level, it can be concluded that hepatic glucose mobilization is the dominant and probably the sole source of the increased amounts of glucose utilized during exercise.

Direct measurements with the hepatic venous-catheter technique have in fact demonstrated an increased production of glucose during physical exercise[15,113] (Fig. 3). The importance of hepatic glucose production for blood glucose homeostasis during physical work and as a substrate for exercising muscle is underscored by the recently demonstrated close agreement between estimated rates of glucose uptake by leg muscle and splanchnic glucose release[121] (Fig. 4). Splanchnic glucose output greatly exceeds leg uptake in the resting state, since it is the brain which

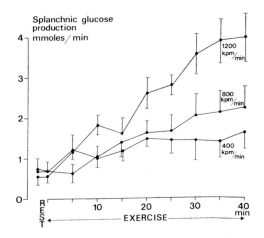

Fig. 3. Comparison of estimated glucose uptake by the legs and splanchnic glucose output in subjects at rest and after 40 minutes of exercise at different work intensities (mean ± SE).

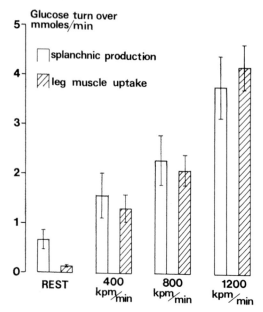

Fig. 4. Estimated splanchnic glucose production at rest and during exercise at different work loads (mean ± SE).

accounts for the major part of total glucose utilization in the basal postabsorptive state. With increasing physical activity the brain's share of total glucose turnover diminishes and splanchnic output corresponds more and more closely to leg glucose uptake.

Theoretically possible rates of hepatic gluconeogenesis, assuming maximum conversion efficiency, can be estimated from the splanchnic uptake of the gluconeogenic substrates lactate, pyruvate, glycerol and glucogenic amino acids. Available data indicate that at rest approximately 20 to 25 per cent of the glucose output may have been derived from these glucose precursors, some 16 per cent from lactate and pyruvate.[36,108] During exercise total substrate extraction by the liver increases at first, primarily as a result of augmented uptake of lactate. As exercise proceeds the hepatic output of glucose rises gradually, whereas the total uptake of glucose precursors remains mainly unchanged at low work intensities and diminishes at heavy work loads, primarily because of a fall in the splanchnic uptake of lactate.[121] Accordingly,

the possible contribution from hepatic gluconeogenesis falls during continued heavy exercise, accounting for perhaps 6 to 11 per cent of total glucose output after 40 minutes of exercise. It is thus apparent that during exercise, particularly of high work intensity, the major part of hepatic glucose production derives from glycogenolysis (Fig. 5).

Among the factors which may be responsible for the increase in glycogenolysis during exercise is the possibility of altered glucagon secretion. Recent reports have indicated a rise in arterial glucagon levels of 30 to 40 per cent during exercise.[38] The elevation of plasma glucagon levels runs parallel to that of hepatic glucose output and the magnitude of the former rise is comparable to the physiological increments seen during prolonged starvation.[1] With regard to the mechanism of exercise-induced hyperglucagonemia, it is noteworthy that an elevation of plasma aminoacid levels, particularly of alanine, stimulates glucagon secretion.[9] Since alanine levels rise markedly during exercise,[37] hyperalaninemia may constitute the secretory stimulus for the hyperglucagonemia in exercise.

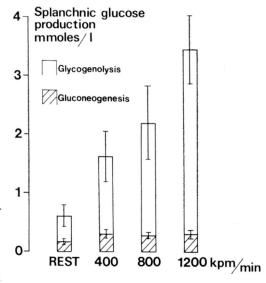

Fig. 5. Estimated contribution by hepatic glycogenolysis and gluconeogenesis to total splanchnic glucose output at rest and after 40 minutes of exercise at different work loads (mean ± SE).

The influence of several other factors is still open to question. Thus, the fall in plasma insulin levels may be significant, since small changes in insulin secretion have been shown to modulate splanchnic glucose balance in intact man during the infusion of glucose.[36] Alternatively, increased adrenergic activity during physical exercise may help to stimulate glycogenolysis, though plasma epinephrine levels fail to increase detectably with exercise.[123] The concentration of norepinephrine rises but the latter is a far less potent stimulus of hepatic glucose release. Hepatic hypoxia has also been proposed as a glycogenolytic stimulus in exhaustive exercise,[112] but this seems unlikely to be important in most forms of exercise, since a rise in hepatic oxygen consumption has been demonstrated during exercise at different work loads on a bicycle ergometer.[121]

Amino-acid Metabolism

Whereas the role of carbohydrate and lipid metabolism in the substrate exchange of resting and exercising muscle has been investigated extensively in man in recent years, little information is available regarding amino-acid metabolism in exercise, although it has long been recognized that physical exertion is associated with a peripheral release of ammonia.[117]

In the basal state, resting muscle shows a net release of most amino acids,[103] reflecting a slow turnover of muscle protein. That this finding does not simply represent a release of stored amino acids is confirmed by its magnitude and persistence during weeks of total starvation.[35] Studies on the pattern of amino-acid exchange across the resting forearm muscle show that alanine is released to a far greater extent than all other amino acids.[103] This primacy of alanine output is unexpected, inasmuch as alanine comprises only 5 to 8 per cent of the amino-acid residues in muscle protein.[85] Moreover, since alanine is quantitatively the most important amino acid to be extracted by the liver in the basal

state[23,34] and is readily converted to glucose by hepatic gluconeogenic processes,[111] it has been suggested that there is a cyclic conversion of glucose and alanine between muscle and liver.[35] The peripheral synthesis and release of alanine would accordingly depend not merely on muscle protein catabolism but also on the rate of glucose metabolism and pyruvate formation and the availability of amino groups for transamination. This hypothesis has recently been studied in man during exercise, a situation in which both glucose utilization[121] and peripheral ammonia formation[117] are augmented, so that an enhanced synthesis of alanine could be expected. The findings are summarized briefly below.[37]

Amino-acid exchange across the leg was evaluated by sampling from the femoral vein and a peripheral artery. At rest there was significant release from the leg of 13 of the 19 amino acids studied (Fig. 6). Alanine release exceeded that of all other amino acids and made up 35 to 40 per cent of the measured total amino-acid output. Small but significant uptakes were noted for citrulline, serine, cystine and α-aminobutyrate. A linear correlation between arterial pyruvate and alanine levels indicated the possibility of interaction between alanine and glucose metabolism. The splanchnic amino-acid exchange was studied by means of the hepatic venous-catheter technique. Significant net uptakes were demonstrable for 10 amino acids, the extraction of alanine exceeding that of all others in agreement with previous reports.[23]

Mild exercise (400 kpm/min) elicited a 20 to 25 per cent increase in arterial alanine levels and more intense exertion caused a rise of 60 to 95 per cent. In contrast, the concentrations of all other amino acids did not change during light exercise, whereas 40 minutes of heavy exercise (1200 kpm/min) elicited increases of 8 to 35 per cent for isoleucine, leucine, methionine, tyrosine and phenylalanine. As in the resting state, alanine was directly proportional to arterial pyruvate.

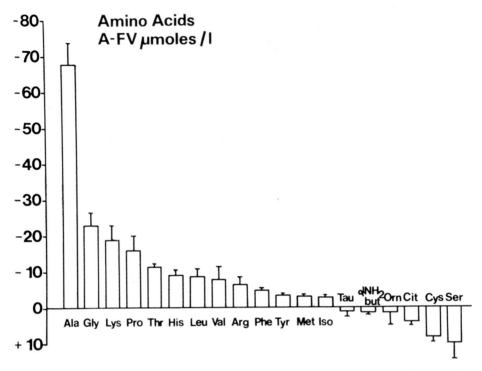

Fig. 6. Net exchange of individual amino acids across the leg (arteriofemoral venous differences, A–FV) in the resting, postabsorptive state (mean ± SE).

Negative arteriofemoral venous differences were noted at all levels of work intensity, indicating a consistent net release from the leg only in the case of alanine. The estimated net alanine release from the leg rose 55 per cent during mild exercise and 90 to 500 per cent during moderate and strenuous exercise. As in the resting state, alanine accounted for the dominant part of splanchnic amino-acid uptake at all levels of work intensity. Net alanine uptake increased 15 to 20 per cent during mild and moderate exercise as a consequence of both augmented arterial concentration and an increased splanchnic fractional extraction (arterial-hepatic venous difference in relation to arterial concentration). A significant release of the branched-chain amino acids valine, leucine and iso-leucine was observed from the splanchnic area during exercise.

Summing up, it appears that alanine has a unique role in splanchnic and muscle amino-acid metabolism. In agreement with findings by Carlsten et al.,[22] alanine is the only amino acid to show an increased arterial concentration during light exercise and a twofold increment with more strenuous exertion. In addition, it is the only amino acid to display a consistent net output from the exercising leg. In this respect exercising skeletal muscle is probably comparable to heart muscle, for which an alanine output also has been demonstrated.[21] The estimated net release of alanine from the exercising leg increased substantially during exercise and in proportion to the severity of the work performed. These findings support the hypothesis that alanine release during exercise does not solely depend on protein catabolism but is also a result of alanine synthesis in muscle, probably by transamination of pyruvate. The interrelationship of alanine and pyruvate metabolism is further emphasized by the significant linear correlations between their arterial concentrations both at rest and during exercise. The carbon skeleton of alanine may thus be an important end-product of glycolysis, particularly in exercise.

Although the fraction of glucose uptake which may be accounted for by alanine formation has not been determined directly, available data permit some approximate calculations. The amino acid lysine does not participate in reversible transamination in muscle tissue, and its release will thus provide an estimate of the rate of muscle protein dissolution. Moreover, the lysine content of muscle protein agrees closely with that of alanine.[85] Under these circumstances the difference in release from muscle tissue between alanine and lysine can be used as an index of glucose-derived alanine. Such calculations indicate that 13 to 18 per cent of the muscle glucose uptake in the resting state may be accounted for by subsequent alanine release. Employing the same assumptions, it may be estimated that production of glucose-derived alanine by muscle occurs at 35 to 60 per cent of the rate at which lactate is produced.[36]

With regard to the mechanism of alanine formation during exercise, the marked augmentation of glycogen utilization and glucose uptake by the leg (see above) points to an increased availability of pyruvate for transamination. As to the amino groups necessary for transamination, these may be supplied in part by catabolism of the branched-chain amino acids, which occurs preferentially in muscle.[92] Aspartate, too, may be a source of amino groups, particularly during exercise, since the formation of oxaloacetate from aspartate increases in association with augmented activity in the tricarboxylic acid cycle.[106] Moreover, exercise is reported to result in a cyclic interconversion of purine nucleotides, accompanied by the conversion of aspartate to fumarate and a liberation of free ammonia;[87] since glutamate is synthesized in part by the reductive amination of α-ketoglutarate and may subsequently undergo transamination with pyruvate to form alanine, the free ammonia formed in exercise may be an important source of amino groups for alanine synthesis. Thus, the flow of both pyruvate and amino groups is likely to be augmented during exercise and thereby enhance the peripheral synthesis of alanine and its release into the general circulation.

The functional importance of peripheral alanine synthesis with respect to body nitrogen metabolism is probably that it provides a nontoxic alternative to ammonia for the transport of amino groups from muscle to the liver. This concept is supported by the finding of hyperalaninemia with exercise, since it is well established that physical exercise is associated with augmented peripheral release of ammonia.[117]

The synthesis of one mole of alanine from pyruvate involving free ammonia is catalyzed in part by glutamate dehydrogenase and is associated with the net conversion of one mole of NADH to NAD. As this is an intra-mitochondrial reaction, alanine formation—unlike the lactate dehydrogenase reaction—probably cannot contribute to the regeneration of oxidized pyridine nucleotides in the cytoplasm. Accordingly, arterial lactate and alanine concentrations differ distinctly in the direction of their respective responses during the course of prolonged submaximal exercise.[37]

The findings regarding splanchnic uptake of amino acids during exercise demonstrate that alanine is not just an end-product of muscle glycolysis but constitutes an important endogenous precursor in hepatic gluconeogenesis. The findings concerning leg muscle and splanchnic amino-acid exchange point to the existence of a glucose-alanine cycle involving muscle and liver (Fig. 7). Alanine may thus be synthesized in muscle from pyruvate and released to the blood. Circulating alanine is then extracted by the liver, where its carbon skeleton is reconverted to glucose. Exercise would seem to influence this cyclic interconversion by increasing the rate of alanine formation in muscle in excess of its net uptake by the liver. As a consequence

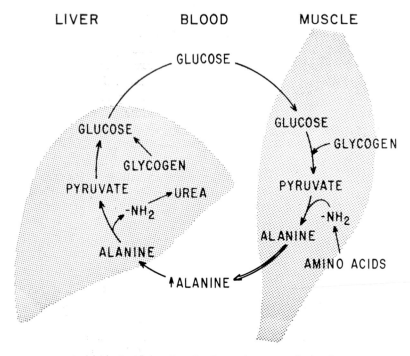

Fig. 7. The glucose-alanine cycle in exercise. In the resting state alanine is synthesized in muscle by transamination of pyruvate, thereby serving to transport amino groups and carbon skeletons to the liver, where the former are converted to urea and the latter to glucose. During exercise an increased availability of pyruvate and amino groups in muscle results in augmented synthesis and greater release of alanine to the circulation. Alanine accumulates in arterial plasma since the rise in release from muscle exceeds the rate of hepatic uptake.

the alanine concentration of arterial plasma rises.

A peripheral formation and hepatic uptake of glutamine have been demonstrated recently in intact man.[90] Arterial glutamine levels apparently do not rise during exercise, however, nor does there seem to be a significant production of glutamine from the leg.[81,82] Thus, while glutamine (like alanine) may well play an important role in the transport of amino groups from the periphery to the liver in the resting state, alanine synthesis and metabolism would appear to be of greater importance during exercise.

LIPID METABOLISM

Adipose Tissue

It has been known for more than a century that fat is the body's principal form of stored energy. Early studies by Benedict on prolonged fasting demonstrated that fat-derived substrates provide the major part of the calories utilized during food deprivation. However, only during the last 15 years has greater insight been gained concerning the physiological mechanisms behind the deposition, mobilization and utilization of lipid substrates.

Man's ability to tolerate marked extremes in caloric intake and fuel consumption is in part a consequence of his ability to store energy in an economical form. While fuel may be accumulated in the body as carbohydrate, protein or fat, the last of these has by far the highest calorie:weight ratio; because of its anhydrous nature, adipose tissue is on this basis approximately eight times more economical as a depot than glycogen and protein tissues. Moreover, the white fat of the body can be expended readily without adverse effects and is capable of meeting the substrate requirements of a large number of the body tissues.

The average 70-kg man has approximately 15 kg of fat in the form of adipose tissue triglycerides, representing about 140,000 kcal —enough to permit survival through 2 to 3 months of total food deprivation. Liver and muscle carbohydrate stores and circulating fuels, although important, are quantitatively insignificant by comparison. Protein, mainly in the form of muscle tissue, has a relatively large caloric potential, approximately 24,000 kcal (Table 1), but only a minor part is available under normal circumstances since (unlike adipose-tissue triglyceride and glycogen in muscle and liver) protein in both muscle and other tissues serves primarily for purposes other than caloric storage. This is emphasized by the body's metabolic adaptation during prolonged fasting, which tends to conserve the protein stores.[96]

Hydrolysis of the adipose-tissue triglycerides (lipolysis) leads to the release of free fatty acids and glycerol to the bloodstream. The insoluble FFA (mainly palmitic, stearic, oleic and linoleic acids) are bound to albumin in plasma and carried as such to their sites of utilization in the body. The regulation of adipose-tissue lipolysis during exercise involves the sympathetic nervous system.[59] Norepinephrine, liberated at sympathetic nerve endings, is a potent stimulus to fat mobilization. Like epinephrine, it activates the adenyl cyclase system to form increased amounts of cyclic $3',5'$-AMP. This substance, in turn, activates a lipolytic system in the adipose-tissue cell which catalyzes the hydrolysis of the stored triglycerides. Plasma levels and the urinary excretion of norepinephrine both increase during exercise, but recent reports suggest that norepinephrine, when transported in plasma, is as effective in eliciting lipolysis as increased activity in sympathetic nerves to adipose tissue.[11] The sympathetic innervation of adipose tissue thus appears to play a greater part

in FFA mobilization during exercise than circulating catecholamines. Regional differences have been described in the sympathetic innervation of adipose tissue[10] and the precise location of the adipose tissue responsible for the augmented FFA mobilization during physical exertion is still not known; subcutaneous tissues of the arms and legs contribute trivial amounts of FFA during exercise[50,63] and the splanchnic area shows a net FFA uptake.[57]

Metabolism of Free Fatty Acids

Albumin-bound plasma FFA function primarily as a means of transporting fuel from adipose-tissue stores to other organs, where they are taken up and utilized as substrates in energy metabolism.[31,44,86] With the exception of the brain, most tissues of the body have the capacity to metabolize FFA; muscle and liver are the major sites of FFA removal under resting conditions. The plasma-FFA pool is small, constituting less than 5 per cent of total plasma fatty acids, but its rate of turnover is high: the half-life of plasma FFA is about 2 to 3 minutes at rest and shorter during exercise.

The study of FFA metabolism in skeletal muscle in man is complicated by the simultaneous uptake and release of FFA both at rest and during exercise.[48,105] The FFA released from muscle may derive from lipolysis in adipose tissue interspersed between the muscle fibers or from hydrolysis of intracellular triglycerides in the muscle tissue itself. This problem has been approached from two angles: (1) lipolysis has been blocked by the infusion of minute amounts of insulin, thereby unmasking the FFA uptake,[105] and (2) isotopic techniques have been used for the measurement of both local FFA uptake and oxidation. The choice of a suitable FFA tracer poses a problem. The individual plasma FFA differ in their rates of release from adipose tissue,[67] their arterial concentrations and patterns of change during exercise[56] and their uptake by muscle and liver.[57] As the use of multiple-tracer FFA tends to introduce methodological difficulties, it is desirable to find a suitable single FFA tracer, one that (1) is present in plasma in a high concentration in relation to other FFA, and (2) shows a metabolic behavior as close as possible to the average for plasma FFA. Oleic and palmitic acids seem to fulfill these requirements. They have the highest concentrations among the individual plasma FFA and their fractional uptakes in both muscle and liver are very similar to that of total FFA.[57] For studies of muscle FFA uptake, oleic acid would seem to be slightly preferable as a tracer; the uptake of palmitic acid by forearm muscle during exercise is about 10 per cent lower than that of total FFA and oleic acid.[50]

At rest about 50 per cent of the FFA entering the forearm or the leg are removed during each circulation.[47,63,105] As approximately the same amount or slightly less is released into the circulation, there is only a small or no net A-V difference for FFA. Most of the FFA taken up are stored for several hours, only a small fraction being oxidized rapidly. In the postabsorptive state the local RQ value for muscle is close to 0.7, indicating that fat substrates almost exclusively are being oxidized.

The FFA uptake by exercising forearm muscle has been examined in healthy subjects in the postabsorptive state[50] and during prolonged starvation.[53] A mixture of labeled palmitic, stearic, oleic and linoleic acids was infused into the brachial artery during rhythmic exercise with a hand ergometer. The individual specific radioactivities of the administered FFA were then determined in samples obtained from the radial artery and a deep forearm vein during the infusion. In addition, blood flow to the forearm was measured using an indicator-dilution technique.[119] It was found that, during exercise, muscle FFA uptake rises in proportion to arterial FFA concentration and also shows a linear relationship to FFA inflow, expressed as the product of arterial concentration and forearm plasma flow.[54] This indicates that

the FFA transport mechanism does not reach a saturation point even under the rather extreme conditions associated with prolonged starvation. Thus it would seem that the magnitude of FFA uptake in muscle is regulated not so much by the muscle itself as by outside factors, such as the rate of FFA mobilization from adipose tissue.

The uptake of FFA during rhythmic forearm exercise is not sufficient to account for the entire fat oxidation of the muscle, as evaluated from the local RQ. During moderately heavy exercise the uptake thus covered only approximately 50 per cent of the simultaneous total fat oxidation,[50] indicating that the muscle may oxidize fatty acids other than those taken up from plasma, as discussed below. During prolonged fasting, when the FFA uptake is larger as a consequence of the higher FFA levels, the rate of fat oxidation during exercise is largely unchanged. Thus in this situation the exercising muscle seems to be capable of covering a larger fraction of its fat metabolism by immediate oxidation of plasma FFA.

The onset of forearm exercise yields an increase in the arterial FFA concentration and a further rise occurs during prolonged exercise,[50] indicating that the mobilization of FFA is increased in excess of the increment to muscle-FFA uptake. At the onset of exercise with larger muscle groups, such as the leg muscles, the increased FFA removal by muscle may outstrip FFA mobilization, giving an abrupt fall in arterial FFA.[20] The mobilization from adipose tissue then increases gradually and arterial FFA levels have usually risen above the resting value after 20 to 30 minutes of work.[22,109] If exercise is continued, the FFA levels rise steadily and reach plateau values 4 to 5 times higher than at rest after 10 to 12 hours of exercise.[126]

In several of the studies reporting a fall in FFA levels during the first 10 to 20 minutes of exercise, the base-line samples were obtained with the subjects supine. The exercise was then performed in the sitting position. In a study in which labeled FFA were infused continuously during the transition from supine to sitting position, FFA specific activity rose markedly but arterial FFA levels fell, indicating a reduced rate of FFA mobilization from adipose tissue.[56] The change in body posture is attended by an increase in sympathetic tone, which affects the lipolytic process in two ways: triglyceride hydrolysis is stimulated but the fatty acids formed are trapped in the adipose tissue as a consequence of vasoconstriction and decreased blood flow.[40] Together with an accelerated uptake of FFA to muscle, these findings may serve to elucidate the fall in arterial FFA during the beginning of an exercise period.

The individual FFA differ markedly in their arterial concentrations during exercise (Fig. 8). The most pronounced increments with prolonged exercise are seen for oleic acid and palmitic acid, while linoleic-acid concentration increases only slightly and

stearic and arachidonic acids not at all.[56] This is probably because palmitic and oleic acids predominate in the exercise-induced increase in FFA mobilization from adipose-tissue triglycerides, whereas very little stearic acid is released. Arachidonic acid occupies an exceptional position among the plasma FFA. Its concentration is independent of the total FFA level, it is not influenced by the administration of nicotinic acid and there is no uptake of this acid to either muscle or liver.[57] The regulation of the plasma arachidonic-acid concentration would thus seem to differ completely from that of the other FFA.

The oxidation of plasma FFA may be studied by measuring the $^{14}CO_2$ output after administering a ^{14}C-labeled tracer. During prolonged, light bicycle exercise 75 to 100 per cent of the FFA uptake to the leg muscles was found to be oxidized immediately.[63] Moderately heavy forearm exercise (10 kpm/

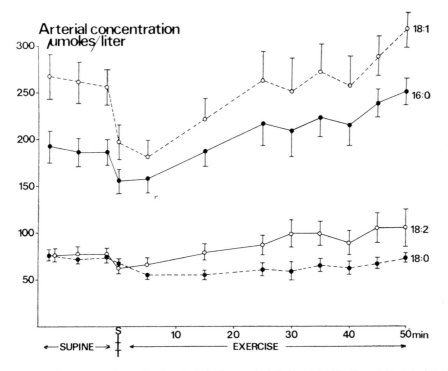

Fig. 8. Arterial concentrations of palmatic (16:0), stearic (18:0), oleic (18:1) and linoleic (18:2) acids at rest in the supine and sitting positions and during upright exercise at 400 kpm/min in healthy subjects (mean ± SE).

min) resulted in the rapid oxidation of an average of 60 per cent of the FFA taken up;[50] at a lower work intensity the FFA oxidation approached 100 per cent.[55] The release of $^{14}CO_2$ from the forearm muscles is rapid, the peak appearing less than two minutes after the tracer infusion has ended. The $^{14}CO_2$ production curve then declines exponentially, with an initial half-time of 2 to 3 minutes. The elimination curve also shows a second phase with a half-time of 10 to 12 minutes, conceivably representing the oxidation of FFA which have passed through an esterified fatty-acid pool in the muscle cell.[50] This hypothetical pool can be estimated to be 0.6 μmoles per gm muscle, thus corresponding in size to the smaller pool of esterified fatty acids in exercising muscle postulated from studies of whole-body FFA oxidation kinetics.[61]

The percentage recovery of $^{14}CO_2$ after infusion of ^{14}C-labeled FFA (the fractional oxidation) showed a positive relation to the oxygen uptake and a negative relation to the lactate production of forearm muscles.[50] A low oxygen consumption and large lactate production thus seem to be associated with a limited ability to oxidize acetyl-CoA. Since 10 kpm/min is a moderately heavy work load for the forearm and the deep venous oxygen saturation seldom falls below 35 per cent, there is no reason to believe that the supply of oxygen to the exercising muscle limits the oxidative process.

In subjects showing less than 100 per cent fractional oxidation the remaining radioactivity could be recovered not in the muscle tissue but as water-soluble metabolites in a perchloric-acid extract of blood. Labeled 3-hydroxybutyrate[52] has been identified among these metabolites, but 20 to 60 per cent of the radioactivity appears to be present in the form of acetate.[55]

The extent to which this loss of labeled material is actually associated with a net release of metabolites is not known, since A-V differences across exercising muscle for the possible metabolites are not available. It is conceivable that the appearance of water-soluble radioactive substances in venous blood during exercise reflects an exchange between metabolites of the FFA tracer and unlabeled material in the arterial inflow. However, the fact that this loss of radioactivity is related to physiological variables such as work load, oxygen uptake and lactate: pyruvate ratio suggests that it is not merely a random process whereby the label is dispersed throughout different metabolic pools. The occurrence of labeled acetate and 3-hydroxybutyrate in the venous blood at a high work intensity may indicate that the production of acetyl-CoA exceeds the simultaneous capacity for its oxidation in the tricarboxylic acid cycle. Such a metabolic situation is likely to develop in skeletal muscle in view of its high capacity for glycolysis and its relative scarcity of mitochondria. Furthermore, the high rate of ATP consumption for muscle contraction may reduce the energy charge of the adenine nucleotides, thereby reducing its inhibitory influence on the breakdown of substrates to acetyl-CoA. The resulting enhanced glycolysis is (because of the cytoplasmic redox state) diverted into production of lactate, while the intramitochondrial overproduction of acetyl-CoA may either result in deacylation, yielding acetate, or be channeled into synthesis of 3-hydroxybutyrate. The above metabolic situation is probably a consequence of insufficient mitochondrial oxidative capacity of the muscle in relation to the work load applied.[68] Support for this formulation is obtained from the finding that physical training is associated with the augmented ability of muscle to oxidize fatty acids.[93]

In an attempt to characterize further the relationship between oxygen supply and FFA oxidation by muscle, patients with impaired arterial circulation of the legs due to obstructive arterial disease were studied during bicycle exercise.[47] Arterial and femoral venous blood was sampled repeatedly during a continuous intravenous infusion of ^{14}C-oleic acid at rest and during a 35- to 55-minute exercise period. The work load was chosen to give mild to moderate symptoms of claudication during the latter part of the exercise. Neither the arterial FFA concentration nor the fractional uptake of FFA differed between the patients and healthy controls, but the estimated lactate production was higher and the FFA fractional oxidation by leg muscles was markedly lower in the patient group. The fractional oxidation of FFA was related linearly to arterial lactate and amounted in some patients to no more than 10 to 20 per cent. Even in these patients, the radioactivity not converted to $^{14}CO_2$ could be recovered in part as labeled acetate. When identical studies were undertaken 3 to 5 months after reconstructive surgery, the fractional oxidation of FFA was found to be normal. It seems that an impairment of the blood-flow capacity of the legs brings about not only a reduced inflow of oxygen and substrates to the leg but also a decreased capacity to oxidize the FFA taken up by the muscles. In these patients the decreased availability of oxygen (as indicated by an oxygen content of femoral venous blood approaching zero and a large lactate production) may well have been a limiting factor for FFA oxidation.

Metabolism of
Acetoacetate and 3-Hydroxybutyrate

In the resting state there is a net uptake of both acetoacetate and 3-hydroxybutyrate to human skeletal muscle,[64] proportional to the arterial concentrations.[51] The fractional uptake for both substances across the forearm muscle is as high as 50 per cent but, because of their relatively low arterial concentrations in the postabsorptive state, the contribution to total substrate exchange is only about 5 to 8 per cent assuming complete oxidation.

During a 60-minute period of forearm exercise the net A-V difference gradually diminished and was even replaced during the second half by a small net release of acetoacetate from the forearm muscle.[51] Failure of the exercising muscle to utilize available ketone bodies may be a consequence of elevated intracellular levels of acetoacetate and 3-hydroxybutyrate, secondary to incomplete FFA oxidation, as discussed above. Moreover, depending on the intramitochondrial $NADH:NAD^+$ ratio during exercise, part of the acetoacetate formed in muscle is reduced to 3-hydroxybutyrate. The changes observed in the ratios of lactate to pyruvate and 3-hydroxybutyrate to acetoacetate indicated that there is a transient rise in the intramitochondrial $NADH:NAD^+$ ratio during the first minutes of exercise while the cytoplasmic ratio remained high for at least 20 minutes.[51] During this time the rate of NADH formation from glycolysis in the cytoplasm evidently exceeded the rate by which it was reoxidized. It is possible that under these conditions the redox pair 3-hydroxybutyrate:acetoacetate acts as a "hydrogen shuttle," transferring reducing equivalents from cytoplasmic NADH to the intramitochondrial respiratory chain. During the latter half of the exercise period, when the redox state in the muscle is returning to normal, part of the acetoacetate release may be derived from the simultaneous uptake of 3-hydroxybutyrate.

The contribution of acetoacetate and 3-hydroxybutyrate to the total substrate supply of exercising muscle is thus negligible in the postabsorptive state. Similar results have been obtained during prolonged fasting, even though the arterial concentrations of both substances are then drastically elevated. In this situation the resting state shows a small uptake to the forearm muscle of acetoacetate and a simultaneous release of 3-hydroxybutyrate;[53,97] for the two combined there is no significant net uptake or release. Furthermore, forearm exercise elicits no significant net exchange for either substance in spite of their markedly elevated arterial levels.[53]

The background to these findings in prolonged fasting is unclear. Although FFA and ketone bodies compete as fuels in muscle metabolism, it has been claimed that the preference for one over the other depends mainly on their relative concentrations.[122] During prolonged fasting, arterial levels of ketone bodies exceed the level of FFA, but the intracellular FFA level is higher in diaphragm muscle than in plasma during starvation.[116] Consequently, it is conceivable that the concentrations of the competitive substrates at the intracellular sites of metabolism are not adequately reflected by their plasma levels and the intracellular FFA concentration during prolonged fasting may in fact be higher than that of either acetoacetate or 3-hydroxybutyrate.

Utilization of Intramuscular Lipids

Several studies in exercising man have emphasized the failure of FFA metabolism to account for the entire fat oxidation as evaluated from the respiratory exchange quotient. In healthy male subjects exercising at a low work intensity on a bicycle ergometer, only 30 to 50 per cent of the exhaled CO_2 could be attributed to the oxidation of plasma FFA, whereas the RQ indicated an almost exclusive utilization of fat substrates.[62] Likewise, direct studies of FFA metabolism in forearm and leg muscle during exercise have demonstrated that FFA uptake and oxidation may account for approximately 50 per cent of the total fat oxidation.[50,63] Quantitative interpretations of substrate exchange based on ventilatory or local RQ values are open to criticism, since several reactions apart from total oxidation influence the production of CO_2, especially in the resting state. During exercise, however, these reactions are much less important, since most metabolic reactions involve complete oxidation of substrates to CO_2 and water in working muscles, particularly during steady-state submaximal exercise. It is probable that changes in body stores of CO_2 invalidate the RQ as an index of fuel utilization during exercise. After an initial period of approximately 10 to 15 minutes, however, the RQ remains stable or falls slightly during exercise, especially at low or moderately heavy work loads with little or no lactate accumulation and steady levels of

P_{CO_2} and body temperature.[24] Under these circumstances the RQ is probably a valid measure of the metabolic mixture involved in oxidative metabolism. The combined findings on FFA oxidation by muscle and local RQ values thus strongly suggest that during exercise skeletal muscle obtains fatty acids from sources other than circulating FFA. It has therefore been suggested that a supply is obtained from triglyceride stores in muscle tissue.

It has long been known that globules of neutral fat occur in skeletal muscle; they are found in close proximity to the mitochondria and are abundant in human muscle, particularly in the red fibers.[41] In an attempt to obtain direct evidence of oxidation of muscle lipid during exercise, Masoro et al.[91] studied the gastrocnemius and soleus muscles of monkey. As no decrease in muscle phospholipid or triglyceride content was noted when leg muscles were stimulated electrically for several hours, it was suggested that intracellular lipids of skeletal muscle do not serve as an energy source for contraction. The relevance of these findings to intact man is uncertain, and it seems difficult to conceive a function other than supply of fuel for the lipid droplets stored in red muscle fibers. Recent results in healthy volunteers exercising to exhaustion on a bicycle ergometer support this view.[18] Muscle biopsy samples were obtained from the lateral portion of the quadriceps muscle before and after prolonged exhaustive exercise. Meticulous dissection of the biopsy was done to remove visible fat and connective tissue before analysis. A 25 per cent reduction in triglyceride content was observed and there was no change in phospholipid content. Intramuscular triglyceride stores contributed an estimated two thirds of the fatty acids for total fat oxidation during this form of exercise, indicating a quantitatively important role for intramuscular lipids in the substrate supply of exercising human muscle.

Finally, some comments are called for on the adipose tissue interspersed between the muscle fibers, particularly the red fibers. It is conceivable that fatty acids may be transported from such tissue stores directly to the working muscle, without traversing plasma. If this is the case, the net fatty-acid utilization by muscle would be greater than that measured by the A-V difference of plasma. Assuming that the fatty-acid content and physiological behavior of this adipose tissue agree with that of such tissue elsewhere in the body, a release of glycerol would be expected during lipolysis. Lack of such release from the exercising human forearm[50] and leg[63] argues against the likelihood of such fatty-acid transport but does not exclude this intriguing possibility, inasmuch as skeletal muscle has the capacity to oxidize glycerol.[50]

INTEGRATED ASPECTS OF SUPPLY AND USE OF FUELS BY MUSCLE

Structure-function Relationships

Normal human muscle is made up of fibers of different histochemical types, and most skeletal muscle contains both red and white fibers. The red fibers are rich in capillaries, oxidative enzymes and lipids. The white fibers show high levels of ATP, creatine phosphate and glycolytic enzymes, while capillary and mitochondrial densities are lower than in red fibers. For human muscle the glycogen content of the two fibers is the same.[42] The proportion of the two types varies between muscles, the biceps brachii having a large component of white fibers and the soleus being relatively red.[33] Considerable evidence indicates that groups of muscle fibers supplied by individual motor units show the same fiber type.[32] The white fibers are innervated by high-threshold motor units discharging phasically, making them suitable for short periods of contraction against large work loads. In man the red fibers predominate in muscles used continuously (heart, diaphragm, postural muscles) and the white fibers in muscles used intermittently. Studies of human tibial muscle indicate that rapid, forceful contraction first activates motor units

with white-fiber characteristics, while slow, less forceful contraction predominantly engages red fibers.[45] These findings suggest that the intensity and duration of the motor-nerve activity may have a bearing on the type of substrate utilized by skeletal muscle. Although the activation pattern for metabolically different types of skeletal muscle fibers may provide a background to the muscle's substrate utilization, it remains to be seen how relevant such factors are to fuel utilization during exercise in man. Preliminary evidence from a study of patients with upper motor lesions and hence white-fiber atrophy indicates that the pattern of muscle substrate utilization in this condition bears no simple relationship to fiber atrophy.[46]

Choice of Fuel at Rest

After an overnight fast the local RQ of the forearm muscle or leg is close to 0.7,[7,49,105] suggesting that fatty acids are the major energy-yielding substrate. Accordingly, FFA uptake by resting muscle is about 50 per cent of the arterial concentration and if oxidized is sufficient to account for approximately 90 per cent of the oxygen consumption.[105] However, only a small fraction of the FFA taken up is released immediately to the venous blood as CO_2, the remainder presumably entering into the intracellular triglyceride pools.[63] Available data suggest a continuous breakdown and resynthesis of stored triglyceride, so that FFA and endogenous fatty acid together provide the bulk of fuel for oxidation. There is a quantitatively minor uptake of acetoacetate and 3-hydroxybutyrate which, if oxidized, may account for 5 to 8 per cent of the oxygen uptake.[51] In addition there is a positive net A-V difference for glucose across the resting forearm and leg vascular beds.[7,121] However, there is also a net production of lactate from these regions as a result of glycolysis in muscle and probably also in erythrocytes in the vascular beds. The fraction of glucose oxidized after being taken up to muscle has not been established; glucose may participate in glycogen synthesis or it may leave the muscle as alanine after transamination of glucose-derived pyruvate.[37] A limited or no terminal oxidation of glucose by muscle is to be expected from the local RQ values and known rates of hepatic glucose output and utilization in brain.[17]

Supply and Use of Fuels during Exercise

During the initial phase of exercise, before blood flow and mobilization of blood-borne substrates have increased, the contracting muscle has to rely on intramuscular stores for energy production. The immediate fuels include the phosphagens ATP and creatine phosphate, of which muscle contains a limited store.[74] Onset of contraction elicits activation of phosphorylase mainly in the white muscle fibers and a resynthesis of ATP and creatine phosphate may be accomplished through degradation of glycogen to lactate. The major part of the rise in blood flow to working muscle occurs within the first 1 to 2 minutes, thereby increasing the oxygen, FFA and glucose available for extraction.

Glycogen degradation, as evidenced by lactate production, occurs even at the onset of exercise at a low work load.[100] The production of lactate gradually diminishes and may cease after the first minutes. During further light exercise which raises the basal oxygen consumption only 2- to 3-fold, the uptake of blood-borne substrates (predominantly FFA) may suffice to supply the fuel required for energy production,[84] but with heavier exercise the degradation of glycogen continues. As the availability of oxygen increases, more and more of the glycogen undergoes terminal oxidation and lactate production gradually diminishes.

The importance of glycogen as an intramuscular fuel depot is attested by studies of exercise tolerance in patients lacking the enzyme responsible for muscle glycogen degradation (myophosphorylase: McArdle's syndrome).[98,102] At the onset of even light work these patients experience intense muscular fatigue, stiffness and swelling of contracting muscles, marked tachycardia and

hyperventilation. After a few minutes the symptoms may subside and the patient can continue exercising for an unlimited period (second-wind phenomenon) but if the work load is raised the symptoms reappear. In accordance with these patients' inability to degrade glycogen, there is no lactate accumulation in blood during exercise. The ability of subjects with this syndrome to exercise can be prolonged by intravenously administering glucose or emulsified fat or by increasing the arterial level of FFA and the local blood flow by the administration of isoproterenol. The subjective symptoms in these patients appear at the time during exercise when the muscle depends to a great extent on glycogen utilization for the resynthesis of energy-rich phosphagens. The ability of these patients to achieve a "second wind" is related to the inflow of blood-borne substrates, inasmuch as an augmentation of local blood flow and/or arterial substrate concentrations, notably FFA, enhances their capacity to continue exercise.[98] These patients' dependence on fuel supply from the blood is further underscored by the finding that they are unable to reach a second wind or to continue exercise if adipose-tissue lipolysis is blocked by infusing nicotinic acid, thereby substantially reducing the availability of plasma FFA.[98]

The glycogen content of muscle gradually falls during prolonged exercise, the rate of utilization being related to the severity of the work performed. The first hour of exercise is accompanied by an increased mobilization of FFA from adipose tissue and of glucose from the liver. The relative importance of these substrates increases if exercise continues, the uptake of FFA from the blood after 1 to 4 hours of moderately heavy bicycle exercise accounting for 25 to 50 per cent of the CO_2 production and almost all FFA taken up by the working muscles being oxidized immediately. The simultaneous uptake of glucose may account for 30 to 35 per cent of total oxidative metabolism and 75 to 90 per cent of estimated carbohydrate oxidation. These findings emphasize the substantial contribution of blood-borne substrates to muscle metabolism during this phase of exercise. Both indirect evidence and specific measurements suggest that intramuscular lipids also contribute fuel in this situation. That muscle glycogen is not essential for the capacity to perform prolonged moderately heavy exercise is indicated by the ability of a subject with McArdle's syndrome to tolerate such exercise for several hours. Moreover, in this subject uptake of substrate from the blood was inadequate to account for the entire oxidative metabolism, thus providing further evidence for the utilization of intramuscular lipids during prolonged exercise of this type.

During prolonged exercise of high work intensity, the relative amount of fuel contributed by blood substrates is less than at low intensity, and the muscle becomes more dependent on local fuel depots. The muscle glycogen content falls gradually and exhaustion generally coincides with depletion of glycogen stores. Blocking FFA release from adipose tissue by the administration of nicotinic acid during this type of exercise results in an accelerated rate of glycogen utilization and probably also of blood glucose uptake by muscle.[16] However, the subjects' ability to perform this type of exercise was not affected. The RQ indicated that fat oxidation continued in spite of low FFA levels.

In an attempt to discover whether FFA availability influences endurance during heavy exercise,[99] the subjects first depleted the glycogen stores of their leg muscles by bicycle exercise to exhaustion and then received a noncarbohydrate diet to decrease the resynthesis of muscle glycogen; they were studied on the following day before and after nicotinic-acid blockade of adipose-tissue lipolysis. With adequate FFA supply but reduced muscle glycogen stores, endurance was markedly shorter than that with the initial exercise. Exclusion of plasma FFA as well as muscle glycogen caused a further substantial impairment. Here, too, there is indirect evidence that fatty acids may be furnished to exercising

muscle without plasma transport from lipid stores within the muscle tissue. However, such lipid stores apparently cannot be utilized to an extent sufficient to obviate the need for glycogen or plasma FFA.

Effects of Physical Training

It has been found that a program of endurance training elicits not only alterations in the capacity of the cardiovascular system to transport and distribute oxygen during exercise but also both structural and functional changes in the exercising muscle; the muscle mass and the size of the muscle cells increase,[88] as does the number of capillaries per muscle fiber.[66,101] Recent studies have emphasized the marked biochemical adaptation in muscle during physical training which results in an increased capacity of skeletal muscle for aerobic metabolism; the sites of these changes are the muscle mitochondria. Electron-microscopic evidence reveals that this adaptation involves an increase in both the size and the number of muscle mitochondria.[43,83] A substantial rise in the total mitochondrial protein fraction has been reported[68] concomitant with augmented levels of activity by the mitochondrial respiratory-chain enzymes, linking the oxidation of NADH and succinate to oxygen.[68] Moreover, the activities of mitochondrial citric-acid cycle enzymes[69] and the rate-limiting enzymes involved in fatty-acid oxidation[93] are markedly enhanced in response to physical training. The mitochondria obtained from trained muscle exhibit tightly coupled oxidative phosphorylation, indicating that the increment to mitochondrial oxidative enzymatic capacity is associated with a parallel rise in aerobic ATP generation.

In contrast, the activity of the enzymes involved in glycolysis and glycogenolysis of muscle does not respond significantly to physical training.[70] Hexokinase is the only exception, its activity being increased in untrained animals by just a few light bouts of exercise; this does not appear to be a training effect in the same sense as the rise in activity of the oxidative enzymes. The lack of effect on the glycolytic enzymes may have to do with the fact that, at submaximal steady-state exercise, the conversion of glycogen and glucose to pyruvate and lactate is determined not so much by the concentrations of the rate-limiting enzymes as by the operation of a number of feedback control mechanisms.

The intracellular stores of glycogen and fat are also influenced by endurance training. Increased glycogen synthetase and glycogen concentration have been observed following physical training.[94] There is likewise an increased incorporation of palmitic acid into intracellular fatty-acid stores, and probably augmented levels of intramuscular triglycerides.[95] Red and white muscle fibers do not appear to be affected differently by training: if anything, the training appears to exaggerate the normal differences between the fiber types.[118]

Considering the increased activity of mitochondrial oxidative enzymes following physical training, it is understandable that the pattern of substrate utilization by muscle also changes. Thus, a greater percentage of the total oxidative metabolism derives from fatty-acid oxidation in trained individuals, compared to untrained, during exercise at the same intensity.[26,114] This difference is referable in part to the adaptive increase in the capacity of muscle to oxidize fatty acids. Furthermore, training appears to be associated with a greater rate of release of fatty acids from adipose tissue.[60,78] This yields elevated levels of FFA in plasma, thereby increasing the availability of FFA to muscle. The muscle's enhanced capacity to oxidize fatty acids thus acts synergistically with the increased rate of FFA mobilization to account for the greater utilization of fat-derived substrates for muscle oxidation in physically trained individuals.

Depletion of muscle glycogen and hypoglycemia have been cited as factors responsible for the development of fatigue during prolonged heavy exercise, making it necessary for an exercising individual to discontinue work or reduce his pace.[3,13,99] The shift in the source of carbon for muscle oxidation toward a greater fatty-acid utilization occurring in response to physical training may contribute to a glycogen-saving effect, thus postponing the depletion of glycogen stores and probably the occurrence of fatigue.

REFERENCES

1. Aguilar-Parada, E., Eisentraut, A. M., and Unger, R. H.: Effects of starvation on plasma pancreatic glucagon in normal man. Diabetes, 18:717, 1969.
2. Ahlborg, B., et al.: Human muscle glycogen content and capacity for prolonged exercise after different diets. Försvarsmedicin, 3:85, 1967.
3. Ahlborg, B., et al.: Muscle glycogen and muscle electrolytes during prolonged physical exercise. Acta Physiol. Scand., 70:129, 1967.
4. Ahlborg, B., et al.: Muscle glycogen consumption during prolonged exercise with and without glucose infusion. To be published.
5. Ahlborg, B., et al.: Muscle metabolism during isometric exercise, performed at constant force. J. Appl. Physiol., 33:224, 1972.
6. Ahlborg, G., Hagenfeldt, L., and Wahren, J.: Glucose metabolism of inactive muscle during physical exertion. Scand. J. Clin. Lab. Invest., in press.
7. Ahlborg, G., and Wahren, J.: Brain substrate utilization during prolonged exercise. Scand. J. Clin. Lab. Invest., 29:397, 1972.
8. Andres, R., Cader, G., and Zierler, K. L.: The quantitatively minor role of carbohydrate in oxidative metabolism by skeletal muscle in intact man in the basal state. Measurements of oxygen and glucose uptake and carbon dioxide and lactate production in the forearm. J. Clin. Invest., 35:67, 1956.
9. Assan, R., Rosselin, G., and Dolais, J.: Effects sur la glucagonémie des perfusions et ingestions d'acides animés. J. Ann. Diabèt. Hôtel Dieu, 7:25, 1967.
10. Ballard, K., and Rosell, S.: The unresponsiveness of lipid metabolism in canine mesenteric adipose tissue to biogenic amines and to sympathetic nerve stimulations. Acta Physiol. Scand., 77:442, 1969.
11. Ballard, K., Cobb, C. A., and Rosell, S.: Vascular and lipolytic responses in canine subcutaneous adipose tissue following infusion of catecholamines. Acta Physiol. Scand., 81: 246, 1971.
12. Bergström, J.: Muscle electrolytes in man. Scand. J. Clin. Lab. Invest., 14 (Suppl. 68), 1962.
13. Bergström, J., et al.: Diet, muscle glycogen and physical performance. Acta Physiol. Scand., 71:140, 1967.

14. Bergström, J., and Hultman, E.: The effect of exercise on muscle glycogen and electrolytes in normals. Scand. J. Clin. Lab. Invest., *18*: 16, 1966.

15. Bergström, J., and Hultman, E.: A study of the glycogen metabolism during exercise in man. Scand. J. Clin. Lab. Invest., *19*:218, 1967.

16. Bergström, J., et al.: The effect of nicotinic acid on physical working capacity and metabolism of muscle glycogen in man. J. Appl. Physiol., *26*:170, 1969.

17. Cahill, G. F., Jr., and Owen, O. E.: Some observations on carbohydrate metabolism in man. In: *Carbohydrate Metabolism and its Disorders* (Dickens, F., Randle, P. J., and Whelan, W. J., Eds.). New York, Academic Press, 1968.

18. Carlson, L. A., Ekelund, L-G., and Fröberg, S. O.: Concentration of triglycerides, phospholipids and glycogen in skeletal muscle and of free fatty acids and β-hydroxybutyric acid in blood in man in response to exercise. Europ. J. Clin. Invest., *1*:248, 1971.

19. Carlson, L. A., and Orö, L.: The effect of nicotinic acid on the plasma free fatty acids. Acta Med. Scand., *271*:641, 1962.

20. Carlson, L. A., and Pernow, B.: Studies on blood lipids during exercise. I. Arterial and venous plasma concentrations of unesterified fatty acids. J. Lab. Clin. Med., *53*:833, 1959.

21. Carlsten, A., et al.: Myocardial metabolism of glucose, lactic acid, amino acids and fatty acids in healthy human individuals at rest and at different work loads. Scand. J. Clin. Lab. Invest., *13*:418, 1961.

22. Carlsten, A., et al.: Arterial concentrations of fatty acids and free amino acids in healthy human individuals at rest and at different work loads. Scand. J. Clin. Lab. Invest., *14*: 185, 1962.

23. Carlsten, A., et al.: Arterio-hepatic venous differences of free fatty acids and amino acids. Studies in patients with diabetes or essential hypercholesterolemia, and in healthy individuals. Acta Med. Scand., *181*:199, 1967.

24. Christensen, E. H., and Hansen, O.: Zur Methodik der Respiratorischen Quotient-Bestimmungen in Ruhe und bei Arbeit. Skand. Arch. Physiol., *81*:137, 1939.

25. Christensen, E. H., and Hansen, O.: Untersuchungen über die Verbrennungsvorgänge bei langdauernder, schwerer Muskelarbeit. Skand. Arch. Physiol., *81*:152, 1939.

26. Christensen, E. H., and Hansen, O.: Arbeitsfähigkeit und Ehrnährung. Skand. Arch. Physiol., *81*:160, 1939.

27. Christensen, E. H., and Hansen, O.: Respiratorischer Quotient und O₂-Aufnahme. Skand. Arch. Physiol., *81*:180, 1939.

28. Corsi, A., Midrio, M., and Granata, A. L.: In situ utilization of glycogen and blood glucose by skeletal muscle during tetanus. Amer. J. Physiol., *216*:1534, 1969.

29. Costill, D. L., et al.: Muscle glycogen utilization during exhaustive running. J. Appl. Physiol., *31*:353, 1971.

30. Danforth, W. H.: Glycogen synthetase activity in skeletal muscle. J. Biol. Chem., *240*:588, 1965.

31. Dole, V. P.: A relation between non-esterified fatty acids in plasma and the metabolism of glucose. J. Clin. Invest., *35*:150, 1956.

32. Edström, L., and Kugelberg, E.: Histochemical composition of distribution of fibres and fatigability of single motor units. J. Neurol. Neurosurg. Psychiat., *31*:424, 1968.

33. Edström, L., and Nyström, B.: Histochemical types and sizes of fibres in normal human muscles. Acta Neurol. Scand., *45*:257, 1969.

34. Felig, P., et al.: Amino acid metabolism during prolonged starvation. J. Clin. Invest., *48*: 584, 1969.

35. Felig, P., et al.: Alanine: Key role in gluconeogenesis. Science, *167*:1003, 1970.

36. Felig, P., and Wahren, J.: Influence of endogenous insulin secretion on splanchnic glucose and amino acid metabolism in man. J. Clin. Invest., *50*:1702, 1971.

37. Felig, P., and Wahren, J.: Amino acid metabolism in exercising man. J. Clin. Invest., *50*: 2703, 1971.

38. Felig, P., et al.: Plasma glucagon levels in exercising man New Eng. J. Med., *287*:184, 1972.

39. Field, R. A.: Glycogen deposition diseases. In: *The Metabolic Basis of Inherited Disease* (Stanbury, J. B., Wyngaarden, J. B., and Fredrickson, D. S., Eds.). New York, McGraw-Hill, 1960.

40. Fredholm, B. B., and Karlsson, J.: Metabolic effects of prolonged sympathetic nerve stimulation in canine subcutaneous adipose tissue. Acta Physiol. Scand., *80*:567, 1970.

41. Gauthier, G. F., and Padykula, H. A.: Cytological studies of fiber types in skeletal muscle. A comparative study of the mammalian diaphragm. J. Cell Biol., *28*:333, 1966.

42. Gollnick, P. D., et al: Enzyme activity and fiber composition in skeletal muscle of untrained and trained men. J. Appl. Physiol., *33*:312, 1972.

43. Gollnick, P. D., and King, D. W.: Effect of exercise and training on mitochondria of rat skeletal muscle. Amer. J. Physiol., *216*:1502, 1969.

44. Gordon, R. S., Jr., and Cherkes, A.: Unesterified fatty acids in human blood plasma. J. Clin. Invest., *35*:206, 1956.

45. Grimby, L., and Hannertz, J.: Recruitment order of motor units on voluntary contraction: Changes induced by proprioceptive afferent activity. J. Neurol. Neurosurg. Psychiat., *31*: 565, 1968.

46. Hagenfeldt, L., Landin, S., and Wahren, J.: Substrate utilization in paretic human forearm muscle during electrically induced exercise. Clin. Sci., *41*:353, 1971.

47. Hagenfeldt, L., Pernow, B., and Wahren, J.: Metabolism of free fatty acids during exercise in patients with occlusive arterial disease of the leg. In: *Muscle Metabolism During Exercise* (Pernow, B., and Saltin, B., Eds.). New York, Plenum Press, 1971.

48. Hagenfeldt, L., and Wahren, J.: Simultaneous uptake and release of individual free fatty acids in human forearm muscle during exercise. Life Sci., 5:357, 1966.

49. Hagenfeldt, L., and Wahren, J.: Human forearm muscle metabolism during exercise. I. Circulatory adaptation to prolonged forearm exercise. Scand. J. Clin. Lab. Invest., 21: 257, 1968.

50. Hagenfeldt, L., and Wahren, J.: Human forearm muscle metabolism during exercise. II. Uptake, release and oxidation of individual FFA and glycerol. Scand. J. Clin. Lab. Invest., 21:263, 1968.

51. Hagenfeldt, L., and Wahren, J.: Human forearm muscle metabolism during exercise. III. Uptake, release and oxidation of β-hydroxybutyrate and observations on the β-hydroxybutyrate/acetoacetate ratio. Scand. J. Clin. Lab. Invest., 21:314, 1968.

52. Hagenfeldt, L. and Wahren, J.: Production of β-hydroxybutyrate from FFA in working muscle during anaerobic conditions. Excerpta Medica Int. Congr. Series, 172S:218, 1969.

53. Hagenfeldt, L., and Wahren, J.: Human forearm muscle metabolism during exercise. VI. Substrate utilization in prolonged fasting. Scand. J. Clin. Lab. Invest., 27:299, 1971.

54. Hagenfeldt, L., and Wahren, J.: Metabolism of free fatty acids and ketone bodies in skeletal muscle. In: *Muscle Metabolism During Exercise* (Pernow, B., and Saltin, B., Eds.). New York, Plenum Press, 1971.

55. Hagenfeldt, L., and Wahren, J.: Human forearm muscle metabolism during exercise. VII. FFA uptake and oxidation at different work intensities. Scand. J. Clin. Lab. Invest., in press.

56. Hagenfeldt, L., et al.: Free fatty acid metabolism of the leg muscles during exercise in patients with obliterative iliac and femoral artery disease before and after reconstructive surgery. J. Clin. Invest., in press.

57. Hagenfeldt, L., et al: Uptake of individual free fatty acids by skeletal muscle and liver in man. J. Clin. Invest., 51:2324, 1972.

58. Harris, P., Bateman, M., and Gloster, J.: The metabolism of glucose during exercise in patients with rheumatic heart disease. Clin. Sci., 23:561, 1962.

59. Havel, R. J.: Autonomic nervous system and adipose tissue. In: *Handbook of Physiology*, Section 5 (Renold, A. E., and Cahill, G. F., Jr., Eds.). Washington, American Physiological Society, 1965.

60. Havel, R. J., et al.: Turnover rate and oxidation of different free fatty acids in man during exercise. J. Appl. Physiol., 19:613, 1964.

61. Havel, R. J., Ekelund, L-G., and Holmgren, A.: Kinetic analysis of the oxidation of palmitate-1-^{14}C in man during prolonged heavy muscular exercise. J. Lipid Res., 8:366, 1967.

62. Havel, R. J., Naimark, A., and Borchgrevink, C. F.: Turnover rate and oxidation of free fatty acids of blood plasma in man during exercise: Studies during continuous infusion of palmitate-1-C^{14}. J. Clin. Invest., 42:1054, 1963.

63. Havel, R. J., Pernow, B., and Jones, N. L.: Uptake and release of free fatty acids and other metabolites in the legs of exercising men. J. Appl. Physiol., 23:90, 1967.

64. Havel, R. J., Segel, N., and Balasse, E. O.: Effect of 5-methylpyrazole-3-carboxylic acid (MPCA) on fat mobilization, ketogenesis and glucose metabolism during exercise in man. Advances Exp. Med. Biol., 4:105, 1969.

65. Hermansen, L., Hultman, E., and Saltin, B.: Muscle glycogen during prolonged severe exercise. Acta Physiol. Scand., 71:129, 1967.

66. Hermansen, L., and Wachtlova, M.: Capillary density of skeletal muscle in well-trained and untrained men. J. Appl. Physiol., 30:360, 1971.

67. Hollenberg, C. H., and Angel, A.: Relation of fatty acid structure to release and esterification of free fatty acids. Amer. J. Physiol., 205:909, 1963.

68. Holloszy, J. O.: Biochemical adaptations in muscle. Effects of exercise on mitochondrial oxygen uptake and respiratory enzyme activity in skeletal muscle. J. Biol. Chem., 242: 2278, 1967.

69. Holloszy, J. O., et al.: Mitochondrial citric acid cycle and related enzymes: Adaptive response to exercise. Biochem. Biophys. Res. Commun., 40:1368, 1970.

70. Holloszy, J. O., et al.: Biochemical adaptations to endurance exercise in skeletal muscle. In: *Muscle Metabolism During Exercise* (Pernow, B., and Saltin, B, Eds.). New York, Plenum Press, 1971.

71. Hultman, E.: Muscle glycogen in man determined in needle biopsy specimens. Method and normal values. Scand. J. Clin. Lab. Invest., 19:209, 1967.

72. Hultman, E.: Studies on muscle metabolism of glycogen and active phosphate in man with special reference to exercise and diet. Scand. J. Clin. Lab. Invest., 94 (Suppl. 19):63, 1967.

73. Hultman, E., and Bergström, J.: Muscle glycogen synthesis in relation to diet studied in normal subjects. Acta Med. Scand., 182:109, 1967.

74. Hultman, E., Bergström, J., and McLennan Andersson, N.: Breakdown and resynthesis of phosphorylcreatine and adenosine triphosphate in connection with muscular work in man. Scand. J. Clin. Lab. Invest., 19:55, 1967.

75. Hultman, E., and Nilsson, L. H.: Liver glycogen in man. Effect of different diets and muscular exercise. In: *Muscle Metabolism During Exercise* (Pernow, B., and Saltin, B., Eds.). New York, Plenum Press, 1971.

76. Hunter, W. M., and Sukkar, M. Y.: Changes in plasma insulin levels during muscular exercise. J. Physiol., *196*:110, 1968.

77. Häggendal, J., Hartley, H., and Saltin, B.: Arterial noradrenaline concentration during exercise in relation to the relative work levels. Scand. J. Clin. Lab. Invest., *3*:337, 1970.

78. Issekutz, B., Jr., et al.: Aerobic work capacity and plasma FFA turnover. J. Appl. Physiol., *20*:293, 1965.

79. Jorfeldt, L., and Wahren, J.: Human forearm muscle metabolism during exercise. V. Quantitative aspects of glucose uptake and lactate production during prolonged exercise. Scand. J. Clin. Lab. Invest., *26*:73, 1970.

80. Karlsson, J., and Saltin, B.: Diet, muscle glycogen, and endurance performance. J. Appl. Physiol., *31*:203, 1971.

81. Keul, J., Doll, E., and Keppler, D.: *Muskelstoffwechsel*. Münich, Johann Ambrosius Barth, 1969.

82. Keul, J., et al.: Über den Stoffwechsel des menschlichen Herzens. Das Verhalten der arteriocoronarvenösen Differenzen der Aminosäuren und des Ammoniak beim gesunden menschlichen Herzen in Ruhe, während und nach Körperlicher Arbeit. Deutsch. Arch. Klin. Med., *209*:717, 1964.

83. Kiessling, K-H., Piehl, K., and Lundquist, C-G.: Effect of physical training on ultrastructural features in human skeletal muscle. In: *Muscle Metabolism During Exercise* (Pernow, B., and Saltin, B., Eds.). New York, Plenum Press, 1971.

84. Klassen, G. A., Andrew, G. M., and Becklake, M. R.: Effect of training on total and regional blood flow and metabolism in paddlers. J. Appl. Physiol., *28*:397, 1970.

85. Kominz, D. R., et al: The amino acid composition of action, myosin, tropomyosin and the meromyosins. Arch. Biochem. Biophys., *50*: 148, 1954.

86. Laurell, S.: Plasma free fatty acids in diabetic acidosis and starvation. Scand. J. Clin. Lab. Invest., *8*:81, 1956.

87. Lowenstein, J., and Tornheim, K.: Ammonia production in muscle: The purine nucleotide cycle. Science, 171:397, 1971.

88. Man-I, M., Ito, K., and Kikuchi, K.: Histological studies of muscular training. Res. Phys. Ed., *11*:153, 1967.

89. Manners, D. J.: Glycogen storage disease, type I. In: *Control of Glycogen Metabolism*. Ciba Foundation Symposium. London, J. & A. Churchill, 1964.

90. Marliss, E. B., et al.: Muscle and splanchnic glutamine and glutamate metabolism in postabsorptive and starved man. J. Clin. Invest., *50*:814, 1971.

91. Masoro, E. J., et al.: Nonutilization of intracellular lipid esters as an energy source for contractile activity. J. Biol. Chem., *241*: 2626, 1966.

92. Miller, L. L.: The role of the liver and the nonhepatic tissues in the regulation of free amino acid levels in the blood. In: *Amino Acid Pools. Proceedings of the Symposium on Free Amino Acids, City of Hope Medical Center* (Holden, J. T., Ed.). Amsterdam, Elsevier, 1962.

93. Mole, P. A., Oscai, L. B., and Holloszy, J. O.: Increase in levels of palmityl CoA synthetase, carnitine palmityltransferase, and palmityl CoA dehydrogenase, and in the capacity to oxidize fatty acids. J. Clin. Invest., *50*:2323, 1971.

94. Morgan, T. E., et al.: Effects of long-term exercise on human muscle mitochondria. In: *Muscle Metabolism During Exercise* (Pernow, B., and Saltin, B., Eds.). New York, Plenum Press, 1971.

95. Morgan, T. E., Short, F. A., and Cobb, L. A.: Effect of long-term exercise on skeletal muscle lipid composition. Amer. J. Physiol., *216*:82, 1969.

96. Owen, O. E., et al.: Liver and kidney metabolism during prolonged starvation. J. Clin. Invest., *48*:574, 1969.

97. Owen, O. E., and Reichard, G. A., Jr.: Human forearm metabolism during progressive starvation. J. Clin. Invest., *50*:1536, 1971.

98. Pernow, B., Havel, R., and Jennings, D. B.: The second wind phenomenon in McArdle's syndrome. Acta Med. Scand., Suppl. *472*: 294, 1967.

99. Pernow, B., and Saltin, B.: Availability of substrates and capacity for prolonged heavy exercise in man. J. Appl. Physiol., *31*:416, 1971.

100. Pernow, B., and Wahren, J.: Lactate and pyruvate formation and oxygen utilization in the human forearm muscles during work of high intensity and varying duration. Acta Physiol. Scand., *56*:267, 1962.

101. Petren, T., Sjöstrand, T., and Sylvén, B.: Der Einfluss der trainings auf die Heufigkeit der Capillaren in Herz- und Skeletmuskulatur. Arbetsphysiol., *9*:376, 1936.

102. Porte, D., Jr., et al.: Cardiovascular and metabolic responses to exercise in a patient with Mc Ardle's syndrome. New Eng. J. Med., *275*:406, 1966.

103. Pozefsky, T., et al.: Amino acid balance across tissues of the forearm in postabsorptive man. Effects of insulin at two dose levels. J. Clin. Invest., *48*:2273, 1969.

104. Pruett, E. D. R.: Plasma insulin concentrations during prolonged work at near maximal oxygen uptake. J. Appl. Physiol., *29*:155, 1970.

105. Rabinowitz, D., and Zierler, K. L.: Role of free fatty acids in forearm metabolism in man quantitated by use of insulin. J. Clin. Invest., *41*:2191, 1962.

106. Randle, P. J., England, P. J., and Denton, R. M.: Control of the tricarboxylate cycle and its interactions with glycolysis during acetate utilization in rat heart. Biochem. J., *117*: 677, 1970.

107. Reichard, G. A., Jr., et al.: Blood glucose metabolism in exercising man. J. Appl. Physiol., *16*:1001, 1961.

108. Reichard, G. A., Jr., et al.: Quantitative estimation of the Cori cycle in the human. J. Biol. Chem., *238*:495, 1963.

109. Rodahl, K., Miller, H. J., and Issekutz, B., Jr.: Plasma free fatty acids in exercise. J. Appl. Physiol., *19*:489, 1964.

110. Rose, I. A., and O'Conell, E. L.: The role of glucose-6-phosphate in the regulation of glucose metabolism in human erythrocytes. J. Biol. Chem., *239*:12, 1964.

111. Ross, B. D., Hems, R., and Krebs, H. A.: The rate of gluconeogenesis from various precursors in the perfused rat liver. Biochem. J., *102*:942, 1967.

112. Rowell, L. B., et al.: Splanchnic blood flow and metabolism in heat-stressed man. J. Appl. Physiol., *24*:475, 1968.

113. Rowell, L. B., Masoro, E. J., and Spencer, M. J.: Splanchnic metabolism in exercising man. J. Appl. Physiol., *20*:1032, 1965.

114. Saltin, B., and Karlsson, J.: Muscle glycogen utilization during work of different intensities. In: *Muscle Metabolism During Exercise* (Pernow, B., and Saltin, B., Eds.). New York, Plenum Press, 1971.

115. Sanders, C. A., et al.: Effect of exercise on the peripheral utilization of glucose in man. New Eng. J. Med., *271*:220, 1964.

116. Schonfeld, G., and Kipnis, D. M.: Glucose-fatty acid interactions in the rat diaphragm in vivo. Diabetes, *17*:422, 1968.

117. Schwartz, A. E., Lawrence, W., Jr., and Roberts, K. E.: Elevation of peripheral blood ammonia following muscular exercise. Proc. Soc. Exp. Biol. Med., *98*:548, 1958.

118. Short, F. A., et al.: Influence of exercise training on red and white rat skeletal muscle. Amer. J. Physiol., *217*:327, 1969.

119. Wahren, J.: Quantitative aspects of blood flow and oxygen uptake in the human forearm during rhythmic exercise. Acta Physiol. Scand., *67* (Suppl. 269):1, 1966.

120. Wahren, J.: Human forearm muscle metabolism during exercise. IV. Glucose uptake at different work intensities. Scand. J. Clin. Lab. Invest., *25*:129, 1970.

121. Wahren, J., et al.: Glucose metabolism during leg exercise in man. J. Clin. Invest., *50*:2715, 1971.

122. Weidemann, M. J., and Krebs, H. A.: The fuel of respiration of rat kidney cortex. Biochem. J., *112*, 149, 1969.

123. Vendsalu, A.: Studies on adrenaline and noradrenaline in human plasma. Acta Physiol. Scand., *49* (Suppl. 173):1, 1960.

124. Villar-Palasi, C., and Larner, J.: Feedback control of glycogen metabolism in muscle. Fed. Proc., *25*:583, 1966.

125. Young, D. R., et al: Glucose oxidation and replacement during prolonged exercise in man. J. Appl. Physiol., *23*:734, 1967.

126. Young, D. R., et al.: Model for evaluation of fatty acid metabolism for man during prolonged exercise. J. Appl. Physiol., *23*:716, 1967.

Chapter 10

THE PHYSIOLOGICAL BACKGROUND TO PHYSICAL TRAINING IN CARDIAC PATIENTS

Gunnar Grimby, M.D.

Physical training in patients may have several purposes and usually several of them influence a particular training program. Our knowledge, however, of ways to design training programs emphasizing different factors is still poor. In this review experiences from training studies of normal persons, especially in middle age, will be summarized as a background to the training of cardiac patients. Different effects of training which can be used therapeutically will be discussed. Some of the experiences from training studies in cardiac patients will be reported.

The aims of physical training in cardiac patients may be to:

1. Increase the physical working capacity by
   A. increasing the aerobic capacity in a similar way as in normal subjects, including central circulatory and peripheral effects.
   B. raising the work load at which certain limiting symptoms appear; of special importance is angina pectoris as a limiting factor for physical exercise. The relationship between the capacity for a short-lasting high-level exercise, as in exercise testing, and the work capacity for longer periods, as in various activities of daily living and professional work, is also important.

2. Reduce the "cost" for a certain physical activity, e.g. reduced cardiac work by reduced heart rate and blood pressure, reduced ventilation volume per liter of oxygen uptake by more efficient ventilation.
3. Produce metabolic effects which may favorably influence the pathogenic processes in ischemic heart disease, such as reduction in plasma lipids or changes in muscle metabolic patterns.
4. Obtain other secondary preventive advantages; these are less specific and include possible effects on vascularization and fibrinolysis.

The effect of training on aerobic work capacity is better known than that on other functions and will be considered first.

TRAINING OF AEROBIC CAPACITY

As a background for training therapy in cardiac patients, work capacity and training in healthy persons, especially the middle aged, will be reviewed.[17,43]

A representative sample (793 men of the total population of men aged 54 years born in 1913 in Goteborg, Sweden) was studied with step-wise increasing work loads on a bicycle ergometer.[17] The aim of the test was to push as many subjects as possible to a maximal work load. Certain contraindications to maximal exercise were adopted, and in some subjects only submaximal work loads were used. Of all the tested subjects, 77 per cent stopped because of general fatigue; only 12 men stopped because of chest pain. The maximal heart rate in the subjects who stopped because of fatigue was 172 and their maximal oxygen uptake was estimated to be 2.3 L/min (30 ml/kg $\times$ min).[23,17]

Thus, the study demonstrated that a high percentage of middle-aged men can perform strenuous exercise. Although a high proportion (around 25 per cent) developed ST-T changes of ischemic type at the maximal exercise test (Bjure et al., to be published), it was concluded that men in this age group can take part in fairly heavy exercise, which might be considered as a possible measure to prevent ischemic heart disease without increased probability of cardiovascular hazards.

The well-known finding[1] of reduction in maximal heart rate and maximal oxygen uptake (aerobic capacity) with age was demonstrated also. While subjects receiving regular physical training have higher aerobic capacities at older ages,[21] even in them reductions with age will occur.

The trainability of healthy persons at different ages can be reviewed only from cross-sectional studies. One important factor here is actual level of fitness when training is begun. In most studies, those in a particular age group who display the greatest percentile and absolute increase in maximal oxygen uptake are those with the lowest initial values[14,34,40,42,43] (Fig. 1). A certain amount of training in early youth appears to result in a greater increase in the various parameters for the circulatory and respiratory system,[14] and accordingly in aerobic capacity, than corresponding training later in life. As summarized by Grimby and Saltin,[22] training in the 20s and 30s may still influence certain circulatory dimensions, such as heart volume and blood volume, while at older ages improved utilization of previously determined parameters is to be expected. The trainability of old men is reduced, and Benestad[4] did not note any significant effect of a training program in 70- to 80-year-old

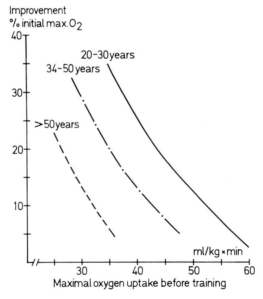

Fig. 1. Improvement in maximal oxygen uptake with 2 to 6 months' physical conditioning calculated in young individuals from the studies by Rowell,[40] Ekblom[14] and Saltin[42] in 34- to 50-year-old subjects and in men over 50 years old from the studies by Kihlbom et al.[34] and Saltin et al.,[43] in relation to the initial level of their maximal oxygen uptake.

men.   In a study on physical training in women, Kihlbom[33] concluded that in the age group above 50 years the training effect was also less pronounced than in younger subjects.   However, no definite difference was found between subjects in their 20s and those in their 30s to 40s.

In addition to the state of training at the start of a controlled training period, the intensity of training is important for the result.   Furthermore, the influence of undefined constitutional factors may have been overemphasized compared to the effect of physical conditioning during early ages.

In recent years, there have been several studies on the effect of various intensities of training.   Increases of maximal oxygen uptake from 0 to 30 per cent, and in extreme situations up to 100 per cent have been reported.[40,42]   As an increase in stroke volume[22] is one of the common circulatory effects of physical training leading to an increased maximal oxygen uptake, a training intensity which produces maximal values for stroke volume during exercise seems to be necessary; this is found at about a 40 per cent utilization of maximal oxygen uptake.[2]   Furthermore, at about this exercise level there is a transition from a predominantly vagal stimulation of the heart to predominantly sympathetic stimulation, and this may be an important stimulus to an increased stroke volume.[15] Training effects have also been noted at training intensities corresponding to about 50 per cent of the individual's maximal oxygen uptake.[33]

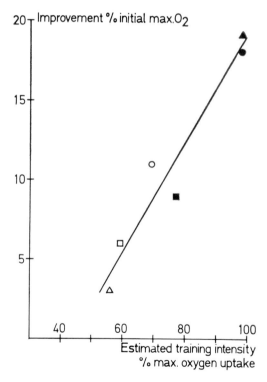

Fig. 2. Improvement in maximal oxygen uptake with about 2 months' training in sedentary middle-aged persons in relation to their training intensity.

Key: Solid circles: 34- to 50-year-old subjects
Solid triangles: 50- to 63-year-old men[43]
Open circles: 34- to 48-year-old women
Solid squares: 51- to 64-year-old women[33]
Open squares: 19- to 45-year-old women[33]

In Figure 2 some of the available studies on the effect of training of various intensities in sedentary middle-aged groups are summarized. The relatively large interindividual differences depending upon the factors mentioned above should, however, be kept in mind. An 11 to 12 per cent increase of a training intensity of 70 per cent was found in young and middle-aged sedentary women by Kihlbom,[33] whereas Siegel et al.[48] in extremely untrained persons (blind men) obtained a 19 per cent increase with a similar training program. It should be pointed out that the effect of a short period of training, usually a few months, is fairly well known, whereas training over a longer period has been less systematically studied. The optimal *length* and *frequency* of the *training sessions*, as well as the *exercise pattern*, have been rather poorly studied. In training programs with normal subjects as well as cardiac patients, sessions of 30 to 60 minutes have often been used. Training three times a week is common, and it appears that training five times a week should not have a substantially greater effect;[36] training less than two times a week is not sufficient, however.[41]

Based primarily on animal experiments, as reviewed by Saltin,[41] the duration or the amount of exercise does not appear to be as critical for the magnitude of improvement as the exercise intensity. Continuous training at a lower intensity but with the same total amount of work as interval training does not give the same result as the latter.[39] There is no satisfactory evidence on whether intermittent exercise with work periods of 3 to 4 minutes (interval training) or continuous exercise on the same high level over a similar total time would be preferable. Thus, at present, practical considerations will dominate the design of the training program. Untrained persons and most patients cannot maintain a fairly heavy or even moderate exercise intensity over a long period, and therefore an interval type of training will be more easily performed. Limiting factors to long-term exercise may not be directly connected to aerobic capacity, but rather to motivation, local muscle fatigue, inexperience with prolonged physical exercise, etc. As demonstrated by Saltin,[41] the long-term work ability under *optimal* conditions is probably uninfluenced by the degree of training as such, but related directly to the individual's maximal oxygen uptake.

The choice of the *types* of exercise should also be made primarily from practical considerations, provided the basic idea that large muscle groups should be engaged is adopted. However, some interesting observations concerning training effects with different muscle groups may influence some aspects of various training programs[10] and will be discussed below.

CIRCULATORY EFFECTS

The hemodynamic effects of training in sedentary, healthy middle-aged Swedish subjects have been studied in men by Hartley et al.[26] and in women by Kihlbom.[33] The men (38 to 55 years of age) were trained at near-maximal intensities for 3 half-hour periods a week during 8 weeks on an interval program. For women in age ranges of 19 to 31, 34 to 48 and 51 to 64 years, training for 7 weeks was performed at intensities around 70 to 75 per cent of maximal oxygen uptake. After training with an increase in maximal oxygen uptake of close to 20 per cent in the men and about 10 per cent in the younger and 6 per cent in the older groups of women (Fig. 2), the heart rate decreased and the stroke volume increased with unchanged oxygen uptake and cardiac output at certain submaximal exercise. At maximal exercise, the stroke volume and cardiac output increased with an unchanged or slightly decreased maximal heart rate. The intra-arterial blood pressure decreased with the reduction in heart rate at a certain work load, and this resulted in a reduction of the contracting work of the left ventricles. The respiratory and circulatory effects of short-time training in healthy middle-aged subjects are summarized in Table 1.

Table 1. Physiological Effects of Conditioning Training in Healthy Middle-aged Subjects

	At Submaximal Exercise	At Maximal Exercise
RESPIRATORY		
Oxygen uptake	0	+
Ventilation	0 or −	+
Respiratory rate	0 or −	+
Tidal volume	0	0
CIRCULATORY		
Heart rate	−	0 (or −)
Stroke volume	+	+
Cardiac output	0	+
Art.-ven. oxygen diff.	0	0 or +
Arterial blood pressure	−	0
Heart volume	0	
Blood volume	+	
METABOLIC		
Blood lactate	−	+?
Oxidative enzymes	+	
(Succinic dehydrogenase)		
Serum cholesterol	0 or −	
Serum triglycerides	−	

− denotes decrease
+ denotes increase
0 denotes no significant change

A reduction in cardiac output at a certain work load, leading to reduced cardiac work, has been observed in some patients with ischemic heart disease.[50,11] This therefore seems to be an important and common effect of physical training, in healthy persons as well as in cardiac patients. The adaptation to training may, however, be different in different groups of patients with ischemic heart disease, for other authors[16] have reported reduced heart rate during exercise combined with increased stroke volume, but with no change in cardiac output.

Among the patients with chest discomfort but no ischemic heart disease, an anxiety syndrome with hyperkinetic circulation due to so-called vasoregulatory asthenia will be found. These patients are further characterized by so-called sympathotonic changes in the ST segment of the electrocardiogram. The hyperkinetic circulation, with increased cardiac output in relation to oxygen uptake as well as ST changes, will tend to normalize with training.[29]

Interest has in recent years been directed also to the peripheral circulatory and metabolic effects of training. The blood flow in working muscles seems to be dependent on the relative work load, as judged from measurements of xenon clearance.[20,51] This implies that, since trained men have more total muscle blood at maximal exercise, the blood flow must be distributed within a greater muscle blood flow. Endurance training for only a few months results in an insignificant increase in muscle mass. Thus, one explanation of the fact that total muscle blood flow can increase with training may be that more motor units are activated in the trained than in the untrained state. There may also be changes in the distribution of blood flow within the muscle and changes in the fiber composition toward slow-twitch red fibers with endurance training.[24]

METABOLIC EFFECTS

In recent years, there has been great interest in studying possible quantitative changes in the skeletal muscle cell with physical training. In animal experiments it has been demonstrated that training can result in changes in the number of mitochondria, in the activity of certain enzymes and in the number of red fibers.[25,28] Also, human subjects studied after endurance training have shown similar effects[32] with an increase in succinic dehydrogenase (SDH) activity.[51] Middle-aged persons with long-term endurance training have larger muscle SDH activity than untrained persons.[8] Even intermittent isometric training can lead to an increase in SDH activity.[18] After training there are increases in aerobic enzymes and in the rates of glycogen synthesis and breakdown. It has also been possible to demonstrate an increased glucose tolerance in well-trained subjects[8] and in convalescents from myocardial infarction taking part in a training program.[7] The plasma insulin values after a glucose tolerance test were also reduced, which indicates high insulin sensitivity of the tissues in trained persons.

Decrease in plasma insulin, low degree of filling of adipose tissue, reduced fasting plasma lipids and rapid removal rate of triglycerides on a lipid tolerance test are seen together in physically well-trained men.[8] There has been great interest in the literature on the effect of physical training on plasma triglycerides and cholesterol. Some studies with short-term training have shown a reduction of about 10 per cent in the cholesterol values[34,33] while others have not been able to demonstrate a significant reduction. In patients with 9 months' training after myocardial infarction, no reduction was seen.[7] A reduction in the plasma triglycerides is a more general finding after physical training, with a fall of 20 to 40 per cent.[27,48] Training in patients after myocardial infarction produced a similar decrease.[7] Acute exercise also reduces the triglycerides, and the effect remains for a few days after a training session.[27] Thus, part of the low triglyceride values in trained persons may be the result of habitual exercise as such, rather than a real training effect. On the other hand, such an explanation does not deny the valuable effect of physical exercise.

The intensity, duration and frequency of training sessions needed to produce the various metabolic effects are not fully known. In most studies, the intensity of training was heavy but submaximal intensity has also been employed, as in the studies by Siegel et al.[48] and Kihlbom.[33] Even if metabolic changes are linked to the improvement in the central circulatory function, the optimal type and intensity of training may not be the same.

The importance of the peripheral capacity for utilization of oxygen for aerobic work capacity has been stressed by Kaijser.[30] By comparing ventilatory and metabolic effects (blood lactate, pH) of arm and leg training respectively during 5 weeks, with heart rates exceeding 170 beats/minute, Clausen et al.[10] concluded that training effects were predominantly peripheral. Further and more extensive training studies with different muscle groups remain to be done. Observations of local metabolic changes with training have led to the idea that dynamic training with relatively small muscle groups might be used in cardiac patients who cannot tolerate a larger increase in total oxygen uptake and cardiac work. At least part of the adaptation of peripheral metabolism may then be achieved, if various muscle groups are successively activated. Whether any changes in the adaptation of central circulation may occur is, however, unclear. On the other hand, arm exercise gives a greater increase in arterial blood pressure than corresponding leg exercise.[3] In this connection, a warning must be given regarding isometric training in cardiac patients with reduced pain tolerance or hypertension: isometric exercise even with small muscle groups produces a substantial rise in arterial blood pressure.[37,35]

RESULTS OF TRAINING STUDIES IN CARDIAC PATIENTS

To study the feasibility of training in patients after myocardial infarction, with its physiological effects and the possibility of secondary preventive effects, a training program for young infarction patients was started in 1967. The results have been reported.[44] Three months after the myocardial infarction, all patients at Sahlgren's Hospital in Goteborg who were born in 1913 or thereafter were tested on a bicycle ergometer with step-wise increased work load. About 50 per cent of the patients stopped the exercise test because of general fatigue, the mean maximal heart rate being 167 beats/min, blood lactate 8.2 mM/L and maximal oxygen uptake 2.0 L/min. This is only slightly lower than the maximal oxygen uptake in 54-year-old healthy men.[23] Thirty per cent of the patients stopped because of angina pectoris at an average work load of 500 kpm/min (85 W) with an oxygen uptake of about 1.3 L/min. In 10 per cent the test was interrupted by the physician for various other clinical reasons. Benestad,[6] in his study on patients under 60 with myocardial infarction, found a maximal oxygen uptake of 2.1 L/min and maximal heart rate of 163 beats/min; these values are lower than those for the healthy population and, with a somewhat reduced maximal arterial blood pressure, suggested impaired chronotropic and inotropic functions. However, a large percentage of young patients after myocardial infarction can perform rather heavy exercise without symptoms and without increased evidence of circulatory failure.

Every second patient in the study by Sanne et al.[44] was then selected for training individually at a relatively high intensity three times a week (those with certain clinical contraindications were excluded). Comparing the training with the nontraining group, a difference in working capacity of 14 per cent was noted after a year. In the group which stopped because of general fatigue and trained adequately, the improvement over the 9-month period was 22 per cent, the training heart rate being about 15 beats/min below the highest achieved heart rate at an exercise test. The highest achieved heart rate did not change after the training. Patients in whom the exercise tolerance was limited by angina pectoris increased their tolerated work load from 3 to 12 months after the infarction, with a larger rise in tolerance in the trained groups. (The long-term clinical effect of a training regimen is outside the scope of this review.)

Thus, training programs can be carried through in unselected groups of postinfarction patients (those with clinical contraindications to training therapy being excluded) with increase in work capacity and exercise tolerance. In large groups of these young patients, only slightly subnormal values for aerobic capacity were found and the effects of training may be similar to those in normal subjects. On the other hand, in patients with impaired myocardial function and low exercise capacity, a different effect of training might be found. Even so, the pain tolerance may be increased.

In a study by Benestad[5] a smaller group of infarction patients showed, after a training period of 6 months, an increase in aerobic capacity of 19 per cent; in the nontraining groups over the same period, the increase was 10 per cent. A training intensity corresponding to 80 per cent of aerobic capacity was used. As in the study by Trap-Jensen and Clausen[49] and in various normal groups, the cardiac work as judged from the product of systolic blood pressure and heart rate (TTI index) was reduced by training. The magnitude of ST-T changes at certain submaximal exercise is reduced after training as an effect of those hemodynamic changes.[12]

The hemodynamic consequences of short-term training in coronary patients have been reported by a number of authors. The common finding is reduced heart rate at submaximal exercise with an increased stroke volume and an unchanged[16] or somewhat reduced cardiac output.[50,49] In the study by Frick et al.[16] an improvement in left ventricular function was demonstrated. As mentioned above, some groups of cardiac patients may show different responses to training as compared to healthy men, emphasizing the peripheral adaptation with redistribution of blood flow and increased oxygen extraction in the working muscles. The metabolic effects of training have already been mentioned.

The effect of training on arterial blood pressure during exercise in healthy persons and in coronary patients has also been discussed. Boyer and Kasch[9] demonstrated a fall in resting systolic and diastolic blood pressures of 12 and 14 mm Hg, respectively, after 6 months of training in patients with essential hypertension. No systematic invesgation on the effect of blood pressure during exercise in these patients has been reported as yet. In a preliminary study, Sannerstedt et al.[46] found that the hyperkinetic circulation at rest and during exercise in patients with mild arterial hypertension can be reduced with physical training.

There is limited experimental evidence on the development of a coronary collateral circulation by physical training in animals,[13] and there is no experimental evidence from studies in patients. Changes in the enzymatic capacity in the myocardium with training have been discussed by Varnauskas and Holmgren.[52]

SOME PRACTICAL ASPECTS OF TRAINING PROGRAMS

Before training is started, the patient's functional capacity should be determined using exercise tests on a bicycle ergometer or treadmill. If the respiratory function is assumed to be impaired, spirometry, and in some patients arterial blood gas studies, should also be performed. The risk of complications must be evaluated. From the clinical history and results of the exercise test, the training intensity can then be prescribed. One tool in planning the training program and in checking tolerance to various exercise, including the detection of arrhythmia, is the use of radio-transmitted electrocardiography.[19]

As mentioned earlier, a number of studies have been performed in healthy persons to evaluate the effect of training with various intensities. It was pointed out that the lower the initial value, the greater is the increase in work capacity. A large group of patients with infarction may respond to training in principle the same way as healthy persons do. Some may have an aerobic capacity similar to normal persons of the same age, while others may have reduced values due to inactivity. The large reduction in aerobic capacity which may occur after a short period of inactivity was demonstrated by Saltin et al.[42] Other groups of infarction patients have impaired myocardial function and show fewer central circulatory effects to training, with reduced arterial blood pressure and predominantly peripheral circulatory and metabolic changes. These groups can, to a certain extent, be differentiated by exercise tests. The optimal safe intensity and type of training are, however, unknown. In the study by Sanne et al.[44] a relatively high intensity (about 15 beats/min below the highest achieved heart rate) was used; practical considerations of this high-intensity training can be found in the authors' paper. In other training programs, intensities up to 70 per cent maximal oxygen uptake[38] or heart rate not above 130 to 140 beats/min[47] have been used. From experience in normal subjects, training can start at a moderate intensity, especially in very inactive patients, and then gradually increase. For patients in whom chest pain or arrhythmia limits the exercise tolerance, fewer guidelines are available as to choice of intensity. According to the experiences of Grimby et al.[19] and Sanne et al.,[44,45] considerable numbers of these patients have markedly reduced exercise tolerance (around 60 per cent of normal aerobic capacity) and the training heart rate must be kept fairly low and often close to the highest heart rate achieved at an exercise test.

Dynamic work should be used and, for central circulatory effects, exercise with large muscle groups is recommended. Bicycle training has its positive value with a standardized and controlled load, but cannot from the clinical point of view be recommended as the only type of training.[44] The possibility of training with different smaller muscle groups to produce peripheral metabolic (and circulatory) changes has been discussed. However, only light work intensities can be used, and no major central circulatory training effects are to be expected as heavier work with smaller muscle groups results in a larger rise in arterial blood pressure.[3]

The optimal intensity and duration for training effects on the metabolic pattern (increased insulin sensitivity and decreased plasma lipids) are still unknown. It may well be that a complete training program for cardiac patients should include exercises of various types and intensities.

The physiological response to exercise should be checked regularly to adjust the training intensity to the actual condition of the patient. The importance of regular training over long periods has been stressed by various authors, for cardiac patients[31] as well as for normal subjects.[41] If the training is not regular, the training effect will soon disappear.

CONCLUSIONS

Exercise studies on middle-aged persons have been reviewed to give the background on physical work capacity and its limiting factors in these age groups. Trainability has been analyzed with respect to training intensity and the state of the person at the start of training. Increased stroke volume and reduced cardiac work are common effects of training in healthy subjects and in some coronary patients. Other groups of patients may show somewhat different training effects. Extensive studies are needed to analyze training effects in patients in different function groups and with various factors limiting exercise tolerance. The mechanisms for the different changes are unknown, as is their clinical importance over a long period. Even so, detailed knowledge obtained from model studies in healthy persons is of great value, as many physiological training effects are identical in principle.

REFERENCES

1. Åstrand, I.: Aerobic work capacity in men and women with special reference to age. Acta Physiol. Scand., 19: (Suppl. 146), 1960.
2. Åstrand, P. O., et al.: Cardiac output during submaximal and maximal work. J. Appl. Physiol., 19:268, 1964.
3. Åstrand, P. O., et al.: Intra-arterial blood pressure during exercise with different muscle groups. J. Appl. Physiol., 20:253, 1965.
4. Benestad, A. M.: Trainability of old men. Acta Med. Scand., 178:321, 1965.
5. Benestad, A. M.: Treningsterapi vid koronare hjertesjukdomar. Oslo, Universitets-forlaget, 1971.
6. Benestad, A. M.: The deteriorative effect of myocardial infarction upon physiological indices of work capacity. Acta Med. Scand., 191:67, 1972.
7. Björntorp, P., et al.: Effects of physical training on glucose tolerance, plasma insulin and lipids and on body composition in men after myocardial infarction. Acta Med. Scand., in press.
8. Björntorp, P., et al.: Carbohydrate and lipid metabolism in middle-aged physically well-trained men. Metabolism, in press.
9. Boyer, J. L., and Kasch, F. W.: Exercise therapy in hypertensive men. JAMA, 211: 1668, 1970.
10. Clausen, J. P., et al.: Effect of strenuous arm and leg training on pulmonary ventilation, metabolism and blood pH during submaximal exercise. Acta Physiol. Scand., 82:8A, 1971.
11. Clausen, J. P., and Trap-Jensen, J.: Effects of training on the distribution of cardiac output in patients with coronary artery disease. Circulation, 42:611, 1970.
12. Detry, J-M., and Bruce, R. A.: Effects of physical training on exertional ST segment depression in coronary heart disease. Circulation, 44:390, 1971.
13. Eckstein, R.: Effect of exercise and coronary artery narrowing on coronary collateral circulation. Circ. Res., 5:230, 1957.
14. Ekblom, B.: Effect of physical training on oxygen transport system in man. Acta Physiol. Scand., Suppl. 328, 1969.
15. Ekblom, B., et al.: Effects of atropin and propranolol on the oxygen transport system at rest and during exercise in man. Scand. J. Clin. Lab. Invest., 30:35, 1972.
16. Frick, M. H., Katila, M., and Sjögren, A-L.: Cardiac function and physical training after myocardial infarction. In: Coronary Heart Disease and Physical Fitness. Copenhagen, Munksgaard, 1971.
17. Grimby, G., et al.: Work capacity and physiological responses to work. The men born in 1913 study. Amer. J. Cardiol., 30:37, 1972.
18. Grimby, G., et al.: Metabolic effects of isometric training. Submitted for publication.
19. Grimby, G., Bjurö, T., and Helander, E.: Radio-transmitted ECG and measurements

of energy expenditure during exercise therapy in patients with myocardial infarction. Mal. Cardiov., *10*, 1, 1969.

20. Grimby, G., Häggendal, E., and Saltin, B.: Local xenon-133 clearance from the quadriceps muscle during exercise in man. J. Appl. Physiol., *22*:305, 1967.

21. Grimby, G., and Saltin, B.: Physiological analysis of physically well-trained middle-aged and old athletes. Acta Med. Scand., *179*:513, 1966.

22. Grimby, G., and Saltin, B.: Physiological effects of physical training. Scand. J. Rehab. Med., *3*:6, 1971.

23. Grimby, G., et al.: Aerobic power and factors in a population study of men aged 54. Scand. J. Clin. Lab. Invest., *26*:287, 1970.

24. Gollnick, P. D., et al.: Enzyme activity and fiber composition in skeletal muscle of untrained and trained men. J. Appl. Physiol., *33*:312, 1972.

25. Gollnick, P. D., and King, D. W.: Effect of exercise and training on mitochondria of rat skeletal muscle. Amer. J. Physiol., *216*:1502, 1969.

26. Hartley, L. H., et al.: Physical training in sedentary middle-aged and older men. III. Cardiac output and gas exchange at submaximal and maximal exercise. Scand. J. Clin. Lab. Invest., *24*:335, 1969.

27. Holloszy, J. O., et al.: Effect of a six month program of endurance exercise on the serum lipids of middle-aged men. Amer. J. Cardiol., *14*:753, 1964.

28. Holloszy, J. O., et al.: Biochemical adaptations to endurance exercise in skeletal muscle. In: *Muscle Metabolism During Exercise*. New York, Plenum Press, 1971.

29. Holmgren, A., et al.: Effect of physical training in vasoregulatory asthenia, in Da Corta's syndrome and in neurosis without heart symptoms. Acta Med. Scand., *165*:89, 1959.

30. Kaijser, L.: Limiting factors for aerobic muscle performance. Acta Physiol. Scand., Suppl. 346, 1970.

31. Katila, M., and Frick, M. H.: A two-year circulatory follow-up of physical training after myocardial infarction. Acta Med. Scand., *187*:95, 1970.

32. Kiessling, K-H., Piehl, K., and Lundquist, C-G.: Effect of physical training on ultrastructural features in human skeletal muscle. In: *Muscle Metabolism During Exercise*. New York, Plenum Press, 1971.

33. Kihlbom, Å.: Physical training in women. Scand. J. Clin. Lab. Invest., *28*: Suppl. 119, 1971.

34. Kihlbom, Å., et al.: Physical training in sedentary middle-aged and older men. I. Medical evaluation. Scand. J. Clin. Lab. Invest., *24*: 315, 1969.

35. Kivowitz, C., et al.: Effects of isometric exercise on cardiac performance. Circulation, *44*: 994, 1971.

36. Knuttgen, H. G., et al.: Physiological effects of physical conditioning on young male adults. Med. Sci. Sports, in press.

37. Lind, A. R.: Cardiovascular responses to static exercise. Circulation, *41*:173, 1970.

38. Merriman, J. E.: The physiological effects on physical activity in cardiac patients. Acta Cardiol., Suppl. *14*:39, 1970.

39. Roskamm, H.: Optimum patterns of exercise for healthy adults. Canad. Med. Assoc. J., *96*:895, 1967.

40. Rowell, L. B.: Factors affecting the prediction of maximal oxygen intake from measurements made during submaximal work. Ph.D. thesis, Univ. of Minnesota, 1962.

41. Saltin, B.: Guidelines for physical training. Scand. J. Rehab. Med., *3*:39, 1971.

42. Saltin, B., et al.: Response to bed rest and training. Circulation, *38*:Suppl. 7, 1968.

43. Saltin, B., et al.: Physical training in sedentary middle-aged and older men. II. Oxygen uptake, heart rate and blood lactate concentration at submaximal and maximal exercise. Scand. J. Clin. Lab. Invest., *24*:323, 1969.

44. Sanne, H., Grimby, G., and Wilhelmsen, L.: Physical training during convalescence after myocardial infarction. In: *Coronary Heart Disease and Physical Fitness*. Copenhagen, Munksgaard, 1971.

45. Sanne, H., and Wilhelmsen, L.: Physical activity as prevention and therapy in coronary heart disease. Scand. J. Rehab. Med., *3*:47, 1971.

46. Sannerstedt, R., et al.: Systemic haemodynamics in mild arterial hypertension before and after physical training. Europ. J. Clin. Invest., in press.

47. Semple, T.: Rehabilitation of patients with coronary disease. Acta Cardiol., Suppl. *14*: 69, 1970.

48. Siegel, W., Blomqvist, G., and Mitchell, J. H.: Effects of a quantitative physical training program on middle-aged sedentary men. Circulation, *41*:19, 1970.

49. Trap-Jensen, J., and Clausen, J. P.: Effect of training on the relation of heart rate and blood pressure to the outset of pain in effort angina pectoris. In: *Coronary Heart Disease and Physical Fitness*. Copenhagen, Munksgaard, 1971.

50. Varnauskas, E., et al.: Hemodynamic effects of physical training in coronary patients. Lancet, *2*:8, 1966.

51. Varnauskas, E., et al.: Effects of physical training on exercise blood flow and succinic dehydrogenase activity in skeletal muscle. Cardiov. Res., *4*:418, 1971.

52. Varnauskas, E., and Holmgren, S.: Myocardial blood flow during exercise in patients with coronary heart disease. Comments on training effects. In: *Coronary Heart Disease and Physical Fitness*. Copenhagen, Munksgaard, 1971.